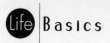
Life | Basics

HERBAL REMEDIES
& HOMEOPATHY

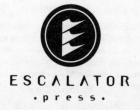
ESCALATOR
· press ·

Published through special arrangement with
Stratthearn Books Ltd

This edition published by Escalator Press
Distributed by Stewart House Publishing Inc.
Etobicoke, Canada

© 2001 Geddes & Grosset, David Dale House,
New Lanark, ML11 9DJ, Scotland

First published in this edition 2002, reprinted 2003

Cover image courtesy of PhotoDisc, Inc.

ISBN 1 55366 276 8

Printed and bound in the UK

Contents

Herbal Remedies: An Introduction

History of the use of herbal remedies

Herbalism is sometimes maligned as a collection of home-made remedies to be applied in a placebo fashion to one symptom or another, provided the ailment is not too serious and provided there is a powerful chemical wonder-drug at the ready to suppress any 'real' symptoms. We often forget, however, that botanical medicine provides a complete system of healing and disease prevention. It is the oldest and most natural form of medicine. Its record of efficacy and safety spans centuries and covers every country worldwide. Because herbal medicine is holistic medicine, it is, in fact, able to look beyond the symptoms to the underlying systemic imbalance; when skilfully applied by a trained practitioner, herbal medicine offers very real and permanent solutions to concrete problems, many of them seemingly intractable to pharmaceutical intervention.

Early civilizations

The medicinal use of herbs is said to be as old as mankind itself. In early civilizations, food and medicine were linked and many plants were eaten for their health-giving properties. In ancient Egypt, the slave workers were given a daily ration of garlic to help fight off the many fevers and infections that were common at that time. The first written records of herbs and their beneficial properties were compiled by the ancient Egyptians. Most of our knowledge and use of herbs can be traced back to the Egyptian priests who also practised herbal medicine. Records dating back to 1500 BC listed medicinal herbs, including caraway and cinnamon.

The ancient Greeks and Romans also carried out herbal medicine, and as they invaded new lands their doctors encountered new herbs and introduced herbs such as rosemary or lavender into new areas. Other cultures with a history of herbal medicine are the Chinese and the Indians. In Britain, the use of herbs developed along with the establishment of monasteries around the country, each of which had

5

its own herb garden for use in treating both the monks and the local people. In some areas, particularly Wales and Scotland, Druids and other Celtic healers are thought to have had an oral tradition of herbalism, where medicine was mixed with religion and ritual.

The first publications

Over time, these healers and their knowledge led to the writing of the first 'herbals', which rapidly rose in importance and distribution upon the advent of the printing press in the 15th century. John Parkinson of London wrote a herbal around 1630, listing useful plants. Many herbalists set up their own apothecary shops, including the famous Nicholas Culpepper (1616–1654) whose most famous work is *The Complete Herbal and English Physician, Enlarged,* published in 1649. Then in 1812, Henry Potter started a business supplying herbs and dealing in leeches. By this time a huge amount of traditional knowledge and folklore on medicinal herbs was available from Britain, Europe, the Middle East, Asia and the Americas. This promoted Potter to write *Potter's Encyclopaedia of Botanical Drugs and Preparations*, which is still published today.

The decline of herbal medicine

It was in this period that scientifically inspired conventional medicine rose in popularity, sending herbal medicine into a decline. In rural areas, herbal medicine continued to thrive in local folklore, traditions and practices. In 1864 the National Association (later Institute) of Medical Herbalists was established, to organize training of herbal medicine practitioners and to maintain standards of practice. From 1864 until the early part of this century, the Institute fought attempts to ban herbal medicine and over time public interest in herbal medicine has increased, particularly over the last 20 years. This move away from synthetic drugs is partly due to possible side effects, bad publicity, and, in some instances, a mistrust of the medical and pharmacological industries. The more natural appearance of herbal remedies has led to its growing support and popularity. Herbs from America have been incorporated with common remedies and scientific research into herbs and their active ingredients has confirmed their healing power and enlarged the range of medicinal herbs used today.

Its rise and relevance today

Herbal medicine can be viewed as the precursor of modern pharmacology, but today it continues as an effective and more natural method of treating and preventing illness. Globally, herbal medicine is three to four times more commonly practised than conventional medicine.

Nowhere is the efficacy of herbalism more evident than in problems related to the nervous system. Stress, anxiety, tension and depression are intimately connected with most illness. Few health practitioners would argue with the influence of nervous anxiety in pathology. Nervous tension is generally acknowledged by doctors to contribute to duodenal and gastric ulceration, ulcerative colitis, irritable bowel syndrome and many other gut-related pathologies.

We know also, from physiology, that when a person is depressed, the secretion of hydrochloric acid—one of the main digestive juices—is also reduced so that digestion and absorption are rendered less efficient. Anxiety, on the other hand, can lead to the release of adrenaline and stimulate the over-production of hydrochloric acid and result in a state of acidity that may exacerbate the pain of an inflamed ulcer. In fact, whenever the voluntary nervous system (our conscious anxiety) interferes with the autonomic processes (the automatic nervous regulation that in health is never made conscious), illness is the result.

Herbalists rely on their knowledge of botanical remedies to rectify this type of human malfunction. The medical herbalist will treat a stubborn dermatological problem using 'alternatives' specific to the skin problem, and then apply circulatory stimulants to aid in the removal of toxins from the area, with remedies to reinforce other organs of elimination, such as the liver and kidneys. Under such natural treatment, free of any discomforting side effects, the patient can feel confident and relaxed—perhaps for the first time in many months.

Curiously, this is an approach that has never been taken up by orthodox medicine. There, the usual treatment of skin problems involves suppression of symptoms with steroids. However, the use of conventional antihistamines or benzodiazepines often achieves less lasting benefit to the patient because of the additional burden of side effects, such as drowsiness, increased toxicity, and long-term drug dependence.

Herbs, on the other hand, are free from toxicity and habituation. Because they are organic substances and not man-made synthetic molecules, they possess an affinity for the human organism. They are extremely efficient in balancing the nervous system. Restoring a sense of wellbeing and relaxation is necessary for optimum health and for the process of self-healing.

Naturally, the choice of a treatment should be based upon a thorough health assessment and the experience and training of a qualified herbal practitioner. The herbalist will then prepare and prescribe herbal remedies in a variety of different forms, such as infusions, loose teas, suppositories, inhalants, lotions, tinctures, tablets and pills. Many of these preparations are available for home use from chemists, health shops and mail-order suppliers.

Herbs for stress management

Chamomile
This has a relaxing effect on the mind and body. It is an excellent sedative for anxiety and muscle tenseness. Many people enjoy its benefits in the form of chamomile tea.

Valerian
This is the ideal tranquillizer. The rhizomes of this plant contain a volatile oil (which includes valerianic acid), volatile alkaloids (including chatinine), and iridoids (valepotriates), which have been shown to reduce anxiety and aggression. So effective is Valerian in relieving anxiety while maintaining normal mental awareness, that it enables us to continue the most complicated mental exercise without drowsiness, loss of consciousness or depression. Valerian has been usefully taken before an examination or a driving test!

Peppermint
This is effective for treating digestive discomfort: it relieves indigestion, flatulence, constipation and nausea. Peppermint is also a good mind tonic, helping to clarify ideas and focus concentration. It is also helpful in alleviating the symptoms of colds and influenza. Peppermint and chamomile tea is thought to be effective in reducing the pain of tension headaches and migraines.

Vervain
This is not only effective against depression but also strongly supports the detoxifying function of the liver. Its French name is still 'Herbe Sacre'; an old English name is 'Holy Wort'—it was one of the seven sacred herbs of the Druids. Today we know that the antispasmodic qualities of Verbena are largely due to the glycoside verbenalin. Recent Chinese research has linked the plant with dilation of arteries in the brain: a likely explanation of its usefulness in treating migraine, especially when this problem is accompanied by liver congestion. It is certainly of use to treat exhaustion and depression.

St John's Wort
Also called *Hypericum perforatum*, St John's wort has analgesic and anti-inflammatory properties, with important local applications to neuralgia and sciatica. Systemically, its sedative properties are based on the glycoside hypericin (a red pigment), which makes it applicable to neurosis and irritability. Many herbalists use it extensively as a background remedy.

Lemon balm
This herb is both carminative and antispasmodic, and is active specifically on that part of the vagus nerve that may interfere with the harmonious functioning of the heart and the stomach. Recent research has indicated that the action of the volatile oil begins within the limbic system of the brain and subsequently operates directly upon the vagus nerve and all the organs that are innervated by it. Accordingly, neurasthenia (complete nervous prostration), migraine, and nervous gastropathy are amenable to its healing power.

Lime flowers
These are thought to be helpful in controlling anxiety and hyperactivity. They are also effective for treating insomnia, high blood pressure and for soothing muscles and nerves.

Borage
This is an effective mind tonic, which helps to alleviate headaches, migraine and depression.

Oats
Oats is one of the great herbal restoratives of the nervous system. The plant contains a nervine alkaloid that is helpful in angina and in cardiac insufficiency. It has also been used in the treatment of addiction to morphine, narcotics, tobacco and alcohol.

Soothing herbal drinks

Warm milk and honey
Perhaps with a dash of cinnamon, this is an ideal drink to take at bedtime. It will help you relax and ward off insomnia.

Hop tea
Three hop cones, or heads, infused in a cup of boiling water whenever

you begin to feel excessively tense, is a marvellous remedy for anxiety and insomnia.

A soothing herb tea to sustain a feeling of equilibrium
> 25g (1 oz) each dried chamomile flowers, lime flowers, hibiscus blossoms and marigold flowers
> 15g (¹/₂ oz) each dried peppermint leaves and vervain
> 1 teaspoon whole fenugreek seeds
> 100g (4 oz) Lapsang Souchong tea

Mix all the ingredients together and store in a dark airtight container. Use 1 teaspoon to 300 ml (¹/₂ pint) of boiling water in a tea pot and leave to infuse for five minutes before straining and serving with a slice of lemon and a teaspoon of honey if desired. This is a very calming tea that soothes feelings of anxiety. It also helps to clear your head and settle an upset tummy. One cup taken morning and night will promote a feeling of wellbeing.

Another calming tea, especially good for the nerves
> 1 teaspoon each grated valerian root and dried mint
> ¹/₂ teaspoon each dried chamomile and lavender flowers
> 600 ml (1 pint) boiling water

Infuse the dry ingredients in the water for 15 minutes then strain and take a glass three times a day for one week only.

Two tonic teas to sip when feeling depressed
Sip either 2 teaspoons of dandelion and 1 of basil infused in 600 ml (1 pint) of boiling water, or 2 teaspoons each of nettle, basil and melissa infused in 600 ml (1 pint) of boiling water.

A tonic tea to relieve stress and anxiety
> 1 tablespoon each fresh dandelion and nettle tops
> 1 teaspoon each fresh blackcurrant and borage leaves
> 600 ml (1 pint) boiling water

Steep the greenery in the water for five minutes. Strain and drink with lemon and honey.

Dock wine
Dock is one of the great tonic herbs because it is extremely high in iron. Here is a recipe for an old-fashioned dock wine.
> 175g (7 oz) dock root
> 15g (¹/₂ oz) liquorice wood

7g ($^1/_4$ oz) juniper berries
100g (4 oz) raw cane sugar
2 litres ($3^1/_2$ pints) organic red wine

Put all the ingredients together in a china container, cover and place either in a very slow oven or in a bain marie. Continue to heat gently until the mixture is reduced by half. Strain, bottle and seal tightly. Drink a sherry glass of the dock wine every morning for two weeks.

Rosemary in wine

Steep 6 sprigs of rosemary in a well-sealed bottle of sweet white wine for 14 days. Take 1 wineglass as a daily tonic.

Sage tonic

Take 100g (4 oz) of fresh sage leaves and put them in a bottle of organic white wine for two weeks. Sweeten to taste with honey and leave for another day. Press and strain through muslin. Bottle, and take 1 sherry glass before lunch and dinner.

You can also infuse sage leaves in boiling water, strain and sweeten with honey for an uplifting sage tea.

A–Z of Herbal Remedies

Aconite *Aconitum napellus.*
COMMON NAME: monkshood, blue rocket, friar's cap, wolfsbane.
OCCURRENCE: indigenous to mountain slopes in the Alps and Pyrenees. Introduced into England very early, before 900 AD.
PARTS USED: the leaves used fresh and the root when dried. It contains alkaloidal material—aconitine, benzaconine and aconine amongst other compounds.
MEDICINAL USES: the plant is poisonous and should not be used except under medical advice. It is an anodyne, febrifuge and sedative. Used for reducing fever and inflammation in the treatment of catarrh, tonsillitis and croup. It may be used in controlling heart spasm.
ADMINISTERED AS: tincture, liniment and occasionally as injection.

Agrimony *Agrimonia eupatoria.*
COMMON NAME: church steeples, cockleburr, sticklewort.
OCCURRENCE: field borders, ditches and hedges throughout England. Found locally in Scotland.
PARTS USED: the herb. Contains a particular volatile oil, tannin and a bitter principle.
MEDICINAL USES: mild astringent, tonic, diuretic, deobstruent. It has a reputation for curing liver complaints and is very good for skin eruptions and blood diseases. Also recommended to treat the sting and bite of snakes.
ADMINISTERED AS: liquid extract.

Alder *Alnus glutinosa.*
COMMON NAME: betula alnus.
OCCURRENCE: commonly found throughout Britain, usually in moist woods or by streams.
PARTS USED: the bark, wood, shoots, catkins and leaves have all been used as dyes. The bark and leaves contain tannic acid.
MEDICINAL USES: tonic and astringent. Used as a decoction to bathe swelling and inflammation, particularly of the throat.
ADMINISTERED AS: decoction.

Aloes *Aloe perryi, Aloe vera.*
OCCURRENCE: indigenous to East and South Africa and introduced into the West Indies.

PARTS USED: the drug aloes is described as the liquid evaporated to dryness which drains from the leaves. It contains two aloin compounds, barbaloin and isobarbaloin, as well as amorphous aloin, resin and aloe-emodin in differing proportions.

MEDICINAL USES: emmenagogue, purgative, vermifuge, anthelmintic. It is generally administered along with carminative and anodyne drugs, and acts on the lower bowel. The liquid form may be used externally to ease skin irritation.

ADMINISTERED AS: fluid extract, powdered extract, decoction, tincture.

Allspice Pimento officinalis.

COMMON NAME: pimento, Jamaica pepper, clove pepper.

OCCURRENCE: indigenous to the West Indies and South America; cultivated in Jamaica and central America.

PARTS USED: the fruit, which contains a volatile oil made up of eugenol, a sesquiterpene and other unknown chemicals.

MEDICINAL USES: aromatic, stimulant, carminative. Allspice acts on the gastro-intestinal tract and is usually added to drinks tonics and purgatives for flavouring. The spice may also be used for flatulent indigestion and hysteria. Allspice is frequently used as a spice and condiment in food or drinks.

ADMINISTERED AS: essential oil, distilled water, powdered fruit, fluid extract.

Almond, Sweet Amygdalus communis var. dulais. *Almond, Bitter* Amygdalus commis var. amara.

OCCURRENCE: native trees of western Asia and North Africa and cultivated in most Mediterranean countries and Great Britain.

PARTS USED: the nut and the oil expressed from it.

MEDICINAL USES: sweet almonds have demulcent and nutritive properties, but since the outer skin can cause irritation of the alimentary canal, almonds are normally blanched and the skin removed before being used as food. The oil produced is emollient, demulcent, nutritive and slightly laxative, and is mainly used in cosmetics but is also taken internally as a medicine. It is of benefit in allaying acrid juices, softening and relaxing solid materials, bronchial diseases, tickling coughs, hoarseness and nephritic pains. Sweet almonds are made into emulsions with barley water or gum arabic to treat gravel, stone, kidney disorders and bladder and biliary duct problems, with more success than almond oil.

Bitter almonds yield a volatile oil upon distillation with water which is used as a flavouring agent. These almonds contain the glucoside amygdalin and the chemical emulsin that acts on the glucoside to produce glucose, prussic acid and benzaldehyde in the presence of water. Prussic acid is poisonous and use of bitter almond oil must be carefully monitored. In the Middle Ages, the oil was used for intermittent fevers, hydrophobia and as an aperient, diuretic and vermifuge drug, but it is seldom administered medicinally now. The cake left after expressing the oil has a special dietary value and is often made into flour for cakes and biscuits for diabetic patients. Almond oil is used in trade as a lubricant for watches, and in soaps and toiletries.

ADMINISTERED AS: expressed oil, bitter almond oil (with prussic acid removed).

Anemone, Wood *Anemone nemorosa.*
COMMON NAME: crowfoot, windflower, smell fox.
OCCURRENCE: found in woods and thickets across Great Britain.
PARTS USED: the root, leaves and juice.
MEDICINAL USES: this species of plant is much less widely used than it has been previously. It used to be good for leprosy, lethargy, eye inflammation and headaches. An ointment made of the leaves is said to be effective in cleansing malignant ulcers.
ADMINISTERED AS: decoction, fresh leaves and root, ointment.

Anemone, Pulsatilla *Anemone pulsatilla.*
COMMON NAME: pasqueflower, meadow anemone, wind flower.
OCCURRENCE: found locally in chalk downs and limestone areas of England.
PARTS USED: the whole herb. It produces oil of anemone upon distillation with water.
MEDICINAL USES: nervine, antispasmodic, alterative and diaphoretic. It is beneficial in disorders of mucous membranes and of the respiratory and digestive passages. Can be used to treat asthma, whooping cough and bronchitis.
ADMINISTERED AS: fluid extract.

Angelica *Angelica archangelica.*
COMMON NAME: garden angelica, *Archangelica officinalis.*
OCCURRENCE: found native to some sites in Scotland although more abundant in Lapland and is a common garden plant in England.
PARTS USED: the root, leaves and seeds. The leaves contain volatile oil, valeric acid, angelic acid, a bitter principle and a resin called angelicin.

The roots contain terebangelene and other terpenes while the seeds also yield two acid compounds.

MEDICINAL USES: angelica has carminative, stimulant, diaphoretic, diuretic, aromatic, stomachic, tonic and expectorant properties and is good for colds, coughs, pleurisy, wind, colic and rheumatism. It is used as a stimulating expectorant and is good for digestion.

ADMINISTERED AS: powdered root, liquid extract, infusion or as a poultice.

Angostura *Galipea officinalis.*
COMMON NAME: cusparia bark, *Cusparia febrifuga*, *Bonplandia trifoliata*, *Galipea cusparia.*
OCCURRENCE: a small tree native to tropical South America.
PARTS USED: the dried bark, which has the active ingredients angosturin, the alkaloids galipine, cusparine, galipidine, cusparidine and cuspareine, as well as a volatile oil and an unidentified glucoside.
MEDICINAL USES: aromatic, bitter, tonic, stimulant, purgative. There is a long history of usage by native South Americans as a stimulant tonic. It is useful in bilious diarrhoea and dysentery, but in large doses it has a purgative and cathartic effect on the body.
ADMINISTERED AS: infusion, powdered bark, tincture, fluid extract.

Anise *Pimpinella anisum.*
COMMON NAME: aniseed.
OCCURRENCE: native to Egypt, Greece, Crete and western Asia, its cultivation spread to central Europe and North Africa.
PARTS USED: the fruit. Upon distillation, the fruit yields a fragrant volatile oil that is made up of anethol, choline, a fixed oil, sugar and mucilage.
MEDICINAL USES: carminative and pectoral. It is very useful against coughs and chest infections and is made into lozenges or smoked to clear the chest. Aniseed tea is good for infant catarrh, and aids digestion in adults. Anise seed is an ingredient of cathartic and aperient pills, to relieve flatulence and lessen the griping caused by purgative herbs. It can also be given in convulsions quite safely.
ADMINISTERED AS: essence, essential oil, tincture, powdered seeds, tea and pills.

Apple *Pyrus malus.*
COMMON NAME: wild apple, *Malus communis,* crab-tree.
OCCURRENCE: native to Great Britain and found throughout the temperate regions of the northern hemisphere.

Apricot

PARTS USED: the fruit and bark. Apples contain water, protein material, carbonaceous matter, vitamins, organic acids, salts of potassium, sodium, carbon and magnesium.

MEDICINAL USES: diuretic, slightly astringent. The organic acids in the fruit benefit sedentary people and ease liver problems, gout and indigestion. Apple juice or cider is drunk frequently in some areas e.g. Normandy, where problems of stone or calculus are unknown because of the diuretic effects of apples. Apples can also help cure constipation, scurvy, sleeplessness or bilious complaints. They act as an excellent dentifrice (tooth cleanser) and are applied as a poultice to sore eyes when rotten. A decoction of the bark is used against intermittent and bilious fevers, while cooked apples are used in sore throats, eye problems, and in skin and tissue infected with the *Streptococcus pyogenes* bacterium. Dropsy is helped by drinking cider in which horseradish was steeped.

ADMINISTERED AS: fresh fruit, expressed juice, fermented drink, infusion, decoction, poultice.

Apricot *Prunus armeniaca.*

COMMON NAME: apricock, *Armeniaca vulgaris.*

OCCURRENCE: originally found in northern China, the Himalaya region and temperate Asia. Now cultivated across temperate regions of Europe. Introduced into England in the sixteenth century.

PARTS USED: the kernels and the oil expressed from them. The oil contains olein and the glyceride of linolic acid. The cake left after oil removal produces an essential oil upon distillation that contains the glucoside amygdalin and is chemically identical to the essential oil from the almond. It is used in confectionery and as a food flavouring.

MEDICINAL USES: apricot oil is substituted for oil of almonds in cosmetics, because of its lower cost. It has a softening action on the skin.

ADMINISTERED AS: expressed oil, essential oil.

Areca Nut *Areca catechu.*

COMMON NAME: betel nut, pinang.

OCCURRENCE: a tree cultivated in the East Indies, India and Sri Lanka.

PARTS USED: the seeds contain a large amount of tannin, gallic acid, a fixed oil, lignin and a volatile oil. They also contain three alkaloids, arcoline, arecain and guracine with the second listed being the active principle.

MEDICINAL USES: aromatic, astringent, taenacide and mydriatic. The native people chew these nuts, which stain the teeth, lips and excrement red. Taken internally, the seeds expel tapeworms and cause contraction of the

pupil of the eye. Areca nut is also made into a toothpaste in Britain.
ADMINISTERED AS: powdered nut, fluid extract.

Arnica *Arnica montana*.

COMMON NAME: mountain tobacco, leopard's bane.
OCCURRENCE: indigenous to central Europe but found in England and southern Scotland.
PARTS USED: the rhizome and flowers. They contain arnicin, tannin, phullin and a volatile oil.
MEDICINAL USES: stimulant, vulnerary and diuretic. It is used in external application to bruises and sprains but is rarely used internally as it irritates the stomach, and may cause severe poisoning. A tincture of arnica has been used to treat epilepsy and seasickness.
ADMINISTERED AS: tincture, poultice.

Arrach *Chenopodium olidum*.

COMMON NAME: stinking motherwort/arrach/goosefoot, dog's arrach, goat's arrach, netchweed.
OCCURRENCE: an annual herb found on waste ground or roadsides throughout Great Britain.
PARTS USED: herb. Contains trimethylamine, osmazome and nitrate of potash.
MEDICINAL USES: nervine, emmenagogue, anti-spasmodic. This is used in female hysteria and was formerly said to cure barrenness.
ADMINISTERED AS: an infusion, fluid extract or injection.

Arrowroot *Maranta arundinacea*.

COMMON NAME: *Maranta indica*, *M. ramosissima*, maranta starch or arrowroot, araruta, Bermuda arrowroot, Indian arrowroot.
OCCURRENCE: indigenous to the West Indies and central America. It is cultivated in Bengal, Java, the Philippines, Mauritius and West Africa.
PARTS USED: the dried, powdered starch from the rhizome.
MEDICINAL USES: nutritive, demulcent, non-irritating. Well suited for infants and convalescents, particularly after bowel complaints. The jelly made of water or milk may be flavoured with sugar, lemon juice or fruit. The fresh rhizomes are mashed and applied to wounds from poisoned arrows, scorpion or spider bites and to stop gangrene. The freshly expressed juice of the rhizome, when mixed with water, is said to be a good antidote against vegetable poisons.
ADMINISTERED AS: fresh root, expressed juice, dietary item.

Asarabacca Asarum europaeum.

COMMON NAME: hazelwort, wild nard.

OCCURRENCE: asarabacca is the only British species of the birthwort family and is very rare. It is found in woodlands.

PARTS USED: the root and herb.

MEDICINAL USES: stimulant, tonic, emetic, purgative, aromatic and sternulatory. As dried powdered leaves of the herb, it is used in the preparation of snuffs, causing sneezing and giving relief to headaches and weak eyes. It has been utilized to remove mucus from the respiratory passages and may be an antidote to the bite of venomous snakes. The herb was formerly used as an emetic or purgative but its use has been replaced by safer drugs.

ADMINISTERED AS: tincture, emulsion.

Asparagus Asparagus officinalis.

COMMON NAME: sparrow grass.

OCCURRENCE: a rare native in Britain, but found wild on the south-west coast of England. It is cultivated as a food crop in parts of Scotland.

PARTS USED: the root.

MEDICINAL USES: this plant has diuretic, laxative, cardiac and sedative effects. It is recommended in cases of dropsy.

ADMINISTERED AS: expressed juice, decoction or made in a syrup.

Avens Geum urbanum.

COMMON NAME: colewort, herb bennet, city Avens, wild rue, way bennet, goldy star, clove root.

OCCURRENCE: a common hedgerow plant in Britain and Europe.

PARTS USED: the herb and root. The herb contains a volatile oil composed of eugenol and a glucoside, while the root also contains tannin.

MEDICINAL USES: an astringent, styptic, febrifuge, sudorific, stomachic, antiseptic, tonic and aromatic. It is useful in diarrhoea, sore throat, chills, fevers and headache amongst other complaints. An infusion may be used for skin problems, as a wash.

ADMINISTERED AS: an infusion, decoction or tincture.

Balm Melissa officinalis.

COMMON NAME: sweet balm, lemon balm, honey plant, cure-all.

OCCURRENCE: a common garden plant in Great Britain, which was naturalized into southern England at a very early period.

PARTS USED: the herb.

MEDICINAL USES: as a carminative, diaphoretic, or febrifuge. It can be made into a cooling tea for fever patients and balm is often used in combination with other herbs to treat colds and fever.

ADMINISTERED AS: an infusion.

Balmony *Chelone glabra*.

COMMON NAME: chelone, bitter herb, snake head, shellflower, turtlehead, turtle bloom, salt-rheum weed, glatte, the hummingbird tree, white chelone.

OCCURRENCE: it grows in swamps, wet woods and rivers in the eastern United States and Canada.

PARTS USED: the whole herb.

MEDICINAL USES: the fresh leaves are anti-bilious, anthelmintic, tonic and detergent in action and are used against consumption, dyspepsia, debility and jaundice. It has a peculiar action on the liver and diseases of that organ, while it is also effective in removing worms from children. When made into an ointment, balmony is recommended for inflamed tumours, ulcers, inflamed breasts and piles.

ADMINISTERED AS: a decoction, powdered herb, fluid extract, tincture.

Balsam of Peru *Myroxylon pereirae*.

COMMON NAME: Peruvian balsam, *Toluifera pereira*, *Myrosperum pereira*.

OCCURRENCE: this comes from a large tree that grows in the forest of El Salvador, central America.

PARTS USED: the balsam is an oleoresinous liquid that exudes from the tree after the bark has been beaten and scorched. It is soaked from the tree and boiled in water.

MEDICINAL USES: stimulant, expectorant, parasiticide. It is used in scabies, irritant skin diseases and acute eczema. The balsam is good in all chronic mucous afflictions, catarrh, leucorrhoea, diarrhoea and dysentery. It stimulates the heart and raises blood pressure. The liquid may be applied to sore nipples and discharges from the ear to effect healing.

ADMINISTERED AS: liquid form.

Baneberry *Actaea spicata*.

COMMON NAME: herb Christopher, bugbane, toadroot.

OCCURRENCE: a rare plant in Britain, found only in limestone districts of the Lake District and Yorkshire.

PARTS USED: the root.

MEDICINAL USES: antispasmodic. The plant is acrid and poisonous. The root is used as a remedy for catarrh and some nervous disorders, but the plant must be used with great caution.

ADMINISTERED AS: infusion, dried or fresh root.

Barberry *Berberis vulgaris.*
COMMON NAME: berbery, pipperidge bush, *Berberis dumetorum.*
OCCURRENCE: a common bush that grows wild in some parts of England but is unlikely to be native to Scotland and Ireland.
PARTS USED: the root, root-bark and berries. The bark contains berberine, a bitter alkaloid, along with several other compounds.
MEDICINAL USES: as a tonic, purgative and antiseptic. It is normally used to treat jaundice and liver complaints, and is an aid to regulating digestion and stopping constipation. The berries are used to produce an acid drink that helps ease diarrhoea and fevers.
ADMINISTERED AS: powdered bark, fluid extract and solid extract.

Barley *Hordeum distichon* and *Hordeum vulgare.*
COMMON NAME: pearl barley, *Perlatum.*
OCCURRENCE: throughout Britain.
PARTS USED: decorticated seeds composed of eighty per cent starch and six per cent proteins, cellulose, etc.
MEDICINAL USES: barley is used to prepare a nutritive and demulcent drink for ill and fevered patients. Barley water is given to sick children suffering from diarrhoea or bowel inflammation etc. Malt extract is also used medicinally.
ADMINISTERED AS: an infusion and beverage.

Basil *Ocimum basilicum.*
COMMON NAME: sweet basil, garden basil.
OCCURRENCE: as a garden plant throughout Britain.
PARTS USED: the herb, which contains a volatile, camphoraceous oil.
MEDICINAL USES: aromatic with carminative and cooling properties. It is used to treat mild nervous disorders, and an infusion of basil is said to be good for obstructions of the internal organs and in stopping vomiting and nausea.
ADMINISTERED AS: a flavouring in food, dried leaves or an infusion.

Bayberry *Myrica corifera.*
COMMON NAME: candleberry, waxberry, tallow shrub, wax myrtle.
OCCURRENCE: widely distributed through America, Europe and Great Britain.

PARTS USED: the bark, which contains volatile oil, starch, lignin, tannic and gallic acids along with lesser compounds.

MEDICINAL USES: a powerful stimulant, astringent and tonic. The powdered bark may be used in poultices, often together with elm. A decoction is used to treat the throat and sore gums.

ADMINISTERED AS: an infusion, decoction, powder and injection.

Bearberry *Archostaphylos uva-ursi.*

COMMON NAME: *Arbutus uva-ursi, uva-ursi.*

OCCURRENCE: on heaths of the Scottish Highlands, south to Yorkshire, and in high mountains of Europe, Asia and America.

PARTS USED: the leaves, which contain arbutin as the chief constituent.

MEDICINAL USES: when made into an infusion, the leaves have a soothing, astringent and diuretic effect. This is of benefit in diseases affecting the bladder, and the kidneys, e.g. urethritis, cystitis, etc.

ADMINISTERED AS: an infusion.

Beech *Fagus Sylvatica.*

COMMON NAME: buche, boke, faggio, fagos.

OCCURRENCE: found in Europe, including Britain, although only indigenous to England.

PARTS USED: the oil of beech nuts, and beech tar.

MEDICINAL USES: beech tar is stimulating and antiseptic so is used internally as a stimulating expectorant to treat chronic bronchitis. It is used externally applied to various skin diseases.

ADMINISTERED AS: beech oil or beech tar.

Beetroot *Beta vulgaris.*

COMMON NAME: spinach beet, sea beet, garden beet, whit beet, mangel-wurzel.

OCCURRENCE: *Beta vulgaris* is native to southern Europe and is derived from the sea beet, *Beta maritima* which grows wild on the coasts of Europe, England, North Africa and Asia. There are many cultivated forms and varieties of beetroot with similar properties.

PARTS USED: the leaves and root. The root contains a pure fruit sugar which is easily taken up by the body, as well as starch and gum.

MEDICINAL USES: the juice of the white beet was said to be of a 'cleansing, digestive quality' to 'open up obstructions of the liver and spleen' and ease headaches. Beetroot is used to produce refined sugar, as a vegetable and to make wine or ale.

ADMINISTERED AS: dietary item, decoction, expressed juice.

Belladonna Atropa belladonna.

COMMON NAME: deadly nightshade, devil's cherries, dwale, black cherry, devil's herb, great morel.

OCCURRENCE: native to central and southern Europe but commonly grows in England.

PARTS USED: the roots and leaves. The root contains several alkaloid compounds, including hyoscyamine, atropine and belladonnine. The same alkaloids are present in the leaves but the amount of each compound varies according to plant type and methods of storing and drying leaves.

MEDICINAL USES: as a narcotic, diuretic, sedative, mydriatic, antispasmodic. The drug is used as an anodyne in febrile conditions, night sweats and coughs. It is valuable in treating eye diseases and is used as a pain-relieving lotion to treat neuralgia, gout, rheumatism and sciatica. Belladonna is an extremely poisonous plant and should always be used under medical supervision. Cases of accidental poisoning and death are well-known. Despite this, it is a valuable drug used to treat a wide range of diseases.

ADMINISTERED AS: a liquid extract that is used to produce alcoholic extracts, plasters, liniment, suppositories, tincture and ointment.

Bergamot Monarda didyma.

COMMON NAME: scarlet monarda, Oswego tea, bee balm.

OCCURRENCE: a plant which is indigenous to North America.

PARTS USED: the oil extracted from the whole plant, and the leaves.

MEDICINAL USES: used in a similar manner to other plants containing thymol as an active chemical. Oil of bergamot has antiseptic, aromatic, carminative, tonic and antispasmodic properties. An infusion of the young leaves was a common beverage in the USA before tea became more common. The infusion is also good for coughs, sore throats, fevers and colds.

ADMINISTERED AS: essential oil, infusion, fluid extract.

Bethroot Trillium pendulum, Trillium erectum.

COMMON NAME: Indian shamrock, birthroot, lamb's quarters, wake-robin, Indian balm, ground lily.

OCCURRENCE: a native North American plant found in the western and middle United States.

PARTS USED: the dried root and rhizome; the leaves.

MEDICINAL USES: antiseptic, astringent, tonic, expectorant, pectoral and alterative. It is useful in all cases of internal bleeding, profuse menstruation and pulmonary complaints. It is used to promote safe childbirth and delivery. The leaves may be applied to ulcers and tumours while the root makes a good antiseptic poultice to stop gangrene spreading or for skin diseases. It was used by the native Americans as a medicine.

ADMINISTERED AS: the powdered root, fresh leaves and infusion.

Betony, Wood *Stachys bentonica, Betonica officinalis.*

COMMON NAME: bishopswort.

OCCURRENCE: found wild in woodlands, or on heath or moorland but less common in Scotland.

PARTS USED: the herb.

MEDICINAL USES: aromatic, astringent and alterative. Betony was thought to be one of the best treatments for headaches and hangovers. It is normally combined with other herbs to produce a tonic for nervous affections, dyspepsia and rheumatism. The dried herb was also used to make a tea substitute and was smoked as tobacco.

ADMINISTERED AS: an infusion.

Bindweed, Greater *Convolvulus sepium.*

COMMON NAME: hedge convolvulus, old man's night cap, hooded bindweed, bearbind.

OCCURRENCE: a native of Britain which is abundant in England but rarer in Scotland.

PARTS USED: the resin produced from the roots.

MEDICINAL USES: the resin is normally made into a tincture. This preparation is then applied internally and has a purgative effect. The effects are not as pronounced as in the related plant species *Convulvus jalapa* (jalap bindweed) and *Convulvus scammonia* (Syrian bindweed).

ADMINISTERED AS: tincture.

Birch, Common *Betula alba.*

COMMON NAME: white birch, bouleau, berke, bereza.

OCCURRENCE: common in Europe, from Sicily to Iceland and also found in northern Asia.

PARTS USED: the bark and leaves. The bark contains tannic acid, behilin and behils camphor while the leaves contain betulorentic acid.

MEDICINAL USES: bitter and astringent. The bark yields oil of birch tar upon destructive distillation, which is very similar to oil of WINTER-GREEN. The oil is used in skin disease ointments, e.g. treating eczema while it is also used as a component of insect repellent. Birch tea made of the leaves is recommended for gout, rheumatism and dropsy and is also said to be good for breaking up kidney stones. Sap from the tree is used to produce beer, wine, spirits and vinegar in various parts of Europe.

ADMINISTERED AS: oil, infusion.

Birthwort *Aristolochia longa.*

COMMON NAME: long-rooted birthwort.

OCCURRENCE: throughout Europe and Great Britain.

PARTS USED: the root, which contains aristolochine.

MEDICINAL USES: aromatic and stimulant. It is useful in treating gout and rheumatism and may be used to clear obstructions after childbirth.

ADMINISTERED AS: powdered root.

Bistort *Polygonum bisorta.*

COMMON NAME: snakeweed, adderwort, twice writhen, osterick, Easter marigiant, English sepentary.

OCCURRENCE: a native of many parts of northern Europe, common in the north of England and southern Scotland.

PARTS USED: the root-stock which contains tannin, starch, gallic acid and gum.

MEDICINAL USES: a strong astringent and is mainly used in external and internal bleeding and haemorrhages from the lungs or stomach. Can be used to treat diarrhoea, dysentery, cholera and bowel complaints. Bistort is important in alleviating diabetes and as a mouth wash or gargle to 'fasten loose teeth' and heal gum problems.

ADMINISTERED AS: a powder, fluid extract, decoction or injection.

Bitter root *Apocynum androsaemifolium.*

COMMON NAME: milkweed, dogsbane, fly-trap, wild cotton.

OCCURRENCE: found in mountainous regions of Europe and North America.

PARTS USED: the dried rhizome and roots. The active chemicals in the plant are a bitter principle called cymarin, and to a lesser extent the glucoside apocynamarin.

MEDICINAL USES: cardiac tonic, hydragogue, alterative. Bitter root is similar to foxglove in action and is very powerful in slowing the pulse and it also has a strong action on the vaso-motor system. It may irritate the mucous membranes, causing nausea and purging of the bowels, so that it cannot be tolerated by all people. As a powerful hydrogogue it is good against fluid accumulation in the abdomen (ascites), particularly when it is linked to liver cirrhosis. It is also highly effective in treating dropsy which is related to heart failure. The plant's alterative powers are used against syphilis, scrofula and rheumatism. Because of irregular absorption of the drug through the gastro-intestinal tract, great care must be taken with the dosage administered and the patient's condition.

ADMINISTERED AS: powdered root, liquid extract.

Bittersweet Solanum dulcamara.

COMMON NAME: woody nightshade, violet bloom, scarlet berry, felonwood, felonwort, dulcamara.

OCCURRENCE: a climbing plant found in hedgerows in Britain.

PARTS USED: the twigs and root-bark. The twigs contain the alkaloid solamine and the glucoside dulcamarine which gives bittersweet its characteristic taste. It also contains sugar, gum, starch and resin.

MEDICINAL USES: narcotic, resolvent, diuretic and alterative. Bittersweet promotes all secretions, particularly of the skin and kidneys, and is generally used to clear up stubborn skin infections and eruptions, scrofula and ulcers and has been recommended in chronic bronchial catarrh, asthma or whooping cough. In large doses, the drug can cause paralysis of the central nervous system and lead to death.

ADMINISTERED AS: a fluid extract, decoction.

Blackberry Rubus fructicosus.

COMMON NAME: bramble, bumble-kite, bramble-kite, bly, brummel, brameberry, scaldhead, brambleberry.

OCCURRENCE: common throughout Britain in hedgerows and ditches.

PARTS USED: the root and leaves, which both contain tannin.

MEDICINAL USES: as astringent and tonic. It is valuable against dysentery and diarrhoea. A decoction of the root was used to treat whooping cough. A cordial or vinegar drink was made and is useful in treating looseness of the bowels, piles or a feverish cold.

ADMINISTERED AS: decoction, fluid extract or cordial, wine or vinegar.

Blackcurrant Ribes nigrum.

COMMON NAME: quinsy berries, squinancy berries.

OCCURRENCE: a common garden plant throughout Britain, but is only truly native to Yorkshire and the Lake District. It is also found in Europe.

PARTS USED: the fruit, leaves, bark and root.

MEDICINAL USES: diuretic, diaphoretic, febrifuge, refrigerant, detergent. The fruit juice is excellent in febrile diseases and can be made to an extract which is good for sore throats. The leaves when infused are cleansing while a root infusion is used in eruptive fevers and has been used to treat cattle. A decoction of the bark is effective against calculus, oedema and haemorrhoids. The fruit was commonly used to make jelly, wine and cheese.

ADMINISTERED AS: juice, infusion or decoction.

Black root Leptandra virginica.

COMMON NAME: culver's root, culver's physic, physic root, leptandrawurzel, *Veronica virginica*, *Veronica purpurea*, *Paederota virginica*, *Eustachya purpurea*, *Eustachya alba*.

OCCURRENCE: found in the eastern United States.

PARTS USED: the rhizome which contains a crystalline principle and an impure resin, which together are called leptandrin and are said to be the active principles.

MEDICINAL USES: violent cathartic, emetic, tonic, antiseptic, diaphoretic. The action of the root on the body depends upon whether the root is dried or fresh. Fresh root is violently cathartic and emetic in action while the dried root has milder effects. It is used to excite the liver and promote the secretion of bile without harming the bowels and it is a good stomach tonic of benefit to diarrhoea, dysentery, cholera and torpid liver problems. The fresh root, however, may induce abortion and gives rise to bloody stools, but a decoction of the fresh root is used for intermittent fevers. The dried root has been used successfully in leprosy, dropsy, cancer, pulmonary tuberculosis and malaria.

ADMINISTERED AS: powdered root, decoction and fluid extract.

Bladderwrack Fucus vesiculosus.

COMMON NAME: bladder fucus, seawrack, kelp ware, black-tang, cutweed, seetang, blasentang, meeriche.

OCCURRENCE: common around the coasts of the North Atlantic Ocean including Britain.

PARTS USED: the root, stem and leaves, the thallus. The seaweed contains a volatile oil, cellulose, mucilage, mannite, soda and iodine along with the bromine compounds of sodium and potassium.

MEDICINAL USES: a deobstruent, antifat. It has been used to cause weight loss and reduce obesity by stimulation of the thyroid gland. The wine made from grapes and dried fucus has been of benefit in diseases of the hip, joints and bones in children. It may also be applied externally as a poultice to treat enlarged glands.

ADMINISTERED AS: a liquid extract, decoction, infusion, fluid extract, or charcoal derived from *Fucus vesiculosus*.

Bloodroot *Sanguinaria candensis.*

COMMON NAME: Indian paint, tetterwort, red pucoon, red root, paucon, coon root, snakebite, sweet slumber.

OCCURRENCE: a spring flower found in woods from Canada to Florida and west to Arkansas and Nebraska in the United States.

PARTS USED: the rhizome. It has the alkaloids sanguinarine, chelery-thrine, protropine and B. homochelidonine as its active components. Protropine is one of the most widely used opium alkaloids.

MEDICINAL USES: emetic, cathartic, expectorant, emmenagogue. The plant is of great benefit in dyspepsia, asthma, bronchitis, croup and pulmonary consumption. It can be used in heart disease, heart weakness and palpitations, nervous irritation, torpid liver, scrofula, dysentery and to lower the pulse rate. Externally, it can be applied to cure ringworm, fungal growths, ulcers, eczema and cancerous growths. Care must be taken as toxic doses of *Sanguinaria* can be deleterious to the person.

ADMINISTERED AS: fluid extract, tincture, powdered root and solid extract.

Bluebell *Scilla nutans, Hyacinthus nonscriptus.*

COMMON NAME: calverkeys, culverkeys, auld man's bell, ring-o'-bells, jacinth, wood bells, *agraphis nutans.*

OCCURRENCE: abundant in western Europe, Great Britain and Italy.

PARTS USED: the bulb, dried and powdered.

MEDICINAL USES: diuretic, styptic. This medicine is little used today but it was considered a very powerful remedy for leucorrhoea. It may also have been used to cure snake bite. The fresh bulbs are poisonous, so the plant is always used when dried.

ADMINISTERED AS: powdered bulb.

Blue flag *Iris versicolor.*

COMMON NAME: poison flag, flag lily, liver lily, snake lily, dragon flower, dagger flower, water flag.

OCCURRENCE: indigenous to North America and was introduced into Britain and Europe and is now a common garden plant.

PARTS USED: the rhizome which contains starch, gum, tannin, isophthalic acid, salicylic acid and oleoresin of which the latter compound contains the medicinal properties.

MEDICINAL USES: alterative, diuretic, cathartic, stimulant. It is chiefly used for its alterative properties being useful as a purgative in disorders of the liver and the duodenum. Also, combined with other herbs as a blood puri-

fier, or used alone against syphilis, scrofula, skin afflictions and dropsy.
ADMINISTERED AS: powdered root, solid extract, fluid extract or tincture.

Bogbean Menyanthes trifoliata.
COMMON NAME: buckbean, marsh trefoil, water trefoil, marsh clover, boonan.
OCCURRENCE: found in spongy bogs, marshes and shallow water throughout Europe and is more common in northern England and Scotland.
PARTS USED: the herb which consists of volatile oil and a glucoside called menyanthin.
MEDICINAL USES: as a tonic, cathartic, deobstruent and febrifuge. A liquid extract is used to treat rheumatism, scurvy and skin complaints. It has also been recommended as an external application to reduce glandular swelling. In the Highlands of Scotland it was used to remedy stomach pains, particularly due to ulcers, and bogbean was also brewed into beer and smoked as herb tobacco. It is thought to cure ague (malaria) where all other cures have failed.
ADMINISTERED AS: the liquid extract, infusion or as tea.

Boneset Eupatonium perfoliatum.
COMMON NAME: thoroughwort, Indian sage, feverwort.
OCCURRENCE: found in meadows in North America and Europe.
PARTS USED: the herb. The important constituents are volatile oil, tannic acid, gum, resin, sugar and the glucoside eupatonin.
MEDICINAL USES: a diaphoretic, tonic, febrifuge, expectorant, stimulant, and laxative. It is used successfully to treat rheumatism, colds and influenza, catarrh and skin diseases. It acts slowly on the stomach, liver, bowel and uterus but it has a persistent beneficial effect. In large doses it has an emetic and purgative effect.
ADMINISTERED AS: powdered herb, fluid extract and solid extract.

Borage Borago officinalis.
COMMON NAME: burrage.
OCCURRENCE: naturalized in Britain and Europe and is found in gardens, rubbish heaps and near houses.
PARTS USED: the leaves and flowers consist of potassium, calcium and mineral acids along with nitrogen salts.
MEDICINAL USES: diuretic, demulcent, emollient, refrigerant. It is effective in treating fevers and pulmonary complaints as it activates the kidneys. It is applied externally as a poultice against inflammation and swelling and

has been developed into a cream which treats itch and skin complaints, e.g. eczema and psoriasis. The flowers may be eaten raw, candied or made into a conserve to strengthen people weakened by prolonged illness.
ADMINISTERED AS: an infusion, poultice or lotion.

Box *Buxus sempervirens*.

COMMON NAME: dudgeon.
OCCURRENCE: native to Europe and western Africa but was introduced into Great Britain and the USA.
PARTS USED: the wood and leaves. The bark contains chlorophyll, wax, resin and tallow along with carbonate, sulphate and phosphate compounds. The leaves contain three alkaloids—buxine, parabuxine and parabuxonidine, as well as tannin.
MEDICINAL USES: the wood is diaphoretic, narcotic and sedative in full doses. It is generally prepared as a decoction for rheumatism and syphilis. The tincture was thought to be a bitter tonic, antiperiodic and cured leprosy. A volatile oil distilled from the wood has been used in epilepsy, piles and toothache. The leaves are sudorific, alterative and cathartic when powdered. The powder is poisonous so thus it makes an excellent purgative, vermifuge and is anthelmintic.
ADMINISTERED AS: powdered leaves, tincture, distilled oil, and decoction.

Brooklime *Veronica beccabunga*.

COMMON NAME: water pimpernel, becky leaves, cow cress, horse cress, housewell grass, limewort, brooklembe, limpwort, wall-ink, water-pumpy, well-ink.
OCCURRENCE: very common in all parts of Great Britain.
PARTS USED: the herb. This plant contains tannin, a bitter principle, a volatile oil and sulphur.
MEDICINAL USES: alterative, diuretic. It is used as an infusion as an antiscorbutic and to treat impurities of the blood.
ADMINISTERED AS: infusion or poultice.

Broom *Cytisus scoparius*.

COMMON NAME: broom tops, Irish tops, basam, bizzom, browne, brum, bream, green broom.
OCCURRENCE: indigenous to England and commonly found on heathland throughout Britain, Europe and northern Asia.
PARTS USED: the young herbaceous tops which contain sparteine and scoparin as the active components.

MEDICINAL USES: diuretic and cathartic. The broom tops may be used as a decoction or infusion to aid dropsy while if the tops are pressed and treated broom juice is obtained. This fluid extract is generally used in combination with other diuretic compounds. An infusion of broom, AGRIMONY and DANDELION root is excellent in remedying bladder, kidney and liver trouble. *Cytisus* should be used carefully as the sparteine has a strong effect on the heart and, depending upon dose, can cause weakness of the heart similar to that caused by HEMLOCK (*Conium maculatum*). Death can occur in extreme cases if the respiratory organ's activity is impaired.

ADMINISTERED AS: fluid extract and infusion.

Bryony, Black *Tamus communis*.

COMMON NAME: blackeye root.

OCCURRENCE: native to Great Britain, common in woods and hedges.

PARTS USED: the root.

MEDICINAL USES: as a rubefacient and diuretic. The drug is seldom used internally now due to its poisonous nature, but was formerly used to treat asthmatic complaints. Externally the fresh root is scraped, pulped and applied as a plaster to areas affected by gout, rheumatism or paralysis. A root pulp poultice was used on bruises and black eyes to remove discolouration from the skin. Chilblains were treated using a tincture made from the roots.

ADMINISTERED AS: a plaster, poultice, tincture, rarely as expressed juice.

Bryony, White *Bryonia dioica, Bryonia alba*.

COMMON NAME: English mandrake, wild vine, wild hops, lady's seal, tetterbury, wild nep, tamus.

OCCURRENCE: a native of Europe, frequently found in England but rare in Scotland.

PARTS USED: the root.

MEDICINAL USES: irritative, hydragogue, cathartic. It was previously used as a purgative drug but these and other uses have been discontinued on account of its highly irritant nature. It is still used in small doses for coughs, influenza, bronchitis and pneumonia. It is useful in cardiac disorders caused by gout or rheumatism and in malarial and contagious diseases. Care should be taken when used, due to its poisonous nature.

ADMINISTERED AS: liquid extract.

Buchu *Barosma betulina*.

COMMON NAME: bucco, *Diosma betulina*.

OCCURRENCE: found at the Cape of Good Hope in South Africa.

PARTS USED: the leaves, which contain volatile oil, mucilage and diosphenol. They are collected from wild plants and this is strictly controlled by the government.

MEDICINAL USES: diuretic, diaphoretic, stimulant. The plant has a direct effect on the urinary organs, benefiting gravel, inflammation and catarrh of the bladder, cystitis, nephritis and urethritis. It has been classed as an official medicine in Great Britain since 1821.

ADMINISTERED AS: fluid extract, tincture and solid extract.

Bugle *Ajuga reptans.*

COMMON NAME: common bugle, carpenter's herb, middle confound, middle comfrey, sicklewort, herb carpenter, bugula.

OCCURRENCE: abundant throughout Great Britain in damp pastures and woods.

PARTS USED: the herb.

MEDICINAL USES: bitter, astringent and aromatic. As an infusion this herb is considered very good in arresting haemorrhages, easing irritation and coughs. It acts in a similar way to that of FOXGLOVE (*Digitalis purpurea*) in lowering the pulse rate and is said to be one of the mildest and best narcotics in existence. It is also considered good for the bad effects of excessive drinking.

ADMINISTERED AS: a decoction and infusion.

Burdock *Artium lappa.*

COMMON NAME: lappa, fox's clote, thorny burr, beggar's buttons, cockle buttons, love leaves, philanthropium, personata, happy major, clot-bur.

OCCURRENCE: freely found in ditches and hedgerows throughout England and Europe but rare in Scotland.

PARTS USED: the root, herb and seeds (fruits). They contain the chemicals inulin, mucilage, sugar and tannic acid along with a crystalline gluco-side, lappin.

MEDICINAL USES: alterative, diuretic and diaphoretic. It is an excellent blood purifier and very effective in remedying all skin diseases. The root is most powerful and has antiscorbutic properties which make it very useful for boils, scurvy and rheumatism. Also used as a wash for ulcers and a poultice for tumours, gouty swellings and bruises. An infusion of the leaves aids the stomach and eases indigestion. The tincture obtained from the seeds is a relaxant, demulcent and a tonic for the skin.

ADMINISTERED AS: a fluid extract, infusion, tincture and solid extract.

Burnet, Greater *Sanguisorba officinalis.*

COMMON NAME: garden burnet, common burnet, salad burnet.

OCCURRENCE: found in moist meadows and shady areas almost all over Europe and in British gardens.

PARTS USED: the herb and root.

MEDICINAL USES: astringent and tonic. Decoction of the whole herb is useful in haemorrhages. Both the herb and root are taken internally to treat abnormal discharges such as diarrhoea, dysentery and leucorrhoea. It is also used to make herb beer.

ADMINISTERED AS: a powder and infusion.

Burr Marigold *Bidens Impartica.*

COMMON NAME: water agrimony.

OCCURRENCE: commonly found in wet places in England but less frequently seen in Scotland.

PARTS USED: the whole plant.

MEDICINAL USES: astringent, diaphoretic, diuretic. This plant has been useful in dropsy, gout, haematuria and fevers. It is very good in treating diseases of the respiratory organs where bleeding occurs and also in uterine haemorrhage.

ADMINISTERED AS: an infusion.

Butcher's Broom *Ruscus aculeatus.*

COMMON NAME: kneeholm, knee holy, jew's myrtle, sweet broom, pettigree.

OCCURRENCE: a low shrubby plant found in woods and waste ground, primarily in the south of England.

PARTS USED: the herb and root.

MEDICINAL USES: diaphoretic, diuretic, deobstruent and aperient. It is used in jaundice, gravel, urinary and female obstructions and is said to be good in clearing phlegm from the chest and relieving difficult breathing.

ADMINISTERED AS: a decoction.

Butterbur *Petasites vulgaris.*

COMMON NAME: langwort, umbrella plant, bog rhubarb, plapperdock, blatterdock, capdockin, bogshorns, butterdock.

OCCURRENCE: in low wet grounds, meadows and riversides in Britain.

PARTS USED: the rhizome or rootstock.

MEDICINAL USES: as a cardiac tonic, a stimulant and diuretic. It is good as a remedy for fevers, asthma, colds, urinary complaints, gravel and plague. It is also taken as a homeopathic remedy for severe neuralgia in the back and loins. Recently, the use of butterbur has been recommended in easing the pain of migraine and painful menstruation. One of the most important developments is the treatment of cancer with *Petasites* when the drug attacks tumours and abnormal cell changes very strongly. In clinical tests, it has been shown to slow or stop the cancer spreading through the body. It has also become an effective remedy for severe asthma.

ADMINISTERED AS: a decoction and tincture.

Buttercup, Bulbous *Ranunculus bulbosus*.
COMMON NAME: St Antony's turnip, crowfoot, frogsfoot, goldcup.
OCCURRENCE: found in meadows and fields throughout Britain.
PARTS USED: the juice and herbs.
MEDICINAL USES: this plant has various uses including easing headaches and as a cure for shingles. The herb inflames and blisters the skin upon contact and is used to aid gout, sciatica and rheumatism. It has also been used as a poultice on the stomach.
ADMINISTERED AS: a poultice, decoction and tincture.

Cacao *Theobroma cacao*.
COMMON NAME: cocoa, chocolate tree.
OCCURRENCE: found in tropical America and cultivated in most tropical countries, e.g. Sri Lanka and Java.
PARTS USED: the seeds, which contain about two per cent of the chemical theobromine and forty to sixty per cent solid fat.
MEDICINAL USES: emollient, diuretic, stimulant and nutritive. The seeds are ground into a paste between hot rollers, with sugar and starch being added to produce cocoa. The cocoa butter (or oil of theobroma) produced forms a hard solid which is used in cosmetics, suppositories and coating pills. It has very good emollient qualities and is used to soften chapped hands and lips. The alkaloid, theobromine, which is contained in the beans is similar to caffeine in action on the central nervous system, but less powerful. It acts on the heart, kidneys and muscle and is used as a diuretic and stimulant of the kidneys. This is useful after fluid has accumulated in the body after heart failure and it is given in conjunction with digitalis (FOXGLOVE). The drug is also of benefit in high blood pressure.
ADMINISTERED AS: expressed oil, theobromine.

Calamint *Calamintha officinalis*.
COMMON NAME: mill mountain, mountain balm, basil thyme, mountain mint.
OCCURRENCE: a bushy plant found in hedgerows and lanes all over Great Britain and Europe.

Calamus

PARTS USED: the herb. This contains a camphoraceous, volatile, stimulating oil similar to those found in other mint plants.
MEDICINAL USES: diaphoretic, expectorant and aromatic. It can be infused into a tea to treat weak stomachs, colic and flatulence. Can also be brewed into a syrup or decoction to heal the spleen, gall bladder and jaundice.
ADMINISTERED AS: an infusion, decoction and syrup.

Calamus *Aconus calamus.*
COMMON NAME: sweet flag, sweet sedge, sweet root, gladdon, sweet rush, sweet cane, myrtle grass, sweet myrtle, cinnamon sedge, myrtle wedge.
OCCURRENCE: grows freely in all European countries except Spain and it is common on river banks in Great Britain.
PARTS USED: the rhizome, which produces a volatile oil after steam distillation, which is made up of pinene and asaryl aldehyde. It also contains alkaloidal material including choline and the glucoside acorin.
MEDICINAL USES: aromatic, carminative, stimulant, tonic and stomachic. It is used to remove the discomfort of flatulence, wind, colic, ague and dyspepsia. It can increase the appetite and aid digestion. Calamus oil is used in inhalations.
ADMINISTERED AS: a fluid extract, infusion, tincture and distilled oil.

Calotrophis *Calotrophis procera, Calotrophis gigantea.*
COMMON NAME: mudar bark, mudar yercum, *Asclepias onocera.*
OCCURRENCE: native to India but is cultivated in the East and West Indies and Sri Lanka.
PARTS USED: the dried bark. This contains several chemicals including madaralbum, madarfluavil, caoutchouc, mudarine, two resins and calatrophin which is an active poison similar to digitalis (FOXGLOVE).
MEDICINAL USES: in India, it is used as a remedy for elephantiasis, leprosy and chronic eczema. It may be taken internally for diarrhoea and dysentery. It has also been used to induce abortion and as a means of suicide. Atropine (from BELLADONNA, *Atropa belladonna*) may be used as an antidote to poisoning with calotrophis.
ADMINISTERED AS: powdered bark, tincture.

Calumba *jateorhiza calumba.*
COMMON NAME: *Cocculus palmatus*, colombo, *jateorhiza palmata.*
OCCURRENCE: indigenous to the forests of Mozambique and found throughout East Africa.
PARTS USED: the dried root. It contains three alkaloids—columbamine,

jateorhizine and palmatine, which are closely related to berberine (from BARBERRY). There is also the crystalline principle, columbine, starch and mucilage in the root.

MEDICINAL USES: bitter tonic, febrifuge. Due to its lack of astringent qualities, it does not cause nausea, headache, sickness or fevers as other similar remedies do. It is very good against pulmonary consumption, weakness of the digestive organs, dysentery and for flatulence in combination with GINGER and SENNA. Calumba can stop sickness in pregnancy and gastric irritation.

ADMINISTERED AS: cold infusion, tincture, fluid extract, powdered root, solid extract.

Camphor *Cinnamonum camphora.*

COMMON NAME: gum Camphor, laurel camphor, camphire, *Laurus camphora*, *Camphora officinarum*.

OCCURRENCE: found in China, Japan and parts of East Asia.

PARTS USED: the gum and distilled oil.

MEDICINAL USES: sedative, anodyne, antispasmodic, diaphoretic, anthelmintic, aromatic. It is mainly used in colds, chills, fevers, inflammatory complaints and for severe diarrhoea. It is taken internally for hysteria, nervousness, neuralgia and is used as an excitant in cases of heart failure due to infections, fevers and pneumonia. Camphor is highly valued in all irritations of the sexual organs. Large doses of camphor should be avoided as they can cause vomiting, palpitations and convulsions due to the effects it has on the human brain.

ADMINISTERED AS: tincture, distilled oil, injection, capsules.

Caraway *Carum Carvi.*

COMMON NAME: caraway seed, caraway fruit, alcaravea.

OCCURRENCE: common in Europe and Asia. Naturalized in Britain.

PARTS USED: the fruit, which produces a volatile oil containing a hydrocarbon, carvene and an oxygenated oil, carvol.

MEDICINAL USES: aromatic, stimulant and carminative. It was widely used as a cordial to ease dyspepsia and hysteria. The oil is applied to treat flatulence and stomach disorders. Distilled caraway water is used to ease flatulent colic in infants and is an excellent children's medicine. The bruised fruits were used to remove pain from bad earache and was also used as a poultice to take away bruises. Caraway is widely used as a flavouring for cheeses and seed-cakes.

ADMINISTERED AS: a liquid extract and poultice.

Cardamom *Elettaria cardamomum.*

COMMON NAME: mysore cardamon seeds, malabar cardamom, ebil, kakelah seghar, capalaga, gujalatti elachi, ilachi, ailum, *Amomum cardamomum, A. repens, Alpina cardamom, matonia Cardamomum, Cardamomum minus, Cardamomi Semina.*

OCCURRENCE: native to southern India and cultivated in Sri Lanka.

PARTS USED: the dried ripe seed containing volatile and fixed oil, starch, mucilage, potassium salts, resin and lignin.

MEDICINAL USES: carminative, stimulant, aromatic. They have a warming aromatic effect which is useful in indigestion and flat-ulence. If chewed, they are said to be good for colic and head-aches. Cardamom is used chiefly as a flavouring for cakes, liqueurs, etc. and forms part of curry powder mixtures used in cookery.

ADMINISTERED AS: powdered seeds, tincture and fluid extract.

Caroba *Jacaranda procera.*

COMMON NAME: carob tree, carobinha, caaroba, *jacaranda caroba, Bignonia caroba.*

OCCURRENCE: found in South America and South Africa.

PARTS USED: the leaves contain many compounds including caroba balsam, caroborelinic acid, carobic acid, steocarobic acid, caroban and carobin.

MEDICINAL USES: alterative, diaphoretic, diuretic. The active principles have proved to be of benefit in treating syphilis and other venereal diseases. The soothing qualities of the herb have also been used to help epilepsy, as it has a sedative effect upon the nervous system. Caroba is rarely used in medicine today.

ADMINISTERED AS: dried, powdered leaves.

Carrot *Daucus carota.*

COMMON NAME: philtron, bird's nest, bee's nest.

OCCURRENCE: a native wild plant common everywhere in Great Britain. The wild and cultivated parts both exist today.

PARTS USED: the whole herb, seeds and root.

MEDICINAL USES: diuretic, stimulant, deobstruent. The herb infused in water is an active remedy in treating dropsy, chronic kidney infections and bladder disorders. Carrot tea was good for gout, while a strong decoction is good against gravel and flatulence. The roots have antiseptic properties and were formerly used as a laxative, vermifuge or a poultice. The wild carrot was particularly well thought of as a poultice for cancerous sores, while the seeds act in a similar manner to CARAWAY in treating stomach and gastric complaints. Carrot seed also has properties as an emmenagogue and in clearing obstructions of the viscera and jaundice. Carrots are made into jam, wine, spirit and can be roasted to produce a coffee substitute.

ADMINISTERED AS: an infusion, tea and poultice.

Cassia Cinnamomum cassia.

COMMON NAME: bastard cinnamon, Chinese cinnamon, cassia bark, canton cassia, *Cassia lignea*, *Cassia aromaticum*.

OCCURRENCE: indigenous to China and cultivated in Japan, Sumatra, Java, South America, Mexico and Sri Lanka.

PARTS USED: the bark. The bark of this tree is regarded as a substitute for cinnamon and it produces a volatile oil similar to oil of cinnamon. Cassia oil contains cinnamic aldehyde, cinnamylacetate, cinnamic acid, tannic acid and starch amongst other compounds.

MEDICINAL USES: stomachic, carminative, tonic, astringent and emmenagogue. The tincture is used in uterine haemorrhage, menorrhagia and to decrease the flow of breast milk. It is also used to assist and flavour other drugs and benefits diarrhoea, vomiting, nausea and flatulence. Cassia oil is a powerful germicide but is not normally used in medicine as such as it is very irritant. It may be used for gastric pain, flatulent colic and gastric debility as it is a strong local stimulant.

ADMINISTERED AS: expressed oil, powdered bark.

Castor oil plant Ricinus communis.

COMMON NAME: palma Christi, castor oil bush.

OCCURRENCE: a native of India, but has been cultivated in many tropical, sub-tropical and temperate countries around the globe.

PARTS USED: the oil expressed from the seeds.

MEDICINAL USES: cathartic, purgative, laxative, vermifuge, galactogogue. Castor oil is regarded as one of the best laxative and purgative preparations available. It is of particular benefit for children and pregnant women due to its mild action in easing constipation, colic and diarrhoea due to slow digestion. The oil expels worms from the body, after other suitable remedies have been given. When applied externally, castor oil eases cutaneous complaints such as ringworm, itch and leprosy, while it is used as a carrier oil for solutions of pure alkaloids, e.g. atropine or cocaine, from BELLADONNA (*Atropa belladonna*), so that these drugs can be used in eye surgery. Castor oil is used for a range of industrial purposes from soap-making to varnishes.

ADMINISTERED AS: expressed oil.

Catmint

Catmint *Nepeta cataria.*

COMMON NAME: catnep, nep.

OCCURRENCE: a wild English plant in hedges, field borders and waste ground. It is found on a localized basis in Scotland.

PARTS USED: the herb.

MEDICINAL USES: carminative, tonic, diaphoretic, refrigerant, mildly stimulating and slightly emmenagogue. This herb is good in treating colds, fevers, restlessness and colic. It is also used in nervousness and insanity and to calm children and soothe nightmares when taken as an infusion or conserve. Catmint can be applied to swellings and bruises as a poultice.

ADMINISTERED AS: an infusion, injection or poultice.

Cayenne *Capsicum minimum, Capsicum frutescens.*

COMMON NAME: African pepper, chillies, bird pepper.

OCCURRENCE: native to Zanzibar but is now cultivated in most tropical and sub-tropical countries, e.g. Sierra Leone, Japan and Madagascar.

PARTS USED: the fruit, both fresh and dried.

MEDICINAL USES: stimulant, tonic, carminative, rubefacient. It is possibly the purest and best stimulant in herbal medicine. It produces natural warmth and helps the blood circulation, and eases weakness of the stomach and intestines. Cayenne is added to tonics and is said to ward off disease and can prevent development of colds and fevers.

ADMINISTERED AS: powdered fruit, tincture, capsules, dietary item.

Cedar, Yellow *Thuja occidentalis.*

COMMON NAME: tree of life, arbor vitae, false white cedar, *Cedrus lycea*, hackmatack, thuia de Canada, Lebensbaum.

OCCURRENCE: the United States and Canada.

PARTS USED: the leaves and twigs. The plant contains the bitter principle pinipicrin, volatile oil, sugar, wax, resin and a colouring principle called thujin. The leaves and twigs yield an essential oil similar to camphor, which contains pinene, fenchone, thujone and carvone.

MEDICINAL USES: aromatic, astringent, diuretic, anthelmintic, irritant, expectorant, emmenagogue. A decoction of the twigs can help intermittent fevers, coughs, gout, amenorrhoea, dropsy and scurvy. When made into an ointment, the leaves ease rheumatism. An infusion is good at removing warts and fungal growths. A preparation of the twigs may induce abortion by reflex action on the uterus from severe gastro-intestinal irritation. This plant should be used with some care.

ADMINISTERED AS: infusion, decoction, injection, poultice, tincture, ointment.

Celandine Chelidonium majus.

COMMON NAME: garden celandine, common celandine, greater celandine.

OCCURRENCE: common all over Great Britain and Europe.

PARTS USED: the herb, which contains the alkaloids chelidanine, chelerythrin (of which the latter is narcotic), homochelidonine A and B. Three other major chemicals are found in the plant.

MEDICINAL USES: alterative, diuretic and purgative. It is of benefit to jaundice, eczema, scrofulous diseases and scurvy. The fresh juice was used to cure warts, ringworm and corns but should not otherwise be allowed to come into direct contact with the skin. In various forms, it has previously been effective against itching, piles, toothache and cancer.

ADMINISTERED AS: infusion, fluid extract, decoction, lotion, poultice.

Celery Apium graveolens.

COMMON NAME: smallage, wild celery.

OCCURRENCE: native to southern Europe and cultivated in Britain.

PARTS USED: the ripe seeds, herb and root of which the seeds contain two oils and apiol.

MEDICINAL USES: carminative, stimulant, diuretic, tonic, nervine and aphrodisiac. It is utilized as a tonic in combination with other herbs, promoting restfulness, sleep and lack of hysteria and is excellent in relieving rheumatism.

ADMINISTERED AS: fluid extract, essential oil and powdered seeds.

Chamomile Anthemis nobilis.

COMMON NAME: Roman chamomile, double chamomile, manzanilla (Spanish), maythen (Saxon).

OCCURRENCE: a low growing plant found wild in the British Isles.

PARTS USED: the flowers and herb. The active principles therein are a volatile oil, anthemic acid, tannic acid and a glucoside.

MEDICINAL USES: tonic, stomachic, anodyne and anti-spasmodic. An infusion of chamomile tea is an extremely effective remedy for hysterical and nervous afflictions in women, as well as an emmenagogue. Chamomile has a powerful soothing and sedative effect which is harmless. A tincture is used to cure diarrhoea in children and it is used with purgatives to prevent griping, and as a tonic it helps dropsy. Externally, it can be applied alone or with other herbs as a poultice to relieve pain, swellings, inflammation and neuralgia. Its strong antiseptic properties make it invaluable for reducing swelling of the face due to abscess or injury. As a lotion, the flowers are good for resolving toothache and earache. The herb itself is an ingredient in herb beers. The use of chamomile can be dated back to ancient Egyptian times when they dedicated the plant to the sun because of its extensive healing properties.

ADMINISTERED AS: decoction, infusion, fluid extract and essential oil.

Cherry laurel *Prunus laurocerasus.*

OCCURRENCE: native to Russia and now cultivated in many temperate European countries.

PARTS USED: the leaves. The main constituent is prulaurasin which resembles amygdalin and hydrocyanic acid.

MEDICINAL USES: sedative, narcotic. The leaves are used to produce a distilled water which is the main herbal preparation used of this herb. It is good against coughs, dyspepsia, indigestion, whooping cough and asthma.

ADMINISTERED AS: cherry laurel water.

Chestnut, Horse *Aesculus hippocastanum.*

COMMON NAME: *Hippocastanum vulgare.*

OCCURRENCE: a tree native to northern and central Asia from which it was introduced into England and Scotland.

PARTS USED: the bark and fruit, from both of which a fluid extract is made.

MEDICINAL USES: tonic, narcotic, febrifuge and astringent. The bark is used in intermittent fevers as an infusion. It is also used externally to treat ulcers. The fruits are employed in easing neuralgia, rheumatism as well as rectal complaints and haemorrhoids.

ADMINISTERED AS: an infusion and fluid extract.

Chestnut, Sweet *Castanea vesca.*

COMMON NAME: *Fagus castanea*, sardia nut, Jupiter's nut, hushed nut, Spanish chestnut, *Castanea vulgaris.*

OCCURRENCE: very common in Britain, Europe and North America.

PARTS USED: the leaves.

MEDICINAL USES: tonic, astringent. It is used in a popular remedy to treat fever and ague. Its reputation is due to the great effectiveness in treating violent and convulsive coughs, particularly whooping cough and in other irritable respiratory organ conditions. The nut is commonly eaten as food or as a stuffing for meat.

ADMINISTERED AS: an infusion.

Chickweed *Stellania media.*

COMMON NAME: starweed, star chickweed, *Alsine media*, passerina.

OCCURRENCE: native to all temperate and North Arctic regions and is naturalized wherever Man has settled. A common weed.

PARTS USED: the whole herb, both fresh and dried.

MEDICINAL USES: demulcent, refrigerant. It is good as a poultice to reduce inflammation and heal indolent ulcers, but is most important as an ointment in treating eye problems and cutaneous diseases. It will also benefit scurvy and kidney disorders as an infusion.

ADMINISTERED AS: an infusion, poultice and ointment.

Chicory *Cichonium intybus.*

COMMON NAME: succory, wild succory, hendibeh, barbe de capucin.

OCCURRENCE: common in England and Ireland but rarer in Scotland.

PARTS USED: the root.

MEDICINAL USES: tonic, diuretic and laxative. A decoction of the root has benefit in jaundice, liver problems, gout and rheumatic complaints. The root, when dried, roasted and ground, may be added to coffee or may be drunk on its own as a beverage.

ADMINISTERED AS: a decoction, poultice, syrup or distilled water.

Chives *Allium schoenoprasum.*

COMMON NAME: cives.

OCCURRENCE: native to temperate and northern Europe and Great Britain. Cultivated over a large area of the northern hemisphere.

PARTS USED: the herb.

MEDICINAL USES: this herb stimulates the appetite and helps digestion during convalescence. It is also said to be effective against infections and to prevent anaemia. They are also widely used in food dishes and add vitamins and colour to many meals.

ADMINISTERED AS: fresh herbs.

Cicely, Sweet *Myrrhis odorata.*

COMMON NAME: smooth cicely, British myrrh, anise, great sweet chervil, smelt chervil, sweet bracken, sweet-fern, sweet humlock, sweets, the Roman plant, shepherd's needle, cow chervil.

OCCURRENCE: native to Great Britain and also found in mountain pastures across Europe.

PARTS USED: the root and herb.

MEDICINAL USES: aromatic, carminative, stomachic, expectorant. The fresh root may be eaten or used as a tonic in brandy. It eases coughs, flatulence, indigestion and stomach upsets. The herb, as an infusion, is good for anaemia and a tonic for young girls. The antiseptic roots have been used for snake or dog bites while the distilled water is diuretic and effective in treating pleurisy. Sweet cicely essence is said to have aphrodisiac properties.

ADMINISTERED AS: a root infusion, herb infusion, decoction, essence and distilled water.

Cinnamon *Cinnamomum zeylanicum.*

COMMON NAME: *Lauris cinnamomum.*

OCCURRENCE: native to Sri Lanka but is cultivated in other Eastern countries.

PARTS USED: the bark.

MEDICINAL USES: carminative, astringent, stimulant, antiseptic, aromatic. It is used as a local stimulant as a powder and infusion, generally combined with other herbs. Cinnamon stops vomiting and nausea, relieves flatulence and diarrhoea and can also be employed to stop haemorrhage of the womb.

ADMINISTERED AS: powder, distilled water, tincture or essential oil.

Clematis *Clematis recta.*

COMMON NAME: upright virgin's bower, *Clammula jovis.*

OCCURRENCE: a perennial plant common to Europe.

PARTS USED: the roots and stem.

MEDICINAL USES: diuretic, diaphoretic. When bruised, the leaves and flowers irritate the eyes and throat prompting tears and coughing. If applied to the skin, it produces inflammation and blisters appear. The herb is used both as a local external application, and internally against syphilis, cancer and other ulcers. It is used by homeopaths for eye complaints, gonorrhoea and inflammatory conditions.

ADMINISTERED AS: dried leaves, fluid extract.

Clivers *Galium aparine.*

COMMON NAME: cleavers, goosegrass, borweed, hedgesheriff, hayriffe, eriffe, grip grass, hayruff, catchweed, scratweed, mutton chops, robin-run-in-the-grass, love-man, goosebill, everlasting friendship.

OCCURRENCE: an abundant hedgerow weed in Europe, Great Britain and North America.

PARTS USED: the herb, which contains chlorophyll, starch, galitannic acid, citric acid and rubichloric acid.

MEDICINAL USES: diuretic, tonic, aperient and alterative. It is successfully administered to treat obstruction of the urinary organs, gravel, suppression of urine, etc. A wash of the herb helps sunburn and freckles, while an ointment provides benefit against cancerous growths and tumours. The expressed juice or infusion will help scurvy, scrofula, psoriasis and other skin complaints as well as stopping insomnia and inducing sleep.

ADMINISTERED AS: an infusion, decoction, ointment, expressed juice or lotion.

Clover, Red *Trifolium pratense.*
COMMON NAME: trefoil, purple clover.
OCCURRENCE: widely distributed in Britain and Europe.
PARTS USED: the flowers.
MEDICINAL USES: alterative, sedative, antispasmodic. The fluid extract or infusion are excellent in treating bronchial and whooping coughs. External applications of the herb in a poultice have been used on cancerous growths.
ADMINISTERED AS: fluid extract and infusion.

Clove *Eugenia caryophyllata.*
COMMON NAME: *Eugenia aromatica*, *Eugenia caryophyllus*, clavos.
OCCURRENCE: grows on the Molucca Islands in the southern Philippines.
PARTS USED: the underdeveloped flowers.
MEDICINAL USES: stimulating, carminative, aromatic. It is given as powder or an infusion for nausea, vomiting, flatulence, languid indigestion and dyspepsia. The volatile oil contains the medicinal properties and it is a strong germicide, antiseptic and a local irritant. It has been used as an expectorant to aid bronchial troubles. Clove oil is often used in association with other medicines.
ADMINISTERED AS: powdered cloves, infusion, essential oil, fluid extract.

Club moss *Lycopodium clavatum.*
COMMON NAME: lycopodium, lycopodium seed, vegetable sulphur, wolf's claw, muscus terrestris repens.
OCCURRENCE: occurs throughout Great Britain being most plentiful on heath or moorland in northern countries and is also found all over the world.
PARTS USED: the fresh plant and spores.
MEDICINAL USES: spores are diuretic, nervine and aperient. The fresh plant has been used as a stomachic and a diuretic herb in calculus and kidney complaints. The spores are currently applied externally to wounds and taken internally for diarrhoea, dysentery, gout and scurvy.
ADMINISTERED AS: dried spores, fresh moss.

Coca, Bolivian: *Erythroxylum coca*; **Peruvian:** *Erythroxylum truxillense.*
COMMON NAME: cuca, cocaine.
OCCURRENCE: native to Peru and Bolivia; cultivated in Java and Sri Lanka.
PARTS USED: the leaves. They contain the alkaloids cocaine, amamyl cocaine and truxilline or cocamine when grown in South America. Eastern-grown plants contain additional chemicals and glucosides.
MEDICINAL USES: nerve stimulant, anodyne, tonic, aphrodisiac. The leaves are used as a cerebral and muscle stimulant during convalescence relieving nausea, vomiting and stomach pains. It is utilized as a general nerve tonic and in treating asthma. In South America, the locals chew the leaves to relieve hunger and fatigue, but this does cause health damage when done over a long period of time. There is a danger of developing an addictive habit to this drug and the possible medicinal benefits are less than the potential health damage. People with a cocaine habit can appear emaciated, suffer loss of memory, sleeplessness and delusions. In Great Britain, the distribution and use of this drug is controlled by the Dangerous Drugs Act.
ADMINISTERED AS: tincture, powdered leaves, fluid extract.

Coffee *Coffea arabica.*
COMMON NAME: caffea.
OCCURRENCE: native to a province of Abyssinia and cultivated throughout the tropics.
PARTS USED: the seed and leaves. When roasted, coffee contains oil, wax, caffeine, aromatic oil, tannic acid, caffetannic acid, gum, sugar and protein.
MEDICINAL USES: stimulant, diuretic, anti-narcotic, anti-emetic. Coffee is commonly used as a beverage but it can also be applied as a medicine. It is a brain stimulant, causing sleeplessness and hence is useful in cases of narcotic poisoning. For this reason it is very good against snake bite in that it helps stop people falling into a coma. Caffeine can be valuable for heart disease and fluid retention and it is used against drunkenness. As a powerful diuretic, it can help ease gout, rheumatism, gravel and dropsy.
ADMINISTERED AS: beverage, caffeine preparation.

Cohosh, Black *Cimicifuga racemosa.*
COMMON NAME: black snakeroot, bugbane, rattleroot, rattleweed, squawroot, *Actaea racemosa, Macrotys actaeoides.*
OCCURRENCE: a native of the United States and Canada and was introduced into England around 1860.
PARTS USED: the rhizome. The main constituents are a resinous substance known as cimicifuga (or macrotin) and racemosin.

MEDICINAL USES: astringent, emmenagogue, diuretic, alterative, expectorant. This root is said to be effective in many disorders including whooping cough and rheumatism. It is supposed to be an antidote to poison and rattlesnake bites. The drug can help ease children's diarrhoea, and in consumption acts by slowing the pulse rate, inducing perspiration and easing the cough. In overdoses, black Cohosh can cause vomiting and nausea.
ADMINISTERED AS: tincture, infusion, decoction, powdered root.

Cohosh, Blue *Caulophyllum thalictroides.*
COMMON NAME: papoose root, squawroot, blueberry root, *Leontice thalichoides.*
OCCURRENCE: found in the United States and Canada.
PARTS USED: the rhizome. It contains gum, starch, salts, soluble resin and a chemical similar to saponin.
MEDICINAL USES: diuretic, antispasmodic, vermifuge, emmenagogue, athelmintic, diaphoretic. This drug has been used in rheumatism, epilepsy, uterine inflammation, hysteria and dropsy. It is also taken to expedite childbirth and induce menstruation.
ADMINISTERED AS: decoction, infusion, tincture, solid extract.

Coltsfoot *Tussilago farfara.*
COMMON NAME: coughwort, hallfoot, horsehoof, ass's foot, foals-wort, fieldhove, bullsfoot, donnhove.
OCCURRENCE: commonly found wild on waste ground and riverbanks in Great Britain.
PARTS USED: the leaves, flowers and root.
MEDICINAL USES: demulcent, expectorant and tonic. Coltsfoot is one of the most popular cough remedies and is generally taken in conjunction with HOREHOUND, MARSHMALLOW or GROUND IVY. It has been called 'nature's best herb for the lungs' and it was recommended that the leaves be smoked to relieve a cough. Today, it forms the basis of British herb tobacco along with BOGBEAN, EYEBRIGHT, WOOD BETONY, ROSEMARY, THYME, LAVENDER and CHAMOMILE which is said to relieve asthma, catarrh, bronchitis and lung troubles.
ADMINISTERED AS: syrup or smoked when dried.

Columbine *Aquilegia vulgaris.*
COMMON NAME: culverwort.
OCCURRENCE: found as both a wild and garden plant in Great Britain.
PARTS USED: the leaves, roots and seeds.
MEDICINAL USES: astringent. It must be administered in small doses where

it is used as a lotion for sore mouths and throats. It was also used for stone, jaundice and liver obstructions. Large doses can cause poisoning, so care must be taken in utilizing this drug.
ADMINISTERED AS: fresh root and infusion.

Comfrey *Symphytum officinale.*
COMMON NAME: common comfrey, knitbone, knitback, bruisewort, slippery root, gum plant, consolida, ass ear, blackwort.
OCCURRENCE: a native of Europe and temperate Asia but common by rivers and ditches throughout England.
PARTS USED: the root and leaves. The roots contain a large quantity of mucilage, choline and allantoin.
MEDICINAL USES: demulcent, mildly astringent, expectorant and vulnerary. It is frequently used in pulmonary complaints, to soothe intestinal trouble and is a gentle remedy for diarrhoea and dysentery. A strong decoction or tea is administered in cases of internal haemorrhage whether it is the lungs, stomach, bowels or haemorrhoids. Externally, the leaves have been used as a poultice to promote healing of severe cuts, ulcers and abscesses and to reduce swelling, sprains and bruises. Allantoin is known to reduce swelling round damaged or fractured bones, thus allowing healing to occur faster and more thoroughly.
ADMINISTERED AS: a decoction, poultice and liquid extract.

Coolwort *Tiarella cordifolia.*
COMMON NAME: foam flower, mitrewort.
OCCURRENCE: found in North America from Canada to Virginia.
PARTS USED: the herb.
MEDICINAL USES: diuretic, tonic. Very good in cases of gravel, suppression of urine and other bladder diseases. It is taken as a tonic in indigestion and dyspepsia where it corrects acidity and aids liver function.
ADMINISTERED AS: infusion, decoction.

Coriander *Coriandrum sativum.*
OCCURRENCE: indigenous to southern Europe and found occasionally in Britain, at riversides, fields and waste ground.
PARTS USED: the fruit and leaves.
MEDICINAL USES: stimulant, aromatic and carminative. It is generally used with active purgatives as flavouring and to lessen their griping tendencies. Coriander water was formerly used for windy colic.
ADMINISTERED AS: powdered fruit, fluid extract.

Corkwood tree _Duboisia myoporoides._
COMMON NAME: duboisia.
OCCURRENCE: found in Australia in the states of New South Wales and Queensland.
PARTS USED: the leaves which contain alkaloidal sulphates, mainly hyoscyamine and hyoscine.
MEDICINAL USES: sedative, hypnotic, mydriatic. The drug aids the activity of the respiratory system and it is sometimes used as a replacement for atropine, from BELLADONNA (_Atropa belladonna_). The tincture of the drug is used in treating eye afflictions and paralysis.
ADMINISTERED AS: tincture.

Cornflower _Centaurea cyanus._
COMMON NAME: bluebottle, bluebow, hurtsickle, blue cap, bluet.
OCCURRENCE: common in cultivated fields and roadsides in Britain.
PARTS USED: the flowers.
MEDICINAL USES: tonic, stimulant and emmenagogue properties. A water distilled from cornflower petals was said to be a remedy for eye inflammation and weak eyesight.
ADMINISTERED AS: distilled water and infusion.

Costmary _Tanacetum balsamita._
COMMON NAME: alecost, balsam herb, costmarie, mace, balsamita.
OCCURRENCE: an old English herb, naturalized from the Orient in the sixteenth century.
PARTS USED: the leaves.
MEDICINAL USES: formerly used as an aperient, antiseptic and astringent herb in treating dysentery. Used as an infusion to heal stomach and head problems. Also flavouring for ale and in salads.
ADMINISTERED AS: infusion and tincture.

Cotton root _Gossypium herbaceum_ (and other species).
OCCURRENCE: indigenous to India and cultivated in Greece, Turkey, Sicily and Malta.
PARTS USED: the root-bark which contains a peculiar acid resin, sugar, gum, chlorophyll, fixed oil and tannin.
MEDICINAL USES: this drug is used to induce abortion or miscarriage as it causes contraction of the uterus. It is useful in treating abnormal uterine bleeding particularly when linked to fibroids, and in cases of difficult or obstructed menstruation. A preparation is given to induce labour (at full

term) to aid safe delivery. It is said to be of use in sexual lassitude.
ADMINISTERED AS: fluid extract, decoction, solid extract.

Couchgrass *Agropyrum repens.*
COMMON NAME: twitchgrass, Scotch quelch, quickgrass, dog's grass, *Triticum repens.*
OCCURRENCE: abundant in fields and waste ground in Britain, Europe, northern Asia and North and South America.
PARTS USED: the rhizome, which contains triticin (a carbohydrate).
MEDICINAL USES: diuretic, demulcent, aperient. Widely used in complaints of the urinary organs and bladder. Also recommended for gout and rheumatism.
ADMINISTERED AS: an infusion, decoction and liquid extract.

Cowslip *Primula veris.*
COMMON NAME: herb Peter, paigle, peggle, key flower, key of heaven, fairy cups, petty mulleins, patsywort, plumrocks, mayflower, Our Lady's keys, arthritica.
OCCURRENCE: a common wild flower in all parts of Great Britain.
PARTS USED: the flower.
MEDICINAL USES: sedative, antispasmodic. It is very good in relieving restlessness and insomnia. Commonly brewed into a wine which was a good children's medicine in small doses.
ADMINISTERED AS: an infusion or wine.

Cramp bark *Viburnum opulus.*
COMMON NAME: guelder rose, snowball tree, king's crown, high cranberry, red elder, rose elder, may rose, whitsun rose, dog rowan tree, silver bells, whitsun bosses, gaitre berries, black haw.
OCCURRENCE: indigenous to Great Britain and North America, although rare in Scotland.
PARTS USED: the bark whose chief constituents are the glucoside viburnine, tannin, resin and valerianic acid.
MEDICINAL USES: antispasmodic, nervine, sedative. This drug is of benefit in all nervous complaints, debility, cramps and spasms of all types, asthma and hysteria. It has been effective in treating convulsions, fits, lockjaw, heart disease, palpitations and rheumatism.
ADMINISTERED AS: tincture, decoction, infusion, fluid extract.

Croton *Croton tiglian.*
COMMON NAME: tiglium, *Tiglium officinale.*

OCCURRENCE: a tree found on the Malabar coast of India and on the Indian archipelago.

PARTS USED: the oil expressed from the seeds, croton oil contains glycerides of stearic, palmitic, myristic, lauric and oleic acids; the glycerin ethers of formic, acetic, isobutyric and isovaleranic acids. The active principle is probably Crotonic acid.

MEDICINAL USES: irritant, rubefacient, cathartic, purgative. A drastic purgative drug which acts quickly, often evacuating the bowels in less than one hour. In large doses, it causes vomiting and severe griping pains which can possibly be fatal. The drug is only used in cases of obstinate constipation where other drugs have failed. It is applied externally as a counter-irritant to relieve rheumatism, gout, neuralgia and bronchitis. The use of this oil should be monitored most carefully, only administered in small doses, and never given to children or pregnant women.

ADMINISTERED AS: expressed oil.

Crowfoot, Upright meadow *Ranunculus acris.*

COMMON NAME: gold cup, grenouillette.

OCCURRENCE: native in meadows, pastures and fields in all parts of northern Europe and Great Britain.

PARTS USED: the whole herb.

MEDICINAL USES: the expressed juice is used to remove warts. A poultice of the fresh herb is good at removing violent, painful headaches or in relieving gout. The fresh herb once formed part of a famous cure for cancer practised in 1794.

ADMINISTERED AS: fresh leaves, expressed juice.

Cuckoopint *Arum maculatum.*

COMMON NAME: lords-and-ladies, starchwort, arum, adder's root, friar's cowl, kings and queens, parson and clerk, ramp, Quaker, wake robin.

OCCURRENCE: the sole British species of the arum, aroidae family and is also widely distributed over Europe.

PARTS USED: the root. This contains starch, albumen, sugar, lignin, saponin and an unidentified alkaloid.

MEDICINAL USES: diaphoretic, expectorant, diuretic, stimulant. The fresh root can be prepared into a tincture and given to remedy sore, feverish throats. The dried root can be stored for long periods, but is rarely employed as a medicine today. An ointment prepared of the fresh root was used to cure ringworm.

ADMINISTERED AS: tincture, expressed juice and ointment.

Cucumber *Cucumis sativa.*
COMMON NAME: cowcumber.
OCCURRENCE: a native of the East Indies,first cultivated in Britain around 1573.
PARTS USED: the whole fruit, peeled or unpeeled, raw and cooked.
MEDICINAL USES: the seeds are diuretic and are an excellent taeniacide and purge. The fruit is very good as a skin cosmetic as it has cooling, healing and soothing effects on irritated skin. Cucumber juice is widely utilized in emollient ointments or creams and is good for sunburn.
ADMINISTERED AS: expressed juice, lotion or ointment.

Cudweed *Graphalium uliginosum.*
COMMON NAME: cottonweed, marsh everlasting, cotton dawes.
OCCURRENCE: found in marshy areas in all parts of Europe.
PARTS USED: the herb.
MEDICINAL USES: astringent. It is a very good remedy for quinsy when used as a gargle and can also be taken internally.
ADMINISTERED AS: an infusion.

Cumin *Cuminum cyminum.*
COMMON NAME: cummin, *Cumino aigro*.
OCCURRENCE indigenous to upper Egypt and is cultivated in Arabia, India, China and Mediterranean countries since early times.
PARTS USED: the fruit. The chief constituents are a volatile oil, a fatty oil with resin, mucilage, gum, malates and albuminous matter.
MEDICINAL USES: stimulant, carminative, antispasmodic. This herb has similar effects to FENNEL and CARAWAY but its use has declined because of its disagreeable taste. It had a considerable reputation in helping correct flatulence caused by languid digestion and as a remedy for colic and dyspeptic headache. Applied externally as a plaster, it eased stitches and pains in the side and has been combined with other herbs to form a stimulating liniment.
ADMINISTERED AS: dried, powdered fruit, whole fruit.

Cup moss *Cladonia pyxidata.*
COMMON NAME: chin cups.
OCCURRENCE: indigenous to north-west America but is also a common weed through Great Britain and Europe.
PARTS USED: the whole plant.
MEDICINAL USES: expectorant—used as a decoction to treat children's coughs and whooping cough with great effectiveness.
ADMINISTERED AS: decoction.

Daffodil Narcissus pseudo-narcissus.

COMMON NAME: porillion, daffy-down-dilly, fleur de coucou, Lent lily.

OCCURRENCE: found wild in most European countries including the British Isles.

PARTS USED: the bulb, leaves and flowers. The bulbs contain an alkaloid called lyconine.

MEDICINAL USES: the flowers, when powdered, have emetic properties and as an infusion are used in pulmonary catarrh. The bulbs are also emetic and, indeed, can cause people to collapse and die as a result of paralysis of the central nervous system caused by the action of lyconine, which acts quickly. Accidents have resulted from daffodil bulbs being mistaken for ONIONS and eaten. Since high temperatures and cooking does not break down the poisonous alkaloid, considerable care should be taken to avoid problems. The bulbs are used externally as an astringent poultice to dissolve hard swellings and aid wound healing.

ADMINISTERED AS: powder and extract.

Daisy, Ox-eye Chrysanthemum leuconthemum.

COMMON NAME: great ox-eye, goldens, marguerite, moon daisy, horse gowan, maudlin daisy, field daisy, dun daisy, butter daisy, horse daisy, maudlinwort, white weed, gowan.

OCCURRENCE: found in fields throughout Europe and northern Asia.

PARTS USED: the whole herb, flowers and root.

MEDICINAL USES: antispasmodic, diuretic, tonic. This herb's main use has been in whooping cough, asthma and nervous excitability. When taken as a tonic, it acts in a similar way to CHAMOMILE flowers and calms night sweats and nightmares. An infusion of ox-eye daisy flowers is good at relieving bronchial coughs and catarrh. It is also used as a lotion for wounds, bruises and ulcers.

ADMINISTERED AS: an infusion and lotion.

Damiana Turnera aphrodisiaca or *Turnera diffusa* var. *aphrodisiaca.*

OCCURRENCE: indigenous to Texas and Mexico; cultivated in other areas of sub-tropical America and Africa.

PARTS USED: the leaves which contain a volatile oil, resins, tannin and the bitter principle damianin.

MEDICINAL USES: mild purgative, diuretic, tonic, stimulant, aphrodisiac. This drug acts as a tonic to the nervous system and has a direct and general beneficial effect on the reproductive organs.

ADMINISTERED AS: fluid extract, solid extract.

Dandelion

Dandelion *Taraxacum officinale.*

COMMON NAME: priest's crown, swine's snout.

OCCURRENCE: widely found across the northern temperate zone in pastures, meadows and waste ground.

PARTS USED: the root and leaves. The main constituents of the root are taraxacin, a bitter substance, and taraxacerin, an acid resin, along with the sugar inulin.

MEDICINAL USES: diuretic, tonic and slightly aperient. It acts as a general body stimulant but chiefly acts on the liver and kidneys. Dandelion is used as a bitter tonic in atonic dyspepsia as a mild laxative and to promote increased appetite and digestion. The herb is best used in combination with other herbs and is used in many patent medicines. Roasted dandelion root is also used as a coffee substitute and helps ease dyspepsia, gout and rheumatism.

ADMINISTERED AS: fluid and solid extract, decoction, infusion and tincture.

Dill *Peucedanum graveolus, Fructus anethi.*

COMMON NAME: dill seed, dill fruit, *Anethum graveolus, Fructus anethi.*

OCCURRENCE: indigenous to Mediterranean districts and South Russia and is cultivated in England and Europe.

PARTS USED: the dried ripe fruit. An oil obtained from the fruit is almost identical to oil of CARAWAY, both containing limonene and carvone.

MEDICINAL USES: stimulant, aromatic, carminative and stomachic. It is usually given as dillwater which is very good for children's flatulence or disordered digestion. Oil of dill is used in medicine in largely the same way, but is also used in perfuming soaps.

ADMINISTERED AS: distilled water, essential oil.

Dock, *Yellow Rumex crispus.*

COMMON NAME: curled dock.

OCCURRENCE: normally found on roadside ditches and waste ground, all over Great Britain.

PARTS USED: the root and whole herb.

MEDICINAL USES: the root has laxative, alterative and a mildly tonic action and is used in rheumatism, bilious complaints and haemorrhoids. It is very useful in treating jaundice, diseases of the blood, scurvy, chronic skin diseases and as a tonic on the digestive system. Yellow dock is said to have a positive effect on slowing the development of cancer, because of its alterative and tonic properties. It has similar effects to that of RHUBARB and has been used in treating diphtheria.

Administered as: dried extract, syrup, infusion, tincture, ointment, fluid extract and solid extract.

Dodder *Cuscuta europea*.
Common name: lesser dodder, dodder of thyme, beggarweed, hellweed, strangle tare, scaldweed, devil's guts.
Occurrence: a parasitic plant found in most areas of the world.
Parts used: the herb.
Medicinal uses: hepatic, laxative, purgative. A decoction made with dodder, GINGER and ALLSPICE has been used against urinary complaints, kidney, spleen and liver disorders. The herb is good in treating sciatica, scorbutic problems, scrofulous tumours and it acts as a purge due to its very bitter taste.
Administered as: decoction, infusion.

Dog-rose *Rosa canina*.
Common name: wild briar, hip tree, cynosbatos.
Occurrence: indigenous to Great Britain.
Parts used: the ripe fruit which contain invert fruit sugars, a range of mineral salts and a large proportion of vitamin C or ascorbic acid.
Medicinal uses: astringent, refrigerant and pectoral. The fruit is used in strengthening the stomach and digestion, as well as easing coughs. It is made into an uncooked preserve, a syrup which is excellent for infants and children and rose-hip tea has very beneficial effects. An infusion of dog-rose leaves has been used as a tea substitute and has a pleasant aroma.
Administered as: an infusion, syrup or dietary item.

Dropwort, Hemlock water *Œnanthe crocata*.
Common name: horsebane, deadtongue, five-fingered root, water lovage, yellow water dropwort.
Occurrence: common in ditches and watering places in England, particularly the southern counties.
Parts used: the roots.
Medicinal uses: the beneficial uses are few because this plant is virulently poisonous. A tincture is used to treat eruptive diseases of the skin, but with very small dosages and great caution. Poultices have been used to heal whitlows or ulcers. This wild plant is the most poisonous of our indigenous plants and many deaths have resulted from adults and children eating the leaves or roots mistakenly.
Administered as: tincture, poultice.

Dropwort, Water *Œnanthe phellandrium.*

COMMON NAME: fine-leaved water dropwort, water fennel, fine-leaved oenanthe, *Phellandrium aquaticum.*

OCCURRENCE: a common plant in ditches and water courses across Europe and Great Britain.

PARTS USED: the fruit, which yields an ethereal oil called water fennel oil. The main chemical in the oil is the terpene, phellandrene.

MEDICINAL USES: expectorant, alterative, diuretic. The fruits are used to ease chronic pectoral conditions like bronchitis, consumption and asthma and also works well against dyspepsia, intermittent fevers and ulcers. Applied externally, the root has been utilized as a remedy for haemorrhoids. When taken in too large amounts, causing an overdose, the fruit prompts vertigo, intoxication and other narcotic effects. If the root is eaten by mistake, it can prove fatal in the same manner as with HEMLOCK WATER DROPWORT (*Oenanthe crocata*) where stomach irritation, circulation failure, giddiness, convulsions and coma can occur.

ADMINISTERED AS: powdered fruit, tincture, essence.

Dwarf elder *Sanbucus ebulus.*

COMMON NAME: danewort, wallwort, ground elder, walewort, blood hilder.

OCCURRENCE: found in ruins and waste ground throughout Europe and the British Isles.

PARTS USED: the leaves, roots and berries.

MEDICINAL USES: expectorant, diuretic, diaphoretic, purgative. The leaves are used internally to ease inflammation of the kidney and liver, and have a healing effect when used as a poultice on swellings and contusions. Dwarf elder tea was prepared from the dried root, when ground, and is one of the finest remedies for dropsy. The fresh root, when used as a decoction, is a drastic purgative. Overall, the dwarf elder is much more drastic in action than the common ELDER (*Sambucus nigra*).

ADMINISTERED AS: fresh root, decoction, poultice, infusion.

Echinacea *Echinacea angustifolia.*

COMMON NAME: black sampson, coneflower, rudbeckia, *Brauneria pallida.*

OCCURRENCE: a native plant of the prairie regions of the United states, west of Ohio. Also cultivated in Britain.

PARTS USED: the dried root and the rhizome. The wood and the bark contain oil, resin and large quantities of inulin, inuloid, sucrose, betaine, two phytosterols and oleic, cerotic, linolic and palmatic fatty acids.

MEDICINAL USES: alterative, antiseptic. This herb is considered sacred by many North American Indian tribes including the Sioux Indians. The herb boosts the immune system and increases bodily resistance to infection. It is used for boils, septicaemia, cancer, syphilis and gangrene. Echinacea is of particular value in treating diphtheria, typhoid and other infectious fevers. The herb can be used to improve appetite and digestion and can ease haemorrhoids when administered via injection.

ADMINISTERED AS: poultice, infusion, injection, fresh herb.

Elder Sambucus nigra.

COMMON NAME: black elder, common elder, European elder, pipe tree, bore tree, bour tree.

OCCURRENCE: frequently seen in Europe and Great Britain.

PARTS USED: the bark, leaves, flowers and berries.

MEDICINAL USES: the bark is a strong purgative and in large doses is emetic. It has been used successfully in epilepsy, and a tincture of the young bark relieves asthmatic symptoms and croup in children. A tea made from elder roots was highly effective against dropsy. The leaves are used both fresh and dried and contain the alkaloid sambucine, a glucoside called sambunigrin, as well as hydrogenic acid, cane sugar and potassium nitrate amongst other compounds. The leaves are used in preparation of green elder ointment which is used domestically for bruises, haemorrhoids, sprains, chilblains and applied to wounds. Elder leaves have the same purgative effects as the bark (but produce more nausea) and have expectorant, diaphoretic and diuretic actions.

The elder flowers are either distilled into elderflower water or dried. The water is used in eye and skin lotions as it is mildly astringent and a gentle stimulant. When infused, the dried flowers make elderflower tea which is gently laxative, aperient and diaphoretic. It is an old-fashioned remedy for colds and influenza when taken hot, before bed. The tea is also recommended to be drunk before breakfast as a blood purifier. Elder flowers would also be made into a lotion or poultice for use on inflamed areas and into an ointment which was good on wounds, scalds and burns. The ointment was used on the battlefields in World War I and at home for chapped hands and chilblains.

ADMINISTERED AS: an infusion, tincture, ointment, syrup, lotion, distilled water, poultice and dried powder.

Elecampane Inula helenium.

COMMON NAME: scabwort, elf dock, wild sunflower, horseheal, velvet dock.

OCCURRENCE: a true native of southern England, temperate Europe and

Asia, but cultivated for medicinal purposes in northern England and Scotland.

PARTS USED: the root. This plant is a rich source of the drug inulin.

MEDICINAL USES: diuretic, tonic, diaphoretic, expectorant, antiseptic, astringent, and gently stimulant. It is used principally in coughs, consumption and pulmonary complaints, e.g. bronchitis. It is also used in acute catarrhal afflictions, dyspepsia ans asthma. Internally, it is normally combined with other herbs, as a decoction. Applied externally, it is rubefacient, and used in treating sciatica and facial neuralgia. The active bitter principle in the herb, helenin, is a very powerful antiseptic and bacterial chemical. This has meant elecampane has been used against the Tubercle bacteria and in surgical dressings.

ADMINISTERED AS: powdered root, fluid extract, tincture, poultice, infusion.

Elm, Common Ulmus campestris.

COMMON NAME: field elm, ulmi cortex, broad-leaved elm.

OCCURRENCE: common in Britain, Europe, Asia and North Africa.

PARTS USED: the dried inner bark.

MEDICINAL USES: tonic, demulcent, astringent and diuretic. It was formerly employed as an antiscorbutic decoction recommended in skin diseases such as ringworm. Also used as a poultice to relieve pain from gout or rheumatism.

ADMINISTERED AS: tincture, fluid extract or tea.

Ephedra Ephedra vulgaris.

COMMON NAME: ephedrine, epitonin, mattuang.

OCCURRENCE: grows in west central China, southern Siberia and Japan.

PARTS USED: the stems, of which ephedrine is the active alkaloidal chemical.

MEDICINAL USES: nerve stimulant, antispasmodic. The herb resembles adrenaline in effect and it relieves swellings of the mucous membranes quickly. It has been used to treat asthma, hay fever and rheumatism as well as being a prophylactic drug to help low blood pressure in influenza or pneumonia.

ADMINISTERED AS: tablets, injection.

Ergot Claviceps purpurea.

COMMON NAME: ergot of rye, smut of rye, spurred rye, *Serale cornutum*.

OCCURRENCE: this herbal remedy is the fungal mycelium which grows parasitically on rye, wheat and other grasses.

PARTS USED: ergot contains two alkaloids—ergotoxine and ergotamine as the active chemicals.

MEDICINAL USES: emmenagogue, haemostatic, uterine, stimulant, and seda-tive. It is normally used as a muscle stimulant in menstrual disorders such as leucorrhoea and painful or lacking menstruation and can be used to stop internal haemorrhage with best results against uterine haemorrhage. It is used as a sedative in cases of delirium, asthma or hysteria and also acts as a galactogogue.

ADMINISTERED AS: extract, infusion, tincture, liquid extract.

Eryngo Eryngicum campestre.

COMMON NAME: sea holly, eringo, sea hulver, sea holme.

OCCURRENCE: found on sandy soils and seashores around England and the rest of Europe's coastline, but rare in Scotland.

PARTS USED: the root.

MEDICINAL USES: diaphoretic, diuretic, aromatic, stimulant, expectorant. It is good in dealing with coughs, consumption, paralysis and chronic nerv-ous diseases. It has effective results against all diseases of the bladder, scorbutic complaints, jaundice and liver problems.

ADMINISTERED AS: decoction.

Eucalyptus Eucalyptus globulus.

COMMON NAME: blue gum tree, stringy bark tree.

OCCURRENCE: native to Australia and Tasmania; now introduced into North and South Africa, India and southern Europe.

PARTS USED: the oil distilled from the leaves. The oil contains eucalyptol, which is the important medically-active chemical.

MEDICINAL USES: antiseptic, antispasmodic, stimulant, aromatic. The oil is used as an antiseptic and stimulant gargle; it increases the action of the heart and is said to have some antimalarial properties. It is taken inter-nally in pulmonary tuberculosis, scarlet, typhoid and intermittent fevers. The oil is used as an inhalant to clear catarrh and used externally to ease croup and throat troubles. However, in large doses it can irritate the kidneys, depress the nervous system and possibly stop respiration and breathing. Despite its harmless appearance, care should be used when administering the drug internally.

ADMINISTERED AS: distilled oil, emulsion.

Euphorbia Euphorbia hirta.

COMMON NAME: asthma-weed, catshair, *Euphorbia pilulifera*.

OCCURRENCE: grows in India and other tropical countries.

PARTS USED: the herb.

Eyebright

MEDICINAL USES: anti-asthmatic, pectoral. It is highly effective in treating paroxysmal asthma, coughs and bronchial and pulmonary disorders. In India it is used against syphilis.

ADMINISTERED AS: tincture, liquid extract.

Evening primrose Oenothera biennis.

COMMON NAME: tree primrose, sun drop.

OCCURRENCE: native to North America but has been naturalized to British and European gardens.

PARTS USED: the bark and leaves.

MEDICINAL USES: astringent, sedative. The drug from this herb is not extensively used but has been of benefit in treating gastro-intestinal disorders, dyspepsia, liver torpor and in female problems in association with pelvic illness. It has also been successfully used in whooping cough and spasmodic asthma.

ADMINISTERED AS: liquid extract.

Eyebright Euphrasia officinalis.

COMMON NAME: euphrasia.

OCCURRENCE: a wild plant growing in meadows and grasslands in England and Europe.

PARTS USED: the herb. This plant contains various chemicals including euphrasia-tannin, mannite and glucose.

MEDICINAL USES: slightly tonic and astringent. As its name suggests, eyebright is recommended in treating diseases of the sight, weak eyes, etc. It is generally used as an infusion in water or milk and is combined in a lotion with GOLDEN SEAL, the pairing said to be highly effective.

ADMINISTERED AS: infusion, ointment or expressed juice.

Fennel Foeniculum vulgare.

COMMON NAME: hinojo, fenkel, sweet fennel, wild fennel.

OCCURRENCE: found wild in most areas of temperate Europe and generally considered indigenous to the shores of the Mediterranean. It is cultivated for medicinal benefit in France, Russia, India and Persia.

PARTS USED: the seeds, leaves and roots. The roots are rarely used in herbal medicine today. The essential oil is separated by distillation with water. Fennel oil varies widely in quality and composition dependent upon where and under what conditions the fennel was grown.

MEDICINAL USES: aromatic, stimulant, carminative and stomachic. The herb is principally used with purgatives to allay their tendency to griping, and the seeds form an ingredient of the compound liquorice powder. Fennel water also acts in a similar manner to DILL water in correcting infant flatulence.

ADMINISTERED AS: fluid extract, distilled water, essential oil.

Fenugreek *Trigonella foenum-graecum.*
COMMON NAME: bird's foot, Greek hay-seed.
OCCURRENCE: indigenous to eastern Mediterranean countries, but is cultivated in India, Africa and England.
PARTS USED: the seeds. These contain mucilage, two alkaloids trigonelline and choline—phosphates, lecithin and nucleoalbumin.
MEDICINAL USES: a preparation where seeds are soaked in water until they swell and form a thick paste is used to prevent fevers, is comforting to the stomach and has been utilized for diabetes. Alcoholic tinctures are used to prepare emollient cream, ointments and plasters while the mucilage is used externally as a poultice for skin infections such as abscesses, boils and carbuncles. It is also good at relieving rickets, anaemia and scrofula, while, combined with the normal dosage of conventional medicine e.g insulin, it is helpful in gout, diabetes and neurasthenia. It is widely used as a flavouring for both human and cattle feed.
ADMINISTERED AS: poultice, ointment, infusion or tincture.

Feverfew *Chrysanthemum parthenium.*
COMMON NAME: featherfew, featherfoil, flirtwort, bachelor's buttons, pyrethrum parthenium.
OCCURRENCE: a wild hedgerow plant found in many areas of Europe and Great Britain.
PARTS USED: the herb.
MEDICINAL USES: aperient, carminative, bitter, stimulant, emmenagogue. It is employed in hysterical complaints, nervousness and low spirits as a general tonic. A decoction is made and is useful in easing coughs, wheezing and difficult breathing. Earache was relieved by a cold infusion while a tincture of feverfew eased the pain and swelling caused after insect or vermin bites. The herb was planted around dwellings to purify the atmosphere and ward off disease. Today, it is used to prevent or ease migraines or headaches.
ADMINISTERED AS: warm or cold infusion, poultice, tincture, decoction.

Fig *Ficus carica.*
COMMON NAME: common fig.
OCCURRENCE: indigenous to Persia, Asia Minor and Syria, but cultivated in most of the Mediterranean countries and England.

Figwort

PARTS USED: the fleshy inflorescence (so-called fruit).
MEDICINAL USES: nutritive, emollient, demulcent, laxative. It is normally utilized in laxative confections and syrups with SENNA and carminatives. Demulcent decoctions are prepared from figs and are used in treating catarrhal afflictions of the nose and throat. Roasted figs, when split open, are used as a poultice to gumboils, dental abscesses, boils and carbuncles. The fruit is used both fresh and dried.
ADMINISTERED AS: poultice, syrup, decoction.

Figwort *Scrophularia nodosa.*
COMMON NAME: rose noble, throatwort, carpenter's square, kernelwort, scrofula plant.
OCCURRENCE: a wild plant of Great Britain and Europe.
PARTS USED: the herb.
MEDICINAL USES: diuretic, anodyne, depurative. Due to this herb's beneficial action on skin abscesses, eruptions and wounds, it has been termed the scrofula plant. The fresh leaves are used as a poultice on sprains, swellings, inflammation, wounds, gangrene and scrofulous sores to great effect.
ADMINISTERED AS: decoction, fresh leaves, dried herb, ointment and fluid extract.

Fireweed *Erechtites hieracifolia* or *Cineraria caradensis.*
COMMON NAME: *Senecio hieracifolius.*
OCCURRENCE: a common weed found in Newfoundland and Canada and south to South America.
PARTS USED: the herb, and the oil of erechtites distilled from the herb. The oil is composed of various terpene chemicals.
MEDICINAL USES: astringent, alterative, tonic, cathartic, emetic. Taken internally, it is good for eczema, diarrhoea, haemorrhages and sore throats. It has also been used for colic, spasms, hiccoughs, dysentery and haemorrhoids. When used externally, the oil gives great relief to gout, rheumatism and sciatica.
ADMINISTERED AS: distilled oil in capsules or emulsion, tincture.

Flax *Linum usitatissimum.*
COMMON NAME: linseed.
OCCURRENCE: grows in most temperate and tropical countries.
PARTS USED: the seeds and oil expressed from the seeds, a cake remains which can be ground up to form linseed meal.
MEDICINAL USES: emollient, demulcent, pectoral. A poultice of linseed meal,

either alone or with mustard, is effective in relieving pain and irritation from boils, ulcers, inflamed areas and abscesses. Flax is normally utilized as an addition to cough medicines, while linseed oil is sometimes given as a laxative or to remove gravel and stones. When mixed with LIME water the oil is excellent on burns and scalds.

ADMINISTERED AS: essential oil, ground seed coats (meal), infusion, syrup and poultice.

Foxglove *Digitalis purpurea.*

COMMON NAME: witch's gloves, dead men's bells, fairy's glove, gloves of Our Lady, bloody fingers, virgin's glove, fairy caps, folk's glove, fairy thimbles, fair women's plant.

OCCURRENCE: indigenous and widely distributed throughout Great Britain and Europe.

PARTS USED: the leaves, which contain four important glucosides—digitoxin, digitalin, digitalein and digitonin—of which the first three listed are cardiac stimulants.

MEDICINAL USES: cardiac tonic, sedative, diuretic. Administering digitalis increases the activity of all forms of muscle tissue, particularly the heart and arterioles. It causes a very high rise in blood pressure and the pulse is slowed and becomes regular. Digitalis causes the heart to contract in size, allowing increased blood flow and nutrient delivery to the organ. It also acts on the kidneys and is a good remedy for dropsy, particularly when it is connected with cardiac problems. The drug has benefits in treating internal haemorrhage, epilepsy, inflammatory diseases and delirium tremens. Digitalis has a cumulative action whereby it is liable to accumulate in the body and then have poisonous effects. It should only be used under medical advice. Digitalis is an excellent antidote in ACONITE poisoning when given as a hypodermic injection.

ADMINISTERED AS: tincture, infusion, powdered leaves, solid extract, injection.

Fringe tree *Chionanthus virginica.*

COMMON NAME: old man's beard, snowdrop tree, poison ash, fringe tree bark, chionanthus.

OCCURRENCE: a small tree, native to the southern United States.

PARTS USED: the dried bark of the root which is thought to contain saponin and a glucoside.

MEDICINAL USES: aperient, diuretic, alterative, tonic. The root is used in typhoid, intermittent or bilious fevers, in liver complaints, jaundice and gallstones. It is taken in conjunction with ANEMONE PULSATILLA and other herbs for women's complaints. Also used as a poultice on wounds and inflammations.

ADMINISTERED AS: infusion, fluid extract.

Frostwort *Helianthemum canadense.*

COMMON NAME: cistus, frostweed, frostplant, rock rose, *Cistus canadensis, Lechea Major, Canadisches Sonnenroschen, Helianthemum ramultoflorum, H. rosmarinifolium, H. michauxii, H. Coprymbosum, Hetraneris canadensis.*

OCCURRENCE: grows in the eastern United States, Great Britain and Europe.

PARTS USED: the dried herb. The main chemical components are a volatile oil, wax, tannin, fatty oil, chlorophyll, gum, inorganic salts and a glucoside.

MEDICINAL USES: antiscrofulous, astringent, alterative, tonic. The herb has a long history of use for diarrhoea, ulcerations, eye complaints, secondary syphilis and any conditions arising from scrofula. It has been beneficial as a poultice for tumours and ulcers and as a gargle in scarlatina. An overdose of the drug is possible and causes nausea and vomiting.

ADMINISTERED AS: liquid extract.

Fumitory *Fumaria officinalis.*

COMMON NAME: earth smoke, beggary, fumus, vapor, nidor, fumus terrae, fumiterry, scheiteregi, taubenkropp, kaphnos, wax dolls.

OCCURRENCE: a common weed plant in Great Britain and Europe, which has been naturalized into North America; originally from Asia and Greece.

PARTS USED: the herb and the expressed juice and fluid extract derived from it.

MEDICINAL USES: weak tonic, diaphoretic, diuretic, aperient. This herb is valuable in all internal obstructions, particularly those of the liver and stomach and is also of benefit in scorbutic afflictions and skin eruptions including leprosy. It is the preferred herb to purify the blood in France and Germany, and in some areas it is smoked as tobacco. It was said to aid removal of skin blemishes and freckles and was also used to ease dyspepsia and headaches.

ADMINISTERED AS: expressed juice, essence, syrup, distilled water, decoction, dried herb, several different tinctures, powdered seed.

Gale, Sweet *Myrica gale.*

COMMON NAME: bayberry, English bog myrtle, Dutch myrtle, gale palustris.

OCCURRENCE: a bushy shrub found in higher latitudes of the northern hemisphere; abundant in Scottish moors and bogs.

PARTS USED: the shrub.

MEDICINAL USES: aromatic, astringent. The leaves have been used as an emmenagogue and an abortifacient (induces abortion or miscarriage).

ADMINISTERED AS: dried leaves and infusion.

Garlic *Allium sativum.*

COMMON NAME: poor man's treacle.

OCCURRENCE: cultivated throughout Europe since antiquity.

PARTS USED: the bulb.

MEDICINAL USES: antiseptic, diaphoretic, diuretic, expectorant, stimulant. It may be externally applied as ointment, lotion, antiseptic or as a poultice. Syrup of garlic is very good for asthma, coughs, difficulty in breathing and chronic bronchitis, while fresh juice has been used to ease tubercular consumption. The essential oil is commonly taken as a supplement in the form of gelatine capsules. Several species of wild garlic are utilized for both medicinal and dietary purposes.

ADMINISTERED AS: expressed juice, syrup, tincture, essential oil, poultice, lotion and ointment.

Gelsemium *Gelsemium sempervirens.*

COMMON NAME: yellow jasmine, *Gelsemium nitridum*, false jasmine, wild woodbine, Carolina jasmine.

OCCURRENCE: a native North American plant found along the sea coast from Virginia, to southern Florida and Mexico.

PARTS USED: the root which contains two alkaloids—gelsemium and gelsemine, as well as gelsemic acid, a volatile oil, resin and starch.

MEDICINAL USES: antispasmodic, arterial sedative, diaphoretic, febrifuge. Used in small doses to treat neuralgic pains, muscular irritability, nervous excitement and hysteria while its antispasmodic qualities aid asthma, whooping cough, croup and convulsions with great success. It relaxes all muscles and acts on the whole body to remove all sense of pain. The root is very good against bowel inflammation, diarrhoea, dysentery, toothache, chorea, epilepsy, insomnia and headaches due to sickness or alcohol consumption. The drug also benefits acute rheumatism, pleurisy, pneumonia, bronchitis, typhoid fever and pelvic disorders in women. This drug is poisonous and so should be administered in small doses, with very careful monitoring of the patient. Death occurs due to the action of the drug on nervous control of the respiratory system, and can occur very quickly after taking the drug—between one and seven hours after ingestion. Treatment of gelsemium poisoning must be rapid with evacuation of the stomach, artificial respiration and the use of atropine, BELLADONNA (*Atropa belladonna*); strychnine, NUX VOMICA (*Strychnos nux-vomica*); or digitalis, FOXGLOVE (*Digitalis purpurea*) to maintain action of the heart being recommended.

ADMINISTERED AS: tincture, solid extract, infusion.

Gentian, Yellow *Gentiana lutea*.

OCCURRENCE: native to alpine regions of central and southern Europe.

PARTS USED: the root. The dried root contains gentian, gentiamarin, bitter glucosides, gentianic acid and various sugars. The fresh root also contains gentiopicrin, another bitter glucoside.

MEDICINAL USES: bitter tonic, stomachic, febrifuge, emmenagogue, anthelmintic and antiseptic. This drug is probably the most effective bitter tonic of use in exhaustion from chronic disease, general debility, weakness of the digestive organs and lack of appetite. It acts to strengthen the whole body and is a very good tonic to combine with purgative drugs in order to temper their debilitating effects. Yellow gentian is useful in many dyspeptic complaints, hysteria, female weakness, intermittent fevers and jaundice. The roots have also been used to make an alcoholic beverage in Germany and Switzerland.

ADMINISTERED AS: infusion, tincture, solid extract, fluid extract.

Germander, Wall *Teucrium chamaedys*.

COMMON NAME: petit chêne, chasse fièvre.

OCCURRENCE: a native of many parts of Europe, the Greek Islands and Syria but is an escape from garden cultivation in England.

PARTS USED: the whole herb, dried.

MEDICINAL USES: stimulant, tonic, diaphoretic, diuretic, aperient. Germander has a reputation as a specific cure for gout, dating back to the sixteenth century. It has been used as a tonic in treating intermittent fevers and uterine obstructions and a decoction of the fresh herb is good against asthmatic afflictions and coughs. The expressed juice is taken for obstructions of the viscera, while the herb has also been used for jaundice, as a vermifuge, ulcers, continual headache and cramps.

ADMINISTERED AS: expressed juice, poultice, decoction, powdered seeds.

Ginger *Zingiber officinale*.

OCCURRENCE: a native of Asia, it is now cultivated in the West Indies, Jamaica and Africa.

PARTS USED: the root, which contains volatile oil, two resins, gum, starch, lignin, acetic acid and asmazone as well as several unidentified compounds.
MEDICINAL USES: stimulant, carminative, expectorant. A valuable herb in dyspepsia, flatulent colic, alcoholic gastritis and diarrhoea. Ginger tea is taken to relieve the effects of cold temperatures including triggering normal menstruation patterns in women. Ginger is also used to flavour bitter infusions, cough mixtures or syrups.
ADMINISTERED AS: infusion, fluid extract, tincture and syrup.

Ginseng *Panax quinquefolium.*
COMMON NAME: *Aralia quinquefolia*, five fingers, tartar root, red berry, man's health, panax, pannag.
OCCURRENCE: native to certain areas of China, eastern Asia and North America. It is largely cultivated in China, Korea and Japan.
PARTS USED: the root which contains a large quantity of gum, resin, volatile oil and the peculiar sweetish compound, panaquilon.
MEDICINAL USES: mild stomachic, tonic, stimulant. The generic name, *panax*, is derived from the Greek for panacea meaning 'all-healing.' The name ginseng is said to mean 'the wonder of the world' and the Chinese consider this herb a sovereign remedy in all diseases. It is good in dyspepsia, vomiting and nervous disorders, consumption and exhaustion. In the West, it is used to treat loss of appetite, stomach and digestive problems, possibly arising from nervous and mental exhaustion. Ginseng is considered to work well against fatigue, old age and its infirmities and to help convalescents recover their health. In healthy people, the drug is said to increase vitality, cure pulmonary complaints and tumours and increase life expectancy. It was also used by the native American Indians for similar problems.
ADMINISTERED AS: tincture, decoction, capsules.

Gladwyn *Iris foetidissina.*
COMMON NAME: stinking gladwyn, gladwin, gladwine, stinking gladdon, spurgewort, spurge plant, roast beef plant.
OCCURRENCE: found in woods and shady parts in southern England.
PARTS USED: the root.
MEDICINAL USES: antispasmodic, cathartic, anodyne. A decoction acts as a strong purge; has been used as an emmenagogue and for removing eruptions. The dried powdered root can be of benefit in hysterical disorders, fainting, nervous problems and to relieve cramps and pain. Taken both internally and as an external poultice, this is an excellent herb to remedy scrofula. The use of this herbal remedy can be dated back to the fourth

century before Christ.

ADMINISTERED AS: decoction, dried root, infusion.

Globe flower *Trollius europaeus.*

COMMON NAME: globe trollius, boule d'or, European globe flower, globe rananculus, globe crow-foot, luchen-gowans.

OCCURRENCE: a native European plant found in moist woods and mountain pastures.

PARTS USED: the whole plant, fresh.

MEDICINAL USES: currently this plant is not used to treat many diseases and it has properties which would benefit from further investigation. It has been used in Russia to treat obstinate scorbutic disorders.

Golden rod *Solidago virgaurea.*

COMMON NAME: verge d'or, solidago, goldruthe, woundwort, Aaron's rod.

OCCURRENCE: normally found wild in woods in Britain, Europe, central Asia and North America but it is also a common garden plant.

PARTS USED: the leaves contain tannin, with some bitter and astringent chemicals which are unknown.

MEDICINAL USES: aromatic, stimulant, carminative. This herb is astringent and diuretic and is highly effective in curing gravel and urinary stones. It aids weak digestion, stops sickness and is very good against diphtheria. As a warm infusion it is a good diaphoretic drug and is used as such to help painful menstruation and amenorrhoea (absence or stopping of menstrual periods).

ADMINISTERED AS: fluid extract, infusion, spray.

Golden seal *Hydrastis canadensis.*

COMMON NAME: orange root, yellow root, yellow puccoon, ground raspberry, wild curcuma, tumeric root, Indian root, eyebalm, Indian paint, jaundice root, warnera, eye root.

OCCURRENCE: a native plant of Canada and eastern United States.

PARTS USED: the rhizome which contains the alkaloids berberine, hydastine and canadine, as well as resin, albumin, starch, fatty matter, sugar, lignin and volatile oil.

MEDICINAL USES: tonic, stomachic, laxative, alterative, detergent. Native American Indians use this plant as a source of yellow dye for clothing and weapons and also as a remedy for sore eyes, general ulceration and disordered digestion. The herb has a special action on the mucous membranes of the body, making it an excellent remedy for catarrh, dyspepsia, gastric catarrh, loss of appetite and liver problems. Given as a tonic, the root is highly effective in easing constipation and is very good at stopping sickness and vomiting. Chronic inflammation of the colon and rectum can be treated by an injection of golden seal, as can haemorrhoids. When taken as an infusion, it may cure night-sweats and passive bleeding from the pelvic tissues. In large doses, *Hydrastis* is very poisonous.

ADMINISTERED AS: injection, infusion, tincture, lotion, fluid extract, dried powdered root, solid extract.

Gooseberry *Ribes grossularia.*
COMMON NAME: fea, feverberry, feabes, carberry, groseille, groset, groser, krusbaar, dewberries, goosegogs, honeyblobs, feaberry.
OCCURRENCE: a well-known shrub native to central and northern Europe, especially Great Britain.
PARTS USED: the fruit and leaves, which contain citric acid, sugar, various minerals and pectose.
MEDICINAL USES: the expressed juice is said to be a cure for all inflammations. The acid red fruit is made into a light jelly which is good for sedentary and bilious complaints as well as in cases of excess body fluid. An infusion of dried leaves is effective in treating gravel and is a useful tonic for menstruating young girls. In the Highlands of Scotland, the prickles were used as charms to remove warts and styes.
ADMINISTERED AS: an infusion, expressed juice, dietary item.

Goutwort *Aegopodium podagraria.*
COMMON NAME: goutweed, goutherb, ashweed, Jack-jump-about, herb gerard, English masterwort, pigweed, eltroot, ground elder, bishops elder, white ash, ground ash, weyl ash, bishopsweed.
OCCURRENCE: a weed plant of Europe, Great Britain and Russian Asia.
PARTS USED: the herb.
MEDICINAL USES: diuretic and sedative. Taken internally for aching joints, gouty and sciatic pain and as an external poultice for inflamed areas. It was thought that carrying some of the herb in a pocket would prevent an attack of gout developing.
ADMINISTERED AS: poultice, liquid extract.

Groundsel *Senecio vulgaris.*
COMMON NAME: common groundsel, grundy, swallow, ground glutton, simson, sention, grounsel.
OCCURRENCE: very common weed throughout Europe and Russian Asia.
PARTS USED: the whole herb and fresh plant. The plant contains senecin

and seniocine.

MEDICINAL USES: diaphoretic, anti scorbutic, purgative, diuretic, anthelmintic. It is good for sickness of the stomach, used as a purgative in a weak infusion and as an emetic when in a strong infusion. This infusion removes bilious trouble and lowers body temperature. A poultice of groundsel is used warm on boils but nursing mothers have cold poultices as a coolant on swollen inflamed or hardened breasts. If boiling water is poured on to the fresh plant, the resulting liquid is a pleasant swab for the skin and helps soften chapped hands.

ADMINISTERED AS: infusion, poultice, lotion.

Guarana Paullinia cupara.

COMMON NAME: paullina, guarana bread, Brazilian cocoa, uabano, uaranzeiro, *Paullina sorbilis*.

OCCURRENCE: native to Brazil and Uruguay.

PARTS USED: the prepared seed, crushed. The seeds are shelled, roasted for six hours and shaken until their outer shell comes off. They are ground to a fine powder, made into a dough with water and formed into cylinders which are dried in the sun or over a fire. The seed preparation is eaten with water by the native people. The roasted seeds contain caffeine, tannic acid, catechutannic acid, starch and a fixed oil.

MEDICINAL USES: nervine, tonic, stimulant, aphrodisiac, febrifuge, slightly narcotic. It is used in mild forms of diarrhoea or leucorrhoea and also for headaches, in particular those linked to the menstrual cycle. guarana stimulates the brain after mental exertion, or after fatigue or exhaustion due to hot temperatures. It may also have diuretic effects where it can help rheumatism, lumbago and bowel complaints. The drug is similar to that of COCA or COFFEE.

ADMINISTERED AS: powder, fluid extract, tincture.

Hair-cap moss Polytrichium juniperum.

COMMON NAME: bear's bed, robin's eye, ground moss, golden maidenhair, female fern herb, robinsrye, rockbrake herb.

OCCURRENCE: found in woods and hedges across Europe and Britain.

PARTS USED: the whole plant.

MEDICINAL USES: powerful diuretic. It is a very important remedy in dropsy, urinary obstructions, gravel and suppression of urine. The herb does not cause nausea and is frequently combined with BROOM or CARROT for best effects.

ADMINISTERED AS: infusion.

Hawthorn Crataegus oxyacantha.

COMMON NAME: may, mayblossom, quick, thorn, whitethorn, haw, hazels, gazels, halves, hagthorn, ladies meat, bread and cheese tree, maybush.

OCCURRENCE: a familiar tree in Great Britain, Europe, North Africa and Western Asia.

PARTS USED: the dried fruits which contain the chemical amyddalin.

MEDICINAL USES: cardiac, diuretic, astringent, tonic. Mainly used as a cardiac tonic in organic and functional heart problems, e.g. hypertrophy, dyspnoea, heart oppression. A decoction of the flowers and berries is good at curing sore throats, and is utilized as a diuretic in dropsy and kidney disorders.

ADMINISTERED AS: liquid extract, decoction.

Heartease Viola tricolor.

COMMON NAME: wild pansy, love-lies-bleeding, loving idol, call-me-to-you, three-faces-under-a-hood, godfathers and godmothers, pink-eyed-John, flower o'luce, Jack-jump-up-and-kiss-me.

OCCURRENCE: abundant all over Great Britain, in cornfields, gardens, waste ground and hedge banks. It is also distributed through Arctic Europe, North Africa, Siberia and North India.

PARTS USED: the whole herb, fresh and dried. The active chemicals within the plant include violine, mucilage, resin, salicylic acid and sugar.

MEDICINAL USES: diaphoretic and diuretic. It was formerly held in high regard as a remedy for epilepsy, asthma and catarrhal infections. It has been utilized in blood disorders and heart diseases, while a decoction of the flowers was recommended for skin diseases. In America, they use heartease as an ointment or poultice in eczema, and it is taken internally for bronchitis. People on the continent have used *Viola tricolor* for its mucilaginous, demulcent and expectorant qualities.

ADMINISTERED AS: decoction, ointment, poultice and tincture.

Hedge-hyssop Gratiola officinalis.

OCCURRENCE: a perennial plant, native to southern Europe and found wild in damp areas in Great Britain.

PARTS USED: the root and herb. The plant contains the glucosides gratiolin and gratiosolin.

MEDICINAL USES: diuretic, cathartic, emetic. Recommended in scrofula, chronic liver complaints and enlargement of the spleen. It is also utilized in relieving dropsy and as a vermifuge.

ADMINISTERED AS: an infusion of powdered root.

Hellebore, Black *Helleborus niger.*

COMMON NAME: Christe herbe, Christmas rose, melampodium.

OCCURRENCE: a native of the mountains in central and southern Europe, Greece and Asia minor, but found in Britain as a garden plant.

PARTS USED: the rhizome and root. The plant has two glucosides within it, helleborin and helleborcin, both of which are powerful poisons.

MEDICINAL USES: the drug has drastic purgative, emmenagogue and anthelmintic properties, but is a violent narcotic. It is of value in treating nervous disorders, hysteria and melancholia and was previously used in dropsy and amenorrhoea. Given externally, the fresh root is violently irritant. The drug must be administered with great care.

ADMINISTERED AS: fluid extract, tincture, solid extract, powdered root or decoction.

Hemlock *Conium maculatum.*

COMMON NAME: herb bennet, spotted conebane, musquash root, beaver poison, poison hemlock, poison parsley, spotted hemlock, vex, vecksies.

OCCURRENCE: common in hedges, meadows, waste ground and stream banks throughout Europe and is also found in temperate Asia and North Africa.

PARTS USED: the leaves, fruits and seeds. The most important con-stituent of hemlock leaves is the alkaloid coniine, which is poison-ous, with a disagreeable odour. Other alkaloids in the plant include methyl-coniine, conhydrine, pseudoconhydrine, ethyl piperidine.

MEDICINAL USES: sedative, antispasmodic, anodyne. The drug acts on the centres of motion and causes paralysis and so it is used to remedy undue nervous motor excitability, e.g. teething, cramp and muscle spasms of the larynx and gullet. When inhaled, hemlock is said to be good in relieving coughs, bronchitis, whooping cough and asthma. The method of action of *Conium* means it is directly antagonistic to the effects of strychnine, from NUX VOMICA (*Strychnos nux-vomica*), and hence it is used as an antidote to strychnine poisoning and similar poisons. Hemlock has to be administered with care as narcotic poisoning may result from internal application and overdoses induce paralysis, with loss of speech and depression of respiratory function leading to death. Antidotes to hemlock poisoning are tannic acid, stimulants, e.g. COFFEE, MUSTARD and CASTOR OIL.

ADMINISTERED AS: powdered leaves, fluid extract, tincture, expressed juice of the leaves and solid extract.

Henbane *Hyoscyamus niger.*

COMMON NAME: hyoscyamus, hog's bean, Jupiter's-bean, symphonica, cassilata, cassilago, deus caballinus.

OCCURRENCE: native to central and southern Europe and western Asia and was introduced to Great Britain, North America and Brazil where it is found on waste ground, ditches and near old buildings.

PARTS USED: the fresh leaves and flowering tops. The chief constituents of henbane leaves are the alkaloids hyoscyamine, atropine and hyoscine. The leaves also contain a bitter principle called hyoscytricin, choline, mucilage, calcium oxalate, potassium nitrate and fixed oil.

MEDICINAL USES: antispasmodic, hypnotic, mild diuretic, mydriatic, anodyne, sedative. The herb has a milder narcotic effect than BELLADONNA or STRAMONIUM and is utilized to lessen muscle spasms, reduce pain and can stop nervous irritation. It is used in cystitis, irritable bladder, hysteria, irritable cough, asthma, gastric ulcers and chronic gastric catarrh. When taken in small doses repeated over time, Henbane tranquillizes people affected by severe nervous irritability, enabling them to sleep without adversely affecting the digestive organs or causing headaches, which opium has the tendency to do. Thus, henbane is given to people with insomnia and to children, to which opium cannot be given. The fresh leaves of henbane can be used as a poultice to relieve local pain from gout, neuralgia, cancerous ulcers, sores and swellings. The solid extract is used to produce suppositories used to relieve haemorrhoids. Henbane is poisonous and should never be used except under medical advice.

ADMINISTERED AS: powdered leaves, tincture, fluid extract, expressed juice, solid extract, suppositories.

Holly *Ilex aquifolium.*

COMMON NAME: holm, hulver bush, hulm, holme chase, holy tree, Christ's thorn.

OCCURRENCE: native to central and southern Europe and grows freely in Great Britain.

PARTS USED: the leaves, berries and bark.

MEDICINAL USES: diaphoretic, febrifuge, cathartic, tonic. Infused holly leaves are used in catarrh, pleurisy and formerly against smallpox. Also in intermittent fevers and rheumatism where the alkaloid ilicin works to good effect. Juice expressed from fresh holly leaves is effective against jaundice. The berries have different properties and are violently emetic and purgative, but they have been utilized in dropsy and as a powder to check bleeding. Holly leaves have been utilized as a tea substitute.

ADMINISTERED AS: infusion of leaves, juice, whole or powdered berries.

Honeysuckle

Honeysuckle *Lonicera caprifolium.*
COMMON NAME: Dutch honeysuckle, goat's leaf, perfoliate honeysuckle.
OCCURRENCE: grows freely in Europe, Great Britain and throughout the northern temperate zone.
PARTS USED: the dried flowers and leaves
MEDICINAL USES: expectorant, laxative. A syrup made of the flowers is used for respiratory diseases and asthma. A decoction of the leaves is laxative and is also good against diseases of the liver and spleen, and in gargles.
ADMINISTERED AS: syrup, decoction.

Hops *Humulus lupulus.*
OCCURRENCE: a native British plant, found wild in hedges and woods from Yorkshire southward. It is considered an introduced species to Scotland but is also found in most countries of the northern temperate zone.
PARTS USED: the flowers, which contain a volatile oil, two bitter principles—lupamaric acid, lupalinic acid- and tannin.
MEDICINAL USES: tonic, nervine, diuretic, anodyne, aromatic. The volatile oil has sedative and soporific effects while the bitter principles are stomachic and tonic. Hops are used to promote the appetite and enhance sleep. An infusion is very effective in heart disease, fits, neuralgia, indigestion, jaundice, nervous disorders and stomach or liver problems. Hop juice is a blood cleanser and is very effective in remedying calculus problems. As an external application, hops are used with CHAMOMILE heads as an infusion to reduce painful swellings or inflammation and bruises. This combination may also be used as a poultice.
ADMINISTERED AS: an infusion, tincture, poultice, expressed juice or tea.

Horehound *Marrubium vulgare.*
COMMON NAME: hoarhound, white horehound.
OCCURRENCE: indigenous to Britain and found all over Europe.
PARTS USED: the herb, which contains the bitter principle marrubium, volatile oil, tannin sugar and resin.
MEDICINAL USES: tonic, expectorant, pectoral, diuretic. It is probably the most popular pectoral herbal remedy. Very valuable in coughs, asthma, consumption and pulmonary complaints. For children, it is given as a syrup to ease croup, stomach upsets and as a tonic. Taken in large doses, Horehound is a gentle purgative and the powdered leaves have been used as a vermifuge. A tea of the herb is excellent for colds. A sweetmeat candy and an ale is also made from horehound.

ADMINISTERED AS: syrup, infusion, tea, powdered leaves, ointment, expressed juice.

Horsemint, American *Monarda punctata.*
OCCURRENCE: native to North America and was introduced into England 1714.
PARTS USED: the herb produces a volatile oil which is composed of thymol and higher oxygenated compounds.
MEDICINAL USES: rubefacient, stimulant, carminative, diuretic. It is used as an infusion for flatulent colic, sickness and urinary disorders and has diaphoretic and emmenagogue actions also. It is principally used externally wherever a rubefacient is required, e.g. chronic rheumatism.
ADMINISTERED AS: a volatile oil.

Horseradish *Cochlearia armoracia.*
COMMON NAME: mountain radish, great raifort, red cole, *Armoracia rusticara.*
OCCURRENCE: cultivated in the British Isles for centuries. The place of origin is unknown.
PARTS USED: the root which contains the glucoside sinigrin, vitamin C, aspargin and resin.
MEDICINAL USES: stimulant, aperient, rubefacient, diuretic, antiseptic, diaphoretic. Horseradish is a powerful stimulant of the digestive organs, and it acts on lung and urinary infections clearing them away. The herb is a very strong diuretic and as such is used to ease dropsy, gravel and calculus, as well as being taken internally for gout and rheumatism. A poultice can be made from the fresh root and applied to rheumatic joints, chilblains and to ease facial neuralgia. Horseradish juice, when diluted with vinegar and glycerine, was used in children's whooping cough and to relieve hoarseness of the throat. An infusion of the root in urine was stimulating to the entire nervous system and promoted perspiration, while it was also used to expel worms in children. Care should be taken when using this herb because over-use of horseradish can blister the skin and is not suitable for people with thyroid troubles.
ADMINISTERED AS: infusion, syrup, expressed juice, fluid extract.

Horsetail *Equisetum arvense.*
COMMON NAME: mare's tail, shave-grass, bottlebrush, paddock-pipes, Dutch rushes, pewterwort.
OCCURRENCE: native to Great Britain and distributed through temperate northern regions.

Hound's tongue

PARTS USED: the herb which is composed of silica, saponin, flavonoids, tannin and traces of alkaloids—nicotine, palustrine and palustrinine.
MEDICINAL USES: diuretic, astringent. Due to the herb's rich store of minerals, horsetail is given for anaemia and general debility and can also work to encourage the absorption and efficient use of calcium by the body, helping prevent fatty deposits forming in the arteries (arteriosclerosis). It helps stop bleeding and hence is good for stomach ulcers and haemorrhage as well as easing dropsy, gravel, cystitis and inflamed prostate glands due to its astringent qualities. The herb can be of benefit in the treatment of bed-wetting in children.
ADMINISTERED AS: infusion, dried herb, syrup.

Hound's tongue *Cynoglossum officinale.*

COMMON NAME: dog's tongue, *Lindefolia spectabilis.*
OCCURRENCE: a common plant in Switzerland and Germany; occasionally found in Great Britain.
PARTS USED: the herb.
MEDICINAL USES: anodyne, demulcent, astringent. Used as pills or as a decoction for colds, coughs, catarrh, diarrhoea and dysentery. Administered both internally and externally to soothe the digestive organs and haemorrhoids.
ADMINISTERED AS: decoction, pills, ointment.

Houseleek *Sempervivum tectorum.*

COMMON NAME: Jupiter's eye, Thor's beard, bullock's eye, sengreen, ayron, ayegreen.
OCCURRENCE: native to the mountains of central and southern Europe and the Greek islands but introduced to Britain many centuries ago.
PARTS USED: the fresh leaves.
MEDICINAL USES: refrigerant, astringent, diuretic. The bruised fresh leaves or its expressed juice are often applied as a poultice to burns, scalds, bumps, scrofulous ulcers and general skin inflammation. The juice is a cure for warts and corns. In large doses, houseleek juice is emetic and purgative. The plant was supposed to guard where it grew against fire, lightning and sorcery, hence it was grown on house roofs.

Hydrangea *Hydrangea aborescens.*

COMMON NAME: wild hydrangea, seven barks, common hydrangea, *Hydrangea vulgaris.*
OCCURRENCE: native to the United States and is cultivated across the world as a garden plant.

PARTS USED: the root which contains two resins, gum, sugar, starch, sulphuric and phosphoric acids and a glucoside called hydrangin.

MEDICINAL USES: diuretic, cathartic, tonic, nephritic. This herb is very good at preventing and removing stones in the urinary system, and relieving the pain due to urinary gravel. The fluid extract is also used to correct alkaline urine, chronic vaginal discharges and irritation of the bladder in older people. This drug was used by native American Indians and its benefits were passed on to European settlers.

ADMINISTERED AS: fluid extract, decoction, syrup.

Iceland moss Cetraria islandica.

COMMON NAME: Iceland lichen, cetraria.

OCCURRENCE: indigenous to a wide area of the northern hemisphere.

PARTS USED: the dried whole lichen. The moss contains a large quantity of starchy mater called lichenin as well as fumaric acid, oxalic acid and iodine.

MEDICINAL USES: demulcent, tonic, nutritive. The lichen has antibiotic properties and used to be given for tuberculosis as it was reputed to kill the tubercle bacillus, and clear phlegm from the lungs. It is used today for asthma, other respiratory problems and to soothe the digestive tract, stopping nausea. It is also used as a food, once the bitter principles are removed by boiling.

ADMINISTERED AS: decoction, dietary item.

Ipecacuanha Cephaelis ipecacuanha.

COMMON NAME: *Psychotria ipecacuanha.*

OCCURRENCE: native to Brazil, Bolivia and parts of South America and was introduced into Europe in the seventeenth century.

PARTS USED: the chief constituents of the root are the alkaloids emetrine, cephaelin and psychotrine, as well as two glucosides, choline, resin, calcium oxalate and a volatile oil among other compounds.

MEDICINAL USES: diaphoretic, emetic, expectorant, stimulant. The effects of the drug on the body are entirely dependent on the dose given. In very small doses, ipecacuanha stimulates the stomach, liver and intestine aiding digestion and increasing appetite while in slightly larger doses it has diaphoretic and expectorant properties which is good for colds, coughs and dysentery. Large doses of the drug are emetic. There is a lot of historical use of this drug against amoebic (or tropical) dysentery where rapid cures can occur. Care should be taken in utilizing this drug as emetine can have a toxic effect on the heart, blood vessels, lungs and intestines and cause severe illness.

ADMINISTERED AS: powdered root, fluid extract, tincture, syrup.

Irish moss *Chondrus crispus.*

COMMON NAME: carrageen, chondrus, carrahan, carragheen.

OCCURRENCE: common at low tide on all shores of the North Atlantic.

PARTS USED: the dried plant which contains mucilage and sulphur compounds.

MEDICINAL USES: demulcent, pectoral, emollient; nutritive. A popular remedy which is made into a jelly for pulmonary complaints, kidney and bladder diseases. It is widely used as a culinary article.

ADMINISTERED AS: dietary item.

Ivy *Hedera helix.*

COMMON NAME: common ivy.

OCCURRENCE: native to many parts of Europe and northern and central Asia.

PARTS USED: the leaves and berries.

MEDICINAL USES: stimulating, diaphoretic, cathartic. The leaves have been used as poultices on enlarged glands, ulcers and abscesses and the berries ease fevers and were used extensively during the Great Plague of London.

ADMINISTERED AS: poultice, infusion.

Ivy, Ground *Glechoma hederacea.*

COMMON NAME: alehoof, gill-go-over-the-ground, haymaids, tun-hoof, hedgemaids, coltsfoot, robin-run-in-the-hedge.

OCCURRENCE: very common on hedges and waste ground all over Britain.

PARTS USED: the whole herb.

MEDICINAL USES: diuretic, astringent, tonic and gently stimulant. It is good in relieving kidney diseases and indigestion. Ground ivy tea is useful in pectoral complaints and in weakness of the digestive organs. The expressed juice, when sniffed up the nose, is said to successfully cure a headache and can be administered externally to ease bruises and black eyes. It also has antiscorbutic qualities.

ADMINISTERED AS: fluid extract, expressed juice and infusion.

Ivy, Poison *Rhus toxicodendron.*

COMMON NAME: poison oak, poison vine.

OCCURRENCE: native to the United States of America.

PARTS USED: the fresh leaves which contain a resin called toxicodendron as the active principle.

MEDICINAL USES: irritant, rubefacient, stimulant, narcotic. This herb is successful in treating obstinate skin eruptions, palsy, paralysis, acute rheumatism and joint stiffness. It has also been good in treating ringworm, allergic rashes and urinary incontinence. In small doses, poison ivy is a very good sedative for the nervous system, but care must be taken in its use as it can trigger gastric and intestinal irritation, drowsiness, stupor and delirium.

ADMINISTERED AS: tincture, fluid extract, infusion.

Jaborandi Pilocarpus microphyllus.

COMMON NAME: arruda do mato, arruda brava, jamguarandi, juarandi.

OCCURRENCE: a native Brazilian plant.

PARTS USED: the dried leaves. The main constituents of the leaves are a volatile oil and three alkaloids—pilocarpine, isopilocarpine, pilocarpidine.

MEDICINAL USES: stimulant, diaphoretic, expectorant. This herb is used as the crude drug and as the purified alkaloid, pilocarpine. Jaborandi is used for psoriasis, deafness, baldness, chronic catarrh, tonsillitis, dropsy and catarrhal jaundice. It can also benefit fat removal from the heart in heart disease, pleurisy, chronic renal diseases and reducing thirst in fevered patients. The extracted alkaloid, Pilocarpine, has an antagonistic effect to atropine, from BELLADONNA, *Atropa belladonna* and other related plants, and causes contraction of the pupil of the eye. It is used as a fast and highly effective diaphoretic drug, increasing gland secretions and the flow of breast milk. Both the jaborandi and pilocarpine can irritate the stomach, causing vomiting even when given as an injection, so care should be advised upon using this drug.

ADMINISTERED AS: powdered leaves, tincture, injection, fluid extract.

Jacob's ladder Polemonicum coeruleum.

COMMON NAME: Greek valerian, charity.

OCCURRENCE: found wild in ditches and streams across England and southern Scotland.

PARTS USED: the herb.

MEDICINAL USES: diaphoretic, astringent, alterative, expectorant. A useful drug in fevers and inflammatory diseases, pleurisy, etc. It induces copious perspiration and eases coughs, colds, bronchial and lung complaints.

ADMINISTERED AS: an infusion.

Jewelweed Impatiens aurea, Impatiens biflora.

COMMON NAME: wild balsam, balsamweed, pale-touch-me-not, slipperweed, silverweed, wild lady's slipper, speckled jewels, wild celandine, quick in the hand, *Impatiens pallida, I. fulva.*

OCCURRENCE: members of the genus *Impatiens* are found distributed across the northern temperate zone and South Africa; mostly natives of mountainous regions in tropical Asia and Africa.

PARTS USED: the herb.

MEDICINAL USES: aperient, diuretic, emetic, cathartic. The diuretic qualities of the herb make it useful against dropsy and jaundice while the fresh juice is reputed to remove warts, corns and cure ringworm. The fresh herb was made into an ointment with lard and used for piles. Due to its acrid taste and strong action, jewelweed is rarely used in herbal medicine today.

ADMINISTERED AS: expressed juice, ointment.

Juniper *Juniperus communis.*

OCCURRENCE: a common shrub native to Great Britain and widely distributed through many parts of the world.

PARTS USED: the berry and leaves.

MEDICINAL USES: the oil of juniper obtained from the ripe berries is stomachic, diuretic and carminative and is used to treat indigestion, flatulence as well as kidney and bladder diseases. The main use of juniper is in dropsy, and aiding other diuretic herbs to ease the disease.

ADMINISTERED AS: essential oil from berries, essential oil from wood, fluid extract, liquid extract, solid extract.

Kamala *Mallotus philippinensis.*

COMMON NAME: *Glandulae rottelerde*, kamcela, spoonwood, *Röttlera tinctoria*, kameela.

OCCURRENCE: native to India, Abyssinia, southern Arabia, China and Australia.

PARTS USED: the powder removed from the capsular fruit, composed of hairs and glands.

MEDICINAL USES: taeniafuge, purgative. The powder kills and expels tapeworms from the body. The worm is usually removed whole. It is a quick and active purgative drug, causing griping and nausea. It is used externally for cutaneous complaints including scabies and herpetic ringworm.

ADMINISTERED AS: powdered kamala, fluid extract.

Kava-kava *Piper methysticum.*

COMMON NAME: ava, ava pepper, kava, intoxicating pepper.

OCCURRENCE: indigenous to Polynesia, Sandwich Islands, South Sea Islands and Australian colonies.

PARTS USED: the peeled, dried rhizome. The plant contains two resins, one called kavine, a volatile oil, starch and an alkaloid termed kavaine methysticcum yangonin.

MEDICINAL USES: tonic, stimulant, diuretic. There is a long history of use against gonorrhoea, vaginitis, leucorrhoea, nocturnal incontinence and other problems of the urinary-genital tract. As a strong diuretic, kava is good for gout, rheumatism, bronchial problems and heart trouble. Kava acts on the nerve centres in a stimulating, then depressing manner, and has been used as a local anaesthetic as it causes paralysis of the respiratory centre. It relieves pain and has an aphrodisiac effect.

ADMINISTERED AS: powdered root, fluid extract, solid extract.

Knapweed, Greater *Centaurea scabiosa.*

COMMON NAME: hardhead, ironhead, hard irons, churls head, logger head, horse knops, mat fellon, bottleweed, bullweed, cowede, bottsede.

OCCURRENCE: a perennial plant frequently seen in field borders and waste ground in England, but rare in Scotland.

PARTS USED: the root and seeds.

MEDICINAL USES: diuretic, diaphoretic and tonic. Formerly greatly appreciated as a vulnerary herb and used to cure loss of appetite. When taken as a decoction, it is good for catarrh; as an ointment for wounds, bruises and sores, etc.

ADMINISTERED AS: decoction and ointment.

Knotgrass *Polyganum ariculare.*

COMMON NAME: centuriode, ninety-knot, nine-joints, allseed, bird's tongue, sparrow tongue, red robin, armstrong, cowgrass, hogweed, pigrush, swynel grass, swine's grass.

OCCURRENCE: native around the globe; abundant on arable land, waste ground and roadside verges.

PARTS USED: the whole herb.

MEDICINAL USES: astringent, diuretic, anthelmintic, vulnerary and styptic. An infusion of the herb was used in diarrhoea, bleeding haemorrhoids and all haemorrhages. As a diuretic, it was said to expel stones and also parasitic worms. The fresh juice stops nosebleeds, if squirted up the nose and applied to the temples. As an ointment, it heals sores very well.

ADMINISTERED AS: expressed juice, infusion, decoction and ointment.

Kola nuts *Kola vera.*

COMMON NAME: guru nut, cola, kola seeds, gurru nuts, bissy nuts, cola seeds, *Cola acuminata*, *Sterculia acuminata*.

OCCURRENCE: native to Sierra Leone and North Ashanti and cultivated in tropical western Africa, West Indies, Brazil and Java.

Laburnum

PARTS USED: the seeds.

MEDICINAL USES: nerve stimulant, diuretic, cardiac tonic. This drug is a good overall tonic, largely due to the caffeine it contains. It has been used as a remedy for diarrhoea and for those with an alcoholic habit.

ADMINISTERED AS: powdered seeds, tincture, fluid and solid extract.

Laburnum *Cytisus laburnam.*

COMMON NAME: yellow laburnum.

OCCURRENCE: indigenous to high mountain regions of Europe and widely cultivated across the globe as a garden plant.

PARTS USED: the alkaloid, obtained from the plant, called cytisine.

MEDICINAL USES: all parts of the laburnum are thought to be poisonous, particularly the seeds. The alkaloid has been recommended in whooping cough and asthma, and also as an insecticide, but it has not been used due to the very poisonous nature of the compound. Laburnum poisoning symptoms include intense sleepiness, vomiting, convulsive movements, coma and unequally dilated pupils. Laburnum is also poisonous to cattle and horses and deaths of both livestock and humans have resulted from ingestion of this plant.

Lady's mantle *Alchemilla vulgaris.*

COMMON NAME: lion's foot, bear's foot, nine hooks, stellaria.

OCCURRENCE: native to mountainous districts of Britain and widely distributed over northern or Arctic Europe, Asia and Greenland.

PARTS USED: the herb.

MEDICINAL USES: astringent, styptic, vulnerary. Herbalists used to say that lady's mantle was one of the best herbs for wounds. In modern times, it is used as a cure for excessive menstruation as an infusion or injection. The root is very good for stopping all bleeding and may also act as a violent purge. The herb is also said to promote quiet sleep.

ADMINISTERED AS: decoction, infusion, injection, tincture, fluid extract, dried root.

Larch *Pinus larix.*

COMMON NAME: *Larix europaea, Abies larix, Larix decidua, Laricus cortex*, European larch, Venice turpentine.

OCCURRENCE: indigenous to hilly regions of central Europe, but was introduced into Britain in 1639.

PARTS USED: the inner bark which contains tannic acid, larixinic acid and turpentine.

MEDICINAL USES: stimulant, diuretic, astringent, balsamic and expectorant.

It is very useful as an external application for eczema and psoriasis. However, it is mainly used as a stimulant expectorant in chronic bronchitis, internal haemorrhage and cystitis. Larch turpentine has also been suggested as an antidote in cyanide or opium poisoning and has been used as a hospital disinfectant.

ADMINISTERED AS: fluid extract or syrup.

Larkspur *Delphinicum consolida.*

COMMON NAME: field larkspur, lark's chaw, lark's heel, knight's spur, lark's toe.

OCCURRENCE: found wild in fields through Europe and Great Britain.

PARTS USED: the seeds. The active principle in the plant is delphinine, an irritant poison also found in STAVESACRE.

MEDICINAL USES: parasiticide, insecticide. The tincture of the seeds is used to destroy lice and nits in the hair and given internally in spasmodic asthma and dropsy. The expressed juice from the leaves was applied to bleeding piles and an infusion of the whole plant was said to benefit colic.

ADMINISTERED AS: infusion, tincture, expressed juice.

Laurel *Laurus nobilis.*

COMMON NAME: bay, sweet bay, true laurel, laurier d'apollon, roman laurel, noble laurel, lorbeer, laurier sauce, daphne.

OCCURRENCE: native to the shores of the Mediterranean and cultivated in Britain.

PARTS USED: the leaves, fruit and essential oil. The volatile oil contains pinene, geraniol, eugenol, cineol, bitter principles and tannin.

MEDICINAL USES: stomachic, narcotic, diaphoretic, emetic. In ancient times, laurel was highly valued as a medicine but now laurel is only selectively utilized. The leaves were formerly used in hysteria, flatulent colic and in treating the absence of menstrual periods, but now are only used to stimulate the digestion. The oil of bays is also used for earache, sprains and bruises and rheumatism.

ADMINISTERED AS: essential oil, infusion.

Lavender, English *Lavandula vera.*

OCCURRENCE: indigenous to mountainous regions in the western Mediterranean and is cultivated extensively in France, Italy, England and Norway.

PARTS USED: the flowers and the essential oil which contains linalool, linalyl acetate, cineol, pinene, limonene and tannin.

MEDICINAL USES: aromatic, carminative, stimulant, nervine. It is mainly used as a flavouring agent for disagreeable odours in ointments or syrups. The essential oil when taken internally is restorative and a tonic against faintness, heart palpitations, giddiness and colic. It raises the spirits, promotes the appetite and dispels flatulence. When applied externally, the oil relieves toothache, neuralgia, sprains and rheumatism. The oil is utilized widely in aromatherapy, often to very beneficial effects.

ADMINISTERED AS: fluid extract, tincture, essential oil, spirit, infusion, tea, poultice, distilled water.

Lemon *Citrus limonica.*

COMMON NAME: limon, *Citrus medica*, *Citrus Limonum*, citronnier, neemoo, leemoo, limoun, limone.

OCCURRENCE: indigenous to northern India and widely cultivated in Mediterranean countries.

PARTS USED: the fruit, rind, juice and oil. Lemon peel contains an essential oil and a bitter principle, while lemon juice is rich in citric acid, sugar and gum. Oil of lemon contains the aldehyde, citral and the oils pinene and citronella.

MEDICINAL USES: antiscorbutic, tonic, refrigerant, cooling. Lemon juice is the best preventative drug for scurvy and is also very valuable in fevers and allaying thirst. It is recommended in acute rheumatism and may be given to counteract narcotic poisons such as opium. It is used as an astringent gargle in sore throats, for uterine haemorrhage after childbirth, as a lotion in sunburn and as a cure for severe hiccoughs. The juice is also good for jaundice and heart palpitations. A decoction of lemon is a good antiperiodic drug and can be used to replace quinine in malarial injections, or to reduce the temperature in typhoid fever. Lemon oil is a strong external rubefacient and also has stomachic and carminative qualities.

ADMINISTERED AS: syrup, decoction, fresh juice, tincture, essential oil, dietary item.

Lettuce, Wild *Lactuca virosa.*

COMMON NAME: lachicarium, strong-scented lettuce, green endive, lettuce opium, acrid lettuce, laitue vireuse.

OCCURRENCE: found in western and southern Europe, including Great Britain.

PARTS USED: the leaves, dried milk juice—lactuarium. Lactuarium is obtained by cutting the stem in sections and collecting the latex juice. It turns reddish-brown in colour when dried.

MEDICINAL USES: anodyne, sedative, narcotic, mild diaphoretic, diuretic. The drug resembles a weak opium, without opium's tendency to upset the digestive system. It is used to allay irritable coughs and as a sedative and narcotic, but only infrequently. It is also used for dropsy, inducing sleep and easing colic.

ADMINISTERED AS: powder, tincture, fluid extract, syrup, alcoholic extract.

Lilac *Syringa vulgaris.*

COMMON NAME: common lilac.

OCCURRENCE: a shrub native to Persia and the mountains of eastern Europe.

PARTS USED: the leaves and fruit.

MEDICINAL USES: as a vermifuge, tonic, antiperiodic and febrifuge. It may be used as a substitute for ALOES (*Aloe vera/Aloe perryi*) and in the treatment of malaria.

ADMINISTERED AS: an infusion.

Lily of the valley *Convallaria magalis.*

COMMON NAME: May lily, convarraria, Our Lady's tears, conval-lily, lily constancy, ladder to heaven, Jacob's ladder.

OCCURRENCE: native to Europe and distributed over North America and northern Asia. A very localized plant in England and Scotland.

PARTS USED: the flowers, leaves and whole herb. The chief constituents are two glucosides—convallamarin (the active principle) and convallarin, as well as tannin and mineral salts.

MEDICINAL USES: cardiac tonic, diuretic. A similar drug to digitalis, from the FOXGLOVE, although it is less powerful. Strongly recommended in valvular heart disease, cardiac debility, dropsy and it slows the action of a weak, irritated heart. Lily of the valley does not have accumulatory effects and can be taken in full and frequent doses without harm. A decoction of the flowers is good at removing obstructions in the urinary canal.

ADMINISTERED AS: fluid extracts, decoction tincture, powdered flowers.

Lily, Madonna *Lilium candidum.*

COMMON NAME: white lily, meadow lily.

OCCURRENCE: a southern European native which has been cultivated in Great Britain and America for centuries.

PARTS USED: the bulb.

MEDICINAL USES: demulcent, astringent, mucilaginous. The bulb is mainly used as an emollient poultice for ulcers, tumours and external inflammation. When made into an ointment, Madonna lily removes corns and eliminates pain and inflammation from burns and scalds, reducing scarring. When used in combination with life root (*Senecio aureus*), Madonnna lily is of great value in treating leucorrhoea, prolapse of the womb and other female complaints. The bulb is eaten as food in Japan.

ADMINISTERED AS: poultice, ointment, decoction.

Lime fruit *Citrus medica* var. *acida*.

COMMON NAME: *Citrus acris*, *Citrus acida*, limettae fructus.

OCCURRENCE: a native Asian tree which is cultivated in many warm countries including the West Indies and Italy.

PARTS USED: the fruit and juice.

MEDICINAL USES: refrigerant, antiscorbutic. The juice of the lime contains citric acid and is a popular beverage, sweetened as a syrup. It is used to treat dyspepsia.

ADMINISTERED AS: fresh juice, syrup.

Lime tree *Tilia europoea*.

COMMON NAME: linden flowers, linn flowers, common lime, tilleul, flores tiliae, *Tilia vulgaris*, *T. intermedia*, *T. cordata*, *T. platyphylla*.

OCCURRENCE: native to the British Isles and the northern temperate zone.

PARTS USED: the lime flowers, bark, powdered charcoal. The flowers contain volatile oil, flavonid glucosides, saponins, condensed tannins and mucilage.

MEDICINAL USES: nervine, stimulant, tonic. An infusion of the flowers is good for indigestion, hysteria, nervous vomiting, colds, 'flu and catarrh. They can also help calm overactive children and relax the nervous system. Lime flower tea eases headaches and insomnia. The flowers are said to lower blood pressure (possibly due to the bioflavonids they contain) and are said to remedy arteriosclerosis. The inner bark of the lime has a diuretic effect and is utilized for gout and kidney stones as well as treating coronary artery disease by dilating the coronary arteries. The powdered charcoal was used in gastric and dyspeptic disorders and applied to burnt or sore areas.

ADMINISTERED AS: infusion, powdered charcoal, dried inner bark, tea.

Liquorice *Glycyrrhiza glabra*.

COMMON NAME: licorice, lycorys, *Liquiriha officinalis*.

OCCURRENCE: a shrub native to south-east Europe and south-west Asia and cultivated in the British Isles.

PARTS USED: the root. The chief compound in the root is glychrrhizin along with sugar, starch, gum, asparagus, tannin and resin.

MEDICINAL USES: demulcent, pectoral, emollient. A very popular and well-known remedy for coughs, consumption and chest complaints. Liquorice extract is included in cough lozenges and pastilles, with sedatives and expectorants. An infusion of bruised root and FLAX (linseed) is good for irritable coughs, sore throats and laryngitis. Liquorice is used to a greater extent as a medicine in China and other eastern countries. The herb is used by brewers to give colour to porter and stout and is employed in the manufacture of chewing or smoking tobacco.

ADMINISTERED AS: powdered root, fluid extract, infusion, solid extract.

Liverwort, English Peltigera canina.

COMMON NAME: lichen caninus, lichen cinereus terrestris, ash-coloured ground liverwort, liverleaf, *Hepatica triloba.*

OCCURRENCE: grows in moist, shady places in Britain and Europe.

PARTS USED: the whole lichen.

MEDICINAL USES: deobstruent, slightly purgative, *Peltigera canina* is held in esteem as a cure for liver complaints and was formerly regarded as a remedy for hydrophobia.

ADMINISTERED AS: infusion and fluid extract.

Lobelia Lobelia inflata.

COMMON NAME: Indian tobacco, asthma weed, pukeweed, jagroot, vomitwort, bladderpod, *Rapuntium inflatum.*

OCCURRENCE: native to North America and grown in British gardens for many years.

PARTS USED: the herb, which contains the alkaloids, lobeline, isolobeline, lobelanidine and lobinaline along with fixed oil, gum, resin and lignin.

MEDICINAL USES: expectorant, emetic, diaphoretic, anti-asthmatic, stimulant. The use of this plant was passed to Europeans from native American Indians and it has been used as a major relaxant remedy used to treat pain caused by muscle spasms. Thus it is highly effective against asthma, bronchial complaints and lung problems. Lobelia may be given to ease convulsive and inflammatory disorders such as epilepsy, tonsillitis, diphtheria and tetanus. Externally, the herb is used for eye complaints, insect bites, POISON IVY irritation, ringworm, sprains, bruises and muscle spasms. The use of lobelia as an emetic is debatable as to whether it would benefit the patient, and its use is encouraged or discouraged by different herbals. Lobelia is a very important herbal remedy in modern usage.

ADMINISTERED AS: tincture, infusion, powdered bark, syrup and fluid extract.

Loosestrife Lysimachia vulgaris.

COMMON NAME: yellow loosestrife, yellow willow herb, herb willow, willow-wort, wood pimpernel.

Lovage

OCCURRENCE: grows in shady banks and riversides in England.
PARTS USED: the herb.
MEDICINAL USES: astringent, expectorant. This herb is good at stopping bleeding of any kind, particularly of the mouth, nose and wounds. It is also used to restrain profuse menstrual bleeding and calm severe diarrhoea. Distilled water made with loosestrife was utilized to clean ulcers and reduce inflammation and to clear spots, marks and scabs from the skin. An infusion was used as a gargle in relaxed throat and quinsy.
ADMINISTERED AS: distilled water, dried herb, infusion and ointment.

Lovage *Levisticum officinale.*

COMMON NAME: *Ligusticum levisticum*, old English lovage, Italian lovage, Cornish lovage, Chinese tang kui, man-mu.
OCCURRENCE: one of the old English herbs which was very generally cultivated; it was not indigenous to Great Britain but native to the Mediterranean region.
PARTS USED: the root, leaves, young stems and seeds. The plant contains a volatile oil, angelic acid, a bitter extract and resin.
MEDICINAL USES: the young stems are used in a similar manner to ANGELICA for flavouring and confectionery. The roots and fruits are aromatic, stimulant, diuretic and carminative in action. They are generally used in stomach disorders, and feverish attacks including those with colic and flatulence. The fresh leaves are eaten as a salad and when dried are infused into a pleasant tea with emmenagogue properties. An infusion of the root was recommended by old herbalists for gravel, jaundice and urinary problems and the sudorific nature of the roots and seeds meant they were highly favoured in treating 'pestilential disorders'.
ADMINISTERED AS: infusion of leaves and root infusion.

Lucerne *Medicago sativa.*

COMMON NAME: purple medick, cultivated lucern, alfalfa, purple medicle.
OCCURRENCE: an ancient herb, of unknown origin. Cultivated in Europe, Great Britain, Peru and Persia for hundreds of years.
PARTS USED: the herb.
MEDICINAL USES: this herb is used, as an infusion, to encourage weight gain and flesh development. It has also been used to feed cattle and horses.
ADMINISTERED AS: infusion.

Lungwort *Sticta pulmonaria.*

COMMON NAME: Jerusalem cowslip, oak lungs, lung moss.

OCCURRENCE: found in Europe, but uncommon in woods in Britain.
PARTS USED: the whole lichen.
MEDICINAL USES: astringent, mucilaginous, pectoral, healing. It is very valuable in treating coughs, lung complaints and asthma. It is also good at reducing inflammation and pain.
ADMINISTERED AS: liquid extract, infusion.

Lupin, White Lupinus albus.
COMMON NAME: lupine, wolfsbohne.
OCCURRENCE: native to southern Europe and parts of Asia and is now extensively cultivated in Italy.
PARTS USED: the seeds, herb. The main compounds within the plant are the glucoside, lupinin; the alkaloids lupinidine and luparine.
MEDICINAL USES: anthelmintic, diuretic, emmenagogue. The bruised seeds, when soaked in water, are applied to ulcers and sores and when taken internally the seeds kill parasitic worms and excite the menstrual discharge. It was used by the Romans as food and can also be used for fibres to make cloth, paper and adhesive.
ADMINISTERED AS: poultice, infusion.

Mace Myristica fragrans.
COMMON NAME: macis, muscadier, *Arillus myristicae*, *Myristica officinalis*, *Myristica moschata*.
OCCURRENCE: native to the Molucca Islands, New Guinea, Bondy Islands and introduced into Sri Lanka and the West Indies.
PARTS USED: the growth outside the shell of the nutmeg seed—called the arillus. The main constituents of mace are a volatile oil, protein, gum, resins, sugars and two fixed oils. The volatile oil contains a lot of pinene and some myristicin.
MEDICINAL USES: stimulant, tonic, carminative, flavouring agent. This herb is used to help digestion and stomach weakness and increase the blood circulation and body temperature. Mace has been used against putrid and pestilential fevers and, combined with other herbs, intermittent fevers.
ADMINISTERED AS: powdered herb.

Magnolia Magnolia Virginiana.
COMMON NAME: cucumber tree, blue magnolia, swamp sassfras, *Magnolia glauca*, *M. acuminata*, *M. tripetata*.
OCCURRENCE: native to the USA but is cultivated in Great Britain.
PARTS USED: the bark of stem and root.

Maidenhair

MEDICINAL USES: mild, diaphoretic, tonic, aromatic, stimulant. The bark is used against rheumatism and malaria, and the cones of the tree are steeped in spirit to make a tonic tincture. A warm infusion of bark is laxative and sudorific while a cold infusion is antiperiodic and tonic in effect.

ADMINISTERED AS: tincture, infusion, fluid extract.

Maidenhair *Adiantum capillus-veneris.*

COMMON NAME: true maidenhair, hair of Venus, rock fern, capillaire common or capillaire de Montpellier.

OCCURRENCE: this grows wild in southern Europe and southern and central Britain.

PARTS USED: the herb, which contains tannin and mucilage but has not yet been fully investigated.

MEDICINAL USES: pectoral, expectorant, mucilaginous. The fern has been used as a remedy in chest complaints, coughs and throat problems. It is an ingredient of cough mixtures, its flavour masked by sugar and ORANGE-FLOWER water. Maidenhair is good at easing pulmonary catarrh and is used in Europe as an emmenagogue.

ADMINISTERED AS: infusion, syrup.

Male fern *Dryopteris felix-mas.*

COMMON NAME: *Aspidium felix-mas*, male shield fern.

OCCURRENCE: grows in all areas of Europe, temperate Asia, North India, North and South Africa, the temperate areas of the United States and the South American Andes.

PARTS USED: the root and the oil extracted from it. The oil is extracted using ether and contains the acid, filmaron, filicic acid, tannin, resin and sugar.

MEDICINAL USES: anthelmintic, vermifuge, taeniafuge. It is probably the best drug against tapeworm, it is normally given at night after several hours of fasting. When followed by a purgative drug in the morning, e.g. CASTOR OIL very good results are obtained. The size of the dose administered must be carefully assessed as male fern is an irritant poison in too large a dose, causing muscle weakness, coma and possible damage to the eyesight.

ADMINISTERED AS: powdered root, fluid extract; oil of male fern.

Mandrake *Atropa mandragora.*

COMMON NAME: mandragora, Satan's apple.

OCCURRENCE: a plant native to southern Europe but it can be cultivated in Great Britain.

PARTS USED: the herb and root.

MEDICINAL USES: emetic, purgative, cooling, anodyne, hypnotic. The fresh root is a very powerful emetic and purgative drug and the dried bark of the root also shares the purgative qualities. Ancient herbalists used mandrake to kill pain and to give rest and sleep to patients, as well as using it for melancholy, convulsions, rheumatic pain and scrofulous tumours. They administered the drug as the bark of the root, expressed juice or as an infusion of the root. In large doses, mandrake was said to cause delirium and madness. The herb was used as an anaesthetic in ancient Greek medicine.

ADMINISTERED AS: infusion, fresh root, powdered bark, expressed juice.

Maple, Red *Acer rubrum.*

COMMON NAME: swamp maple, curled maple.

OCCURRENCE: a native American tree, introduced into Britain in 1656 as an ornamental tree.

PARTS USED: the bark.

MEDICINAL USES: astringent. The native American Indians used an infusion of the bark as an application for sore eyes.

ADMINISTERED AS: an infusion.

Mare's tail *Hippuris vulgaris.*

COMMON NAME: female horsetail, marsh barren horsetail.

OCCURRENCE: a native British aquatic flowering plant found in shallow ponds, rivers, ditches and lake margins.

PARTS USED: the herb.

MEDICINAL USES: vulnerary. Old herbalists viewed mare's tail as good for stopping bleeding, be it internal or external. It was said to be used to heal ulcers, green wounds in children, ruptures and urinary stones. The herb was also used to strengthen the intestinal system, for head colds and as a warm poultice on skin eruptions and inflammations.

ADMINISTERED AS: poultice, decoction.

Marigold *Calendula officinalis.*

COMMON NAME: *Caltha officinalis*, golds, ruddes, marg gowles, oculus Christi, marygold, garden marigold, solis sponsa.

OCCURRENCE: a native of southern Europe and a common garden plant in Great Britain.

PARTS USED: the petals and herb. Only the deep orange-flowered variety is of medicinal use.

Marjoram

MEDICINAL USES: stimulant, diaphoretic. Mainly used as a local remedy. Taken internally, an infusion of the herb prevents pus formation and externally is good in cleaning chronic ulcers and varicose veins. Formerly considered to be of benefit as an aperient and detergent to clear visceral obstructions and jaundice. A marigold flower, when rubbed onto a bee or wasp sting, was known to relieve pain and reduce swelling, while a lotion from the flowers was good for inflamed and sore eyes. The expressed juice of the plant was used to clear headaches and remove warts.
ADMINISTERED AS: infusion, distilled water and lotion.

Marjoram *Origanum vulgare*
OCCURRENCE: generally distributed over Asia, Europe and North Africa and also found freely in England.
PARTS USED: the herb and volatile oil.
MEDICINAL USES: the oil has stimulant, carminative, diaphoretic, mildly tonic and emmenagogue qualities. As a warm infusion, it is used to produce perspiration and bring out the spots of measles as well as giving relief from spasms, colic and dyspeptic pain. The oil has been used externally as a rubefacient and liniment, and on cotton wool placed next to an aching tooth it relieves the pain. The dried herb may be utilized as a hot poultice for swellings, rheumatism and colic, while an infusion of the fresh plant will ease a nervous headache.
ADMINISTERED AS: essential oil, poultice and infusion.

Marjoram, Sweet *Origanum marjorana.*
COMMON NAME: knotted marjoram, *Majorana hortensis*.
OCCURRENCE: native to Portugal and grown as an annual plant through the rest of Europe and Great Britain.
PARTS USED: the herb and leaves. The plant contains tannic acid, mucilage, bitter substances and an essential oil.
MEDICINAL USES: tonic, stimulant, emmenagogue. The essential oil, oleum majoranae when extracted from the leaves, makes a good external application for sprains and bruises, and acts as an emmenagogue when taken internally. Sweet marjoram is widely used in cookery and aids digestion of food.
ADMINISTERED AS: essential oil, dried or fresh leaves.

Marshmallow *Althaea officinalis.*
COMMON NAME: mallards, mauls, schloss tea, cheeses, mortification, root, guimauve.

OCCURRENCE: a native of Europe, found in salt marshes, meadows, ditches and riverbanks. It is locally distributed in England and has been introduced to Scotland.

PARTS USED: the leaves, root and flowers. Marshmallow contains starch, mucilage, pectin, oil, sugar, asparagin, glutinous matter and cellulose.

MEDICINAL USES: demulcent, emollient. Very useful in inflammation and irritation of the alimentary canal and the urinary and respiratory organs. A decoction of the root is effective against sprains, bruises of any muscle aches. When boiled in milk or wine marshmallow relieves diseases of the chest, e.g. coughs, bronchitis or whooping cough and it eases the bowels after dysentery without any astringent effects. It is frequently given as a syrup to infants and children.

ADMINISTERED AS: infusion, decoction, syrup, fluid extract.

Masterwort *Imperatoria ostruthium*.

OCCURRENCE: native to central Europe and alpine regions; cultivated in Great Britain for many years.

PARTS USED: the rhizome.

MEDICINAL USES: stimulant, antispasmodic, carminative. Masterwort has been used in asthma, stroke, dyspepsia and menstrual problems. A decoction of the herb in urine was considered beneficial against dropsy, cramp, epilepsy, flatulence, gout and kidney and uterine problems.

ADMINISTERED AS: distilled water, decoction, fluid extract.

Mastic *Pistacia lentiscus*.

COMMON NAME: mastich, lentisk.

OCCURRENCE: indigenous to the Mediterranean regions of Spain, Portugal, France, Greece, Turkey, tropical Africa and the Canary Islands.

PARTS USED: the resin, which contains a volatile oil, an alcohol-insoluble resin and an alcohol-soluble resin.

MEDICINAL USES: stimulant, diuretic. Similar to TURPENTINE in effect, but its use in medicine has declined. In some areas it is used for diarrhoea in children, or chewed to sweeten the breath. Today, mastic is mainly used as a filling for carious teeth.

ADMINISTERED AS: resin.

Matico *Piper angustifolium*.

COMMON NAME: soldier's herb, thoho-thoho, moho-moho, *Artanthe elongata, Stephensia elongata, Piper granulosium,* matica.

OCCURRENCE: native to Peru and spread over much of tropical America. It has been grown in England.

PARTS USED: the dried leaves which contain a volatile oil, artanthic acid, tannin and resin.

MEDICINAL USES: astringent, stimulant, styptic, diuretic. It is recommended for chronic mucous discharges, leucorrhoea, haemorrhoids, diarrhoea, dysentery and urinary and genital complaints. The leaves stop bleeding from most sites, and are used as an application to slight wounds, ulcers, bites from leeches or after teeth extraction.

ADMINISTERED AS: dried leaves, fluid extract.

Mayweed *Anthemis cotula.*

COMMON NAME: maroute, cotula, dog chamomile, wild chamomile, foetid or stinking chamomile (or mayweed), dog's fennel, maithes, mathor, *Maruta cotula, Maruta foetida, Manzilla loca, Camomille puante.*

OCCURRENCE: frequently grows in fields and wild places in Great Britain and Europe.

PARTS USED: the flowers and leaves. The flowers contain volatile oil, oxalic, valeric and tannic acids, a bitter extractive and salts of iron, potassium, calcium and magnesium.

MEDICINAL USES: tonic, antispasmodic, emmenagogue and emetic. The smell of the flowers is still repulsive, but is less offensive than that of the rest of the plant, so the flowers are mainly used in medicine. It is used in hysteria, as a poultice for haemorrhoids and as an infusion in the bath. The flowers have also been used in headaches, menstrual problems, gastric troubles; to induce sleep in asthma and in convalescence after fevers.

ADMINISTERED AS: fluid extract, poultice, infusion, decoction.

Meadowsweet *Spiraea ulmaria.*

COMMON NAME: meadsweet, dolloff, queen of the meadow, bridewort, lady of the meadow.

OCCURRENCE: common in the British Isles in meadows or woods.

PARTS USED: the herb.

MEDICINAL USES: aromatic, astringent, diuretic, alterative. This herb is good against diarrhoea, stomach complaints and blood disorders. It is highly recommended for children's diarrhoea and dropsy and was used as a decoction ir wine to reduce fevers. Meadowsweet makes a pleasant everyday drink when infused and sweetened with honey.

ADMINISTERED AS: infusion, decoction.

Melilot *Melilotus officinalis, Melilotus alba, Melilotus arvensis.*
COMMON NAME: king's clover, king's chafer, yellow melilot, white melilot, corn melilot, sweet clover, plaster clover, sweet lucerne, wild laburnham hart's tree.
OCCURRENCE: naturalized in all parts of the British Isles.
PARTS USED: the dried herb containing coumarin, hydrocoumaric acid, orthocoumaric acid and melilotic anhydride.
MEDICINAL USES: aromatic, emollient, carminative. When applied as a plaster, ointment or poultice, the herb is good at relieving abdominal or rheumatic pain. It is taken internally to relieve flatulence. The herb was formerly used for clearing the eyesight, headaches, wounds, ulcers and inflammation.
ADMINISTERED AS: poultice, expressed juice, infusion.

Mercury, Dog's *Mercurialis perennis.*
OCCURRENCE: a common plant in woods in Europe and Russian Asia.
PARTS USED: the herb.
MEDICINAL USES: purgative. Recommended for use externally to treat sore, watery eyes, deafness, pains in the ear, ague, jaundice and women's diseases. The fresh juice of the plant is used to remove warts and to cleanse sores and swellings. A lotion is made for antiseptic external dressings while the juice is used as a nasal douche for catarrh.
ADMINISTERED AS: expressed juice, lotion, fresh herb.

Mescal buttons *Anhalonicum lewinii.*
COMMON NAME: *Lopophora lewinii, Analonium williamsii, Echinacactus lewinii, Echinocactus williamsii,* pellote, muscal buttons.
OCCURRENCE: Mexico and Texas.
PARTS USED: the tops of the cacti plant. The drug contains four alkaloids—anhalonine, mescaline, anhalonidine and lophophorine—as well as the chemicals pellotine and anhalamine.
MEDICINAL USES: cardiac, tonic, narcotic, emetic. The drug is useful in head injuries, asthma, gout, neuralgia and rheumatism. The extracted compound pellotine has been used to induce sleep in people with insanity as it has no undesirable reactions. Large doses of mescal buttons produce an odd cerebral excitement, with visual disturbances. The physical effects include muscular relaxation, wakefulness, nausea, vomiting and dilation of the pupil. The ancient Aztec Indians believed mescal buttons to have divine properties and included its use to produce exaltation in their religious ceremonies.
ADMINISTERED AS: fluid extract, tincture, extracted alkaloid.

Mezereon

Mezereon *Daphne mezereum.*

COMMON NAME: spurge olive, spurge laurel, camolea, wolt schjeluke, kellernals, dwarf bay, flowering spurge, wild pepper, *Mezerei cortex*, *Mezerei officinarum*, *Laureole gentile*.

OCCURRENCE: indigenous to Britain, Europe and Siberia and was naturalized into the United States and Canada.

PARTS USED: the root, berries, the bark of the stem and root. The bark tastes acrid and this is due to a resin called mezeen. The other active chemicals are a fixed oil, a bitter glucoside called daphnin and a substance similar to euphorbone.

MEDICINAL USES: alterative, diuretic, stimulant, vesicant. An ointment of the bark is used to promote discharge from indolent ulcers, and it is also used for snake and other venomous bites. It is taken internally for chronic rheumatism, scrofula, syphilis, skin diseases and dropsy. The tincture is used to ease neuralgic pain and toothache. In large doses, it acts as an irritant poison and purgative drug causing vomiting, so care should be taken in monitoring the dose used.

ADMINISTERED AS: infusion, tincture, ointment.

Mistletoe *Viscum album.*

COMMON NAME: European mistletoe, bird lime mistletoe, herbe de la croix, mystyldene, lignum crucis.

OCCURRENCE: an evergreen, true parasitic plant found on several tree species including fruit and oak trees. It is found throughout Europe and Britain except in Scotland, where it is very rare.

PARTS USED: the leaves and young twigs. They contain mucilage, sugar, fixed oil, tannin and viscin, the active part of the plant.

MEDICINAL USES: nervine, antispasmodic, tonic and narcotic. It is highly recommended for epilepsy and other convulsive disorders, along with stopping internal haemorrhage. It has also been used in delirium, hysteria, neuralgia, nervous debility, urinary disorders and many other complaints arising from a weakened state of the nervous system. The berries are taken to cure severe stitches in the side, and the plant produces a sticky substance called bird-lime which is applied to ulcers and sores. Mistletoe is excellent for reducing blood pressure and has been indicated to be a successful cure for chronic arthritis and in treating malignant tumours in the body.

ADMINISTERED AS: tincture, powdered leaves, infusion, fluid extract.

Motherwort *Leonurus cardiaca.*

COMMON NAME: lion's ear, lion's tail.

OCCURRENCE: a native plant in many parts of Europe, but only rarely found in the wild in Britain.

PARTS USED: the dried herb which contains the alkaloids leonurinine and stachydrine; the bitter glucosides leonurine and leonuridin, tannins and a volatile oil.

MEDICINAL USES: diaphoretic, antispasmodic, tonic, nervine, emmenagogue, sedative. An important use of the herb is in easing the anxiety after childbirth or at the menopause by lowering the blood pressure. It is excellent for female complaints by allaying nervous irritability, regulating menstruation and treating functional infertility. As a tonic, the herb acts well and is effective in treating fevers and allowing good recovery from them. Throughout history, Motherwort has been used to treat palpitations and rapid heart beat, particularly when they develop from anxiety or hysteria. As the name suggests, motherwort acts on the uterine system and the alkaloid stachydrine has the effect of hastening childbirth so this herb should not be used by pregnant women. It is beneficial, however, in causing the uterus to contract after delivery and in this manner is more effective than ERGOT.

ADMINISTERED AS: powdered herb, infusion, decoction, conserve.

Mountain flax *Linum catharticum.*

COMMON NAME: purging flax, dwarf flax, fairy flax, mill mountain.

OCCURRENCE: a common plant in meadows and pastures across Europe and Great Britain.

PARTS USED: the herb which contains a bitter resin and a crystalline principle called linin.

MEDICINAL USES: purgative, laxative, cathartic. It is a gentle cathartic drug with a laxative action preferred to SENNA. As an infusion, the dried herb has been used internally to treat muscular rheumatism and catarrhal infections. It can also be beneficial in liver complaints and jaundice.

ADMINISTERED AS: infusion, dried herb.

Mugwort *Artemisia vulgaris.*

COMMON NAME: felon herb, St. John's plant, moxa, cirigulum Sancti Johannis.

OCCURRENCE: this grows wild in Great Britain on roadsides and hedgerows.

PARTS USED: the leaves, which contain volatile oil, flavonoids, tannin and a bitter principle called absinthin; the roots.

MEDICINAL USES: emmenagogue, stimulant, tonic, nervine, diuretic, diaphoretic. As a nervine, this herb is good in palsy, fits, epilepsy and for people with a feeble constitution. An infusion of the herb is used for intermittent fevers and the ague and given as a tonic. Mugwort's main use is as an emmenagogue to provoke delayed or absent periods and therefore it should not be used during pregnancy, except under the guidance of a qualified herbal practitioner. However, it does help during and after childbirth in speeding up the birth process and to expel the afterbirth. Mugwort acts on the digestive process and stimulates the liver and is used to treat gout and rheumatism. In China, the dried herb is burnt on or near the skin to stop rheumatic pain caused by damp and cold conditions. Also in China, mugwort is taken during pregnancy to prevent miscarriage, differing from the Western viewpoint.

ADMINISTERED AS: dried herb, fluid extract.

Mulberry *Monus nigra.*

COMMON NAME: common mulberry, black mulberry, purple mulberry.
OCCURRENCE: a native of Turkey, Armenia, Persia and is cultivated throughout Europe and Britain.
PARTS USED: the fruit which contains glucose, protein, pectin, tartaric and malic acids and ash.
MEDICINAL USES: laxative, refrigerant, nutritive. The fruit juice is a beneficial drink for convalescent people, as it checks the thirst and cools the blood after fevers. The fruits are made into wine, jam and conserve. The bark of the tree has a purgative and vermifuge effect on the body.
ADMINISTERED AS: syrup, expressed juice, infusion of bark.

Mullein *Verbascum thapsus.*

COMMON NAME: blanket herb, beggar's blanket, Aaron's rod, lady's foxglove, donkey's ears, torches, candlewick plant, wild ice leaf, Jupiter's staff, clown's lungwort, velvet plant, clot.
OCCURRENCE: widely distributed through Europe, temperate Asia, North America, Ireland and Great Britain.
PARTS USED: the leaves and flowers. The plant contains saponins, mucilage, gum volatile oil, flavonoids and glucosides.
MEDICINAL USES: demulcent, emollient, astringent, sedative, narcotic. This herb is very useful in pectoral complaints, hoarseness, bronchitis, asthma, whooping-cough, wasting diseases and bleeding of the lungs and bowels. It can also be good for diarrhoea, mild catarrh, colic, inflammation of the urinary system, and as a poultice for boils and sores. The dried leaves may be smoked to remove irritation of the mucous membranes, the cough associated with consumption and spasmodic coughs in gen-

eral. After placing bruised mullein leaves in olive oil and leaving it for a period, the oil can be used for relieving pain from bruises, frostbite and earache. Water distilled from the flowers was recommended for gout, burns and the condition called erysipelas, where the skin and tissue is infected with the bacterium *Streptococcus pyogenes* and the affected areas are red and swollen.

ADMINISTERED AS: fluid extract, distilled water, poultice, tincture, decoction.

Musk seed Hibiscus abelmoschus.

COMMON NAME: ambretta, Egyptian alcée, bisornkorner, target-leaved hibiscus, galu gastrin, *Abelmoschus moschatus*.

OCCURRENCE: native to India and grown in Egypt and the East and West Indies.

PARTS USED: the seeds. They contain fixed oil, a resin and a volatile body.

MEDICINAL USES: antispasmodic, aromatic, stomachic, nervine, aphrodisiac, insecticide. An emulsion of the seeds is regarded as anti-spasmodic and the seeds were chewed to benefit the nerves and stomach. The seeds are dusted over woollens to protect the fibre from moths.

ADMINISTERED AS: whole seeds, emulsion.

Mustard, Black Brassica nigra, Siriapis nigra.

COMMON NAME: *Brassica sinapioides*.

OCCURRENCE: it grows wild throughout Europe, South Siberia, Turkey and North Africa and is cultivated in England, Italy, Germany and the Netherlands as a condiment.

PARTS USED: the seeds which contain an acrid, volatile oil, an active principle, the glucoside sinigrin and the enzyme myrosin. When the seeds are crushed with water, these latter two chemicals come into contact and form oil of mustard.

MEDICINAL USES: irritant, stimulant, diuretic and emetic. Mainly used as a poultice to relieve acute local pain, e.g. pneumonia, bronchitis and other respiratory organ diseases. The herb draws blood to the skin surface, easing congestion of the organs, headaches, neuralgia and spasms. The oil of mustard is a powerful irritant and rubefacient when undiluted, but is very useful when dissolved in spirit for chilblains, rheumatism and colic. A hot infusion of the seed is a stimulating footbath and aids removal of colds or headaches. Mustard flour, when taken internally, can act as an emetic, aperient and alterative herb and may also cure hic-cups. It is also a very good antiseptic and sterilizing agent and deodorizer.

ADMINISTERED AS: poultice, infusion, essential oil, seed flour, leaves.

Myrrh *Commiphora molmol.*

COMMON NAME: *Balsamodendron myrrha, Commiphora myrrha* var. *molmol*, mira, morr.

OCCURRENCE: obtained from bushes in North-East Africa and in Arabia.

PARTS USED: the oleo-gum-resin which contains volatile oil, resins and gum.

MEDICINAL USES: stimulant, tonic, healing, antiseptic, astringent, expectorant, emmenagogue. Myrrh has a long history of use in countering poisons and putrid tissues throughout the body. It is used in leucorrhoea, chronic catarrh, thrush, athlete's foot, absence of menstrual periods, ulcers and as a vermifuge. The resin acts as a tonic in dyspepsia, stimulates the circulation, appetite and the production of gastric juices. It makes a very good gargle or mouth-wash for an inflamed sore throat, spongy gums and mouth ulcers.

ADMINISTERED AS: fluid extract, tincture, pills.

Nettle *Urtica dioica, Urtica urens.*

COMMON NAME: common nettle, stinging nettle.

OCCURRENCE: widely distributed throughout temperate Europe and Asia, Japan, South Africa and Australia.

PARTS USED: the whole herb, which contains formic acid, mucilage, mineral salts, ammonia and carbonic acid.

MEDICINAL USES: astringent, stimulating, diuretic, tonic. The herb is anti-asthmatic and the juice of the nettle will relieve bronchial and asthmatic troubles, as will the dried leaves when burnt and inhaled. The seeds are taken as an infusion or in wine to ease consumption or ague. Nettles are used widely as a food source and can be made into puddings, tea, beer, juice and used as a vegetable. A hair tonic or lotion can also be made from the nettle. In the Highlands of Scotland, they were chopped, added to egg white and applied to the temples as a cure for insomnia.

ADMINISTERED AS: expressed juice, infusion, decoction, seeds, dried herb, dietary item.

Nightshade, Black *Solarum nignum.*

COMMON NAME: garden nightshade, petty morel.

OCCURRENCE: a common plant in south England, seen less frequently in northern England and Scotland.

PARTS USED: the whole plant, fresh leaves. Both contain the active principle, solanine which is found in variable quantities within the plant, throughout the year.

MEDICINAL USES: the bruised fresh leaves are used external to the body to ease pain and reduce inflammation. Juice of the leaves has been used for ringworm, gout and earache and is supposed to make a good gargle or mouthwash when mixed with vinegar. This species of plant is reputed to be very poisonous, narcotic and sudorific, so is only utilized in very small doses, under careful supervision.

ADMINISTERED AS: infusion, expressed juice and fresh leaves.

Nutmeg *Myristica fragrans.*

COMMON NAME: nux moschata, *Myristica officinalis*, *M. aromata*, myristica.
OCCURRENCE: native to the Banda Islands, Malay Archipelago and the Molucca Islands. It is cultivated in Java, West Indies, Sumatra and French Guiana.
PARTS USED: the dried kernel of the seed which contains a volatile and a fixed oil, starch, gum, various acids and terpenes.
MEDICINAL USES: carminative, stomachic, stimulant. The grated or powdered kernel is used to relieve flatulence, vomiting and nausea. It is mainly used as an ingredient of various medicines and as a culinary spice. Nutmeg has similar properties to MACE but mace has a stronger flavour. Large doses of nutmeg can be toxic, producing disorientation, double vision and convulsions.

ADMINISTERED AS: expressed oil, powdered kernel.

Nux vomica *Strychnos Nux-vomica.*

COMMON NAME: poison nut, semen strychnox, Quaker buttons.
OCCURRENCE: a tree indigenous to India and now grown in Burma, China, Australia and the Malay Archipelago.
PARTS USED: the dried ripe seeds. They contain the alkaloids, strychnine, brucine and strychnicine, fatty matter, caffeotannic acid and the glucoside, loganin.
MEDICINAL USES: tonic, bitter, stimulant. Nux vomica is utilized as a general tonic, mainly when combined with other herbal remedies, to treat neuralgia, dyspepsia, impotence, chronic constipation and general debility. This drug can also be of benefit in cardiac failure, surgical shock or poisoning by chloroform where it raises blood pressure and increases pulse rate, but it can also cause violent convulsions. Nux vomica should only be used in limited circumstances and under strict control as strychnine is very poisonous.

ADMINISTERED AS: fluid extract, tincture.

Oak *Quercus robur.*

COMMON NAME: common oak, tanner's bark.

Oats

OCCURRENCE: a tree widely dispersed over Europe.
PARTS USED: the bark.
MEDICINAL USES: slightly tonic, strongly astringent, antiseptic. It is very good in chronic diarrhoea, dysentery as a decoction and used as a gargle for sore throats. May also be used as an injection for leucorrhoea and applied locally for piles and bleeding gums. Water distilled from the oak buds was said to be good on any kind of inflammation.
ADMINISTERED AS: fluid extract, infusion, tincture, injection.

Oats *Avena sativa.*

COMMON NAME: groats, oatmeal.
OCCURRENCE: distributed across Europe, Britain and the USA.
PARTS USED: the seeds which are made up of starch, gluten, albumen and other proteins, sugar, gum oil and salts.
MEDICINAL USES: nervine, stimulant, antispasmodic, *Avena* forms a nutritious and easily digested food for convalescent patients and exhaustion after fevers. It can be made into a demulcent enema, or a good emollient poultice. Oat extract or tincture is useful as a nerve and uterine tonic.
ADMINISTERED AS: fluid extract, tincture, enema, dietary item.

Olive *Olea Europea.*

COMMON NAME: *Olea oleaster*, *Olea larcifolia*, *Olea gallica*, oliver.
OCCURRENCE: native to the Mediterranean countries, Syria and Turkey. Now cultivated in Chile, Peru and Australia.
PARTS USED: the oil expressed from the ripe fruit, the leaves.
MEDICINAL USES: the oil is emollient, demulcent, laxative and aperient. It is a good substitute for CASTOR OIL when given to children, but its value in clearing parasitic worms or gallstones is unsure. The oil is a good ingredient in liniments or ointment and is used for bruises, sprains, cutaneous injuries and rheumatic prob-lems. It is also utilized externally in joint, kidney and chest com-plaints or for chills, typhoid and scarlet fevers, plague and dropsy. When combined with alcohol, the oil is good as a hair tonic. Olive leaves have astringent and antiseptic properties, and an infusion of these leaves has proved beneficial in obstinate fevers.
ADMINISTERED AS: expressed oil, infusion, ointment.

Onion *Allium cepa.*

OCCURRENCE: originally native to south-west Asia and now cultivated around the globe.
PARTS USED: the bulb.

MEDICINAL USES: diuretic, expectorant, antiseptic. Although onions are extensively used in cookery, they also have medicinal uses. A roasted onion is applied to tumours or earache to remove the pain and onions steeped in gin produce a fluid extract which is given for gravel and dropsy. A homeopathic remedy is made from red onions and is useful in neuralgic pain, colds, hay fever, toothache and in the early stages of laryngitis with hoarseness.

ADMINISTERED AS: poultice, tincture.

Orange, Bitter *Citrus aurantium* subsp. *amara*. **Orange, Sweet** *Citrus vulgaris*.

COMMON NAME: (bitter orange) *Citrus bigaradia*, *Citrus vulgaris*, *Bi garadier*, bigarade orange, Seville orange, naranja; (sweet orange) Portugal orange, China orange, *Citrus dulcis*.

OCCURRENCE: the bitter orange originated from northern India but is now grown in Mediterranean countries. The sweet orange is grown in Sicily, Africa and the West Indies.

PARTS USED: the fruit, peel and flowers. Oil is extracted from the peel of both types of orange—bitter orange produces oil of bigarde and the sweet orange oil is oil of Portugal. Distillation of the bitter orange flowers with water produces orange flower water and an essential oil called neroli.

MEDICINAL USES: tonic, stomachic, carminative, aromatic. Both sweet and bitter orange oils are used as flavouring agents for medicinal compounds but may be used in a similar manner to oil of TURPENTINE in treating chronic bronchitis. An infusion of dried flowers can be taken as a mild nervous stimulant and a tonic may be given of bitter orange peel, either on its own or as an infusion. In China, the dried peel of the sweet orange is used as a diuretic and to aid digestion. Oil of neroli is used in aromatherapy for treating anxiety and nervous depression.

ADMINISTERED AS: infusion, dried peel, essential oil, distilled water.

Orris *Iris florentina* (and other species).

COMMON NAME: Florentine orris, orris root.

OCCURRENCE: grown in Italy and Morocco and to a smaller extent in England.

PARTS USED: the root, which contains oil of orris, fat, resin, starch, mucilage, a glucoside called iridin and a bitter extractive substance.

MEDICINAL USES: Orris root is rarely used in medicine today. The fresh root has emetic, diuretic and cathartic properties and was formerly used against congested headache, dropsy, bronchitis and chronic diarrhoea. It is more generally used in perfumery, as it strengthens the odour of other fragrant herbs and acts as a fixative in perfumes and pot pourri. It is also part of dusting powders, toilet powders and tooth powders.

Paraguay Tea *Ilex paraguayensis.*
COMMON NAME: Paraguay herb, maté, yerba maté, jesuit's tea, Brazil tea, gón gouha, ilex maté, houx maté.
OCCURRENCE: largely cultivated in South America.
PARTS USED: the leaves, which contain caffeine, tannin ash and insoluble matter.
MEDICINAL USES: tonic, diuretic, diaphoretic, powerful stimulant. The leaves are infused in a similar manner to TEA and drunk with lemon juice and sugar by the local people in South America. There is a huge consumption of this herb as it is taken at every meal. In large doses, it can cause purging and vomiting.
ADMINISTERED AS: infusion.

Paris, Herb *Paris quadrifolia.*
COMMON NAME: herba Paris, true love, one berry, *Solarum quadrifolium*, *Aconitum pardalianches*.
OCCURRENCE: found in Europe, Russian Asia and locally distributed in Great Britain.
PARTS USED: the whole plant picked as it is just coming into bloom.
MEDICINAL USES: narcotic. In large doses, the herb induces nausea, vertigo, vomiting, profuse sweating, delirium, dry throat and convulsions. Overdoses can be fatal, particularly in children. If administered in small doses, the herb can relieve spasmodic cough, rheumatism, bronchitis, cramp, heart palpitation and colic. Juice expressed from the leaves is good for green wounds, tumours and inflammation while the juice from the berries eases inflammation of the eyes. In Russia, the leaves are proposed to ease madness and its effects. As it has a similar set of qualities to opium, it has been used as an aphrodisiac. Herb Paris has also been utilized as an antidote against mercury and arsenic poisoning.
ADMINISTERED AS: tincture, expressed juice of leaves, expressed juice of berries, ointment, powdered root, decoction.

Parsley *Carum petroselinum.*
COMMON NAME: *Apium petroselinum*, *Petroselinum lativum*, petersylinge, persely, persele.
OCCURRENCE: this was first cultivated in Britain in 1548, now completely naturalized through England and Scotland.

PARTS USED: the root, seeds and leaves. The root is slightly aromatic and contains starch mucilage, sugar, volatile oil and apiin. Parsley seeds contain more volatile oil, which consists of terpenes and apiol, an allyl compound.
MEDICINAL USES: carminative, tonic, aperient, diuretic. A strong decoction of the root is used in gravel, stone, kidney congestion, jaundice and dropsy. Bruised parsley seeds used to be given against plague and intermittent fevers, while the external application of the leaves may help to dispel tumours. A poultice of the leaves is effective against bites and stings of poisonous insects.
ADMINISTERED AS: fluid extract, essential oil, infusion, ointment and poultice.

Parsley piert *Alchemilla arvensis.*
COMMON NAME: parsley breakstone, parsley piercestone, field lady's mantle.
OCCURRENCE: common across Great Britain, Europe and North Africa and was introduced into North America.
PARTS USED: the herb.
MEDICINAL USES: diuretic, demulcent, refrigerant. This herb is mainly employed in gravel, stone, dropsy and in bladder and kidney problems. It can effect results even in seemingly incurable cases. It can also help jaundice and clearing obstructions of the liver. To limit its irritancy, it is sometimes combined with demulcent or diuretic herbs for best effect, e.g. BROOM, JUNIPER, CARROT, COMFREY or MARSHMALLOW.
ADMINISTERED AS: fresh herb or infusion.

Parsnip *Pastinaca sativa.*
COMMON NAME: le panais, die pastinake.
OCCURRENCE: native European, cultivated commercially as food.
PARTS USED: the root.
MEDICINAL USES: nutritive. The parsnip exceeds almost all other vegetables in terms of food value (except potatoes) and is very nourishing for humans and animals alike. They are preferred to carrots for fattening pigs and given to cattle. Some old herbalists saw parsnips as a cure for asthma, cancer and consumption and used bruised parsnip roots as an application on bruises. In many areas, parsnips were made into a preserve, a beer or wine. They are also used extensively in salads, soups, as a vegetable and in cakes.

Passionflower *Passiflora incarnata.*
COMMON NAME: passion vine, granadilla, maracoc, maypops.
OCCURRENCE: a native of Virginia in the United States.
PARTS USED: the flower and the dried vine. The plant contains flavonoids,

sugars, sterols and gum as well as the alkaloids harmone, harmol, harmaline, harmine and harmalol.

MEDICINAL USES: antispasmodic, sedative, narcotic. This drug relaxes the nervous system and the sedative effects are good as well. It is non-addictive. It is a very good remedy for anxiety, tension, insomnia, diarrhoea, dysentery, neuralgia and painful menstruation. The alkaloids have tranquillizing effects and it is used to reduce high blood pressure.

ADMINISTERED AS: fluid extract.

Peach *Prunus persica.*

COMMON NAME: *Persica vulgaris, Amygdalus persica.*

OCCURRENCE: cultivated in Asia for centuries and introduced into Europe from Persia.

PARTS USED: the bark, leaves and the oil expressed from the weeds.

MEDICINAL USES: demulcent, sedative, diuretic, expectorant. The leaves or bark, when used as an infusion, are almost a specific for irritation and congestion of the gastric surfaces. The infusion is also good for chronic bronchitis, whooping cough and ordinary coughs. A syrup or infusion made of the peach flowers was thought to be a mild acting purgative for children, as well as good for jaundice and giving health to a poorly child. The kernel oil was thought to induce sleep and rest if rubbed on to the temples. The oil is also used as a substitute for the more expensive ALMOND oil.

ADMINISTERED AS: infusion, fresh leaves, powdered leaves, oil.

Pellitory *Anacyclus pyrethrum.*

COMMON NAME: Roman pellitory, pellitory of Spain, Spanish chamomile, pyrethre, *Matricaria pyrethrum, Anthemis pyrethrum, Pyrethrum officinarum, Pyrethri radix.*

OCCURRENCE: cultivated in Spain, Algeria and other Mediterranean countries.

PARTS USED: the root, which contains two oils, a brown resin thought to contain peletonin, tannin, gum, lignin and various mineral salts. The alkaloid, pyrethrine is the active chemical.

MEDICINAL USES: local irritant, rubefacient. The main use of this herb is to relieve toothache and promoting the flow of saliva. This eases conditions such as dryness of the throat and partial paralysis of the lips and tongue. The powdered root is used as snuff to clear chronic catarrh of the head, exciting the flow of nasal mucous and tears. The herb is added to many dental toothpowders.

ADMINISTERED AS: powdered root, infusion, tincture.

Pellitory-of-the-wall *Parietaria officinalis.*

COMMON NAME: *Parietaria diffusa*, lichwort, paritary.

OCCURRENCE: a common wild plant in Europe and Great Britain.

PARTS USED: the herb, which contains a bitter glucoside, tannin, sulphur, mucilage and flavones among its chemical constituents.

MEDICINAL USES: diuretic, laxative, refrigerant, demulcent. It is given as an infusion or decoction to treat urine retention, cystitis, nephritis, dropsy, prostate inflammation, urinary stones and gravel. In the form of an ointment, this herb was used for haemorrhoids, gout and fistulas. The fresh herb is more effective than the dried herb.

ADMINISTERED AS: infusion, syrup, poultice, decoction.

Pennyroyal *Mentha pulegium.*

COMMON NAME: pulegium, run-by-the-ground, pudding grass, lurk-in-the-ditch, piliolerial.

OCCURRENCE: a native plant of most of Europe and parts of Asia and commonly grown in gardens.

PARTS USED: the herb and the oil distilled from the herb called oil of pulegiam.

MEDICINAL USES: carminative, diaphoretic, stimulant, emmenagogue. The herb is mainly used to bring on menstruation which has been obstructed by cold or chills. It is also beneficial in spasms, flatulence, hysteria, sickness, colds, headaches and is a blood purifying herb. Pennyroyal is supposed to encourage sleep and was hung in bedrooms for that purpose. The oil has been used to prevent mosquito and gnat bites for many years. If taken internally, the oil can be highly toxic and death can result. This herb should not be taken by pregnant women as it promotes menstruation and may cause haemorrhage and death.

ADMINISTERED AS: dried herb, infusion, distilled oil.

Peony *Paeonia officinalis.*

COMMON NAME: paeony, paeonia, common peony, piney, *Paeonia lactifloria*, *Paeonia corrallina*.

OCCURRENCE: introduced into Great Britain some centuries ago.

PARTS USED: the root, which contains benzoic acid, asparagin, an alkaloid and an essential oil.

MEDICINAL USES: antispasmodic, tonic. In the past, peony has been used successfully in spasmodic nervous problems such as epilepsy and spasms as well as lunacy. An infusion of the powdered root is recommended for liver obstructions, and helps kidney and gall bladder diseases. Since this

plant is poisonous, it is rarely utilized in modern herbal medicine.
ADMINISTERED AS: infusion.

Pepper *Piper nigrum.*
COMMON NAME: black pepper, piper.
OCCURRENCE: grows wild in South India and Cechin-China; now cultivated in the East and West Indies, Malay Archipelago, the Philippines,
Java, Sumatra and Borneo.
PARTS USED: the dried unripe fruits. White pepper comes from the same
plant, except that the pericarp of the fruit has been removed prior to drying. The active chemicals in black or white pepper are piperine, volatile
oil, starch, cellulose and a resin called chavicin.
MEDICINAL USES: aromatic, stimulant, carminative, febrifuge. The herb
is useful in treating constipation, gonorrhoea, prolapsed rectum, paralysis of the tongue and acts on the urinary organs. The stimulant
properties of pepper work on the gastro-intestinal system to aid digestion, ease dyspepsia, torbid stomach conditions, and relieve flatulence and nausea. Pepper has also been recommended in diarrhoea,
cholera, scarlatina, vertigo and paralytic and arthritic disorders. Pep-
percorns, as the dried fruit is known, are used both whole and ground
in many culinary dishes and are used as a condiment. In the Siege of
Rome in 408 AD, pepper was so highly priced that it was used as a
form of currency.
ADMINISTERED AS: powdered dried fruits, gargle.

Peppermint *Mentha piperita.*
COMMON NAME: brandy mint, curled mint, balm mint.
OCCURRENCE: found across Europe, was introduced into Britain and grows
widely in damp places and waste ground.
PARTS USED: the herb and distilled oil. The plant contains peppermint oil,
which is composed of menthol, menthyl acetate and isovalerate, menthone,
cineol, pinene and limonene. The medicinal qualities are found in the
alcoholic chemicals.
MEDICINAL USES: stimulant, antispasmodic, carminative, stomachic, oil
of peppermint is extensively used in both medicine and commerce. It is
good in dyspepsia, flatulence, colic and abdominal cramps. The oil al-
lays sickness and nausea, is used for chorea and diarrhoea but is normally used with other medicines to disguise unpalatable tastes and effects.
Peppermint water is in most general use and is used to raise body temperature and induce perspiration. Peppermint tea can help ward off colds

and influenza at an early stage, can calm heart palpitations and is used to reduce the appetite.

ADMINISTERED AS: infusion, distilled water, spirit, essential oil and fluid extract.

Pimpernel, Scarlet *Anagallis arvensis.*

COMMON NAME: shepherd's barometer, poor man's weatherglass, adder's eyes, bipinella.

OCCURRENCE: a very widely distributed plant found in all the temperate regions, in both hemispheres.

PARTS USED: the whole herb, of which little is known of the active chemicals within it. It does contain the compound, saponin.

MEDICINAL USES: diuretic, diaphoretic, expectorant. This plant has an ancient reputation for healing, particularly dealing with diseases of the brain and mental illness. It is considered beneficial in dropsy, liver obstruction, disorders of the spleen, gravel, rheumatic complaints and gout, but caution should be taken as in experiments extracts from this plant have been found to be poisonous to animals and its full effects on humans are not yet known.

ADMINISTERED AS: infusion, dried herb, tincture, fluid extract.

Pine oils there are several kinds: **Siberian pine oil,** from *Abies Sibirica*; **Pumilio pine oil,** from *Pinus muge*; **Sylvestris pine oil,** from *Pinus sylvestris.*

PARTS USED: the oil produced from when pine wood is distilled using steam under pressure.

MEDICINAL USES: rubefacient, aromatic. These oils are mainly used as inhalants for bronchitis or laryngitis or as liniment plasters.

ADMINISTERED AS: distilled oil.

Pine, White *Pinus strobus.*

COMMON NAME: Weymouth pine, pin du lord, *Pinus alba*, deal pine.

OCCURRENCE: widely distributed in the northern hemisphere, especially in North America.

PARTS USED: the bark.

MEDICINAL USES: expectorant, diuretic, demulcent. Used for the relief of coughs, colds and chest diseases. It has a beneficial effect on the bladder and kidney systems. A compound syrup is the most commonly administered form of the drug, but it contains morphine so care must be taken that morphine dependence does not develop.

ADMINISTERED AS: compound syrup and fluid extract.

Pink root *Spigelia marylandica.*

COMMON NAME: Indian pink, wormgrass, carolina pink, Maryland pink, American wormroot, starbloom.

OCCURRENCE: grows in the southern states of the United States of America.

PARTS USED: the whole plant or the root. This plant contains a poi-sonous alkaloid called spigeline, volatile oil, resin, mucilage, lignin, a bitter principle and salts of calcium potassium and sodium.

MEDICINAL USES: very active vermifuge. This plant has very beneficial effects on removing tapeworms and roundworms, and is safe enough to give to children as long as a saline aperient is given after pinkroot, to temper the unpleasant side effects. These side effects include disturbed vision, muscular spasms, increased heart action and dizziness and are increased in severity as the dose given rises. This can lead to convulsions and death if care is not taken with this drug.

ADMINISTERED AS: fluid extract, powdered root.

Pipsissewa *Chinaphila umbellata.*

COMMON NAME: winter green, butter winter, prince's pine, king's cure, ground holly, love in winter, rheumatism weed, *Pyrola umbellata.*

OCCURRENCE: grows in Europe, Asia, the United States and Siberia.

PARTS USED: the leaves, which contain chinaphilin, arbutin gum, resin, pectic acid, starch, chlorophyll, tannic acids and several mineral salts.

MEDICINAL USES: diuretic, astringent, tonic, alterative. A decoction of the leaves is good for fluid retention, chronic gonorrhoea, dropsy and catarrh of the bladder. Applied to the skin, it acts as a rubefacient and vesicant which is good in kidney and cardiac diseases, scrofular and chronic rheumatism. It is also of value in skin diseases and may be a effective against diabetes.

ADMINISTERED AS: fresh leaves, decoction, fluid extract, syrup.

Plantain, Common *Plantago major.*

COMMON NAME: broad-leaved plantain, ripple grass, waybread, snakeweed, cuckoo's bread, Englishman's foot, white man's foot, waybroad.

OCCURRENCE: a familiar weed all over Europe, Great Britain and other parts of the world.

PARTS USED: the root, leaves and flowers.

MEDICINAL USES: refrigerant, diuretic, deobstruent, astringent, cooling, alterative. The plant has been used in inflammation of the skin, malignant ulcers, intermittent fever, applied to sores and as a vulnerary. The fresh leaves can stop bleeding of minor wounds, relieve the pain of insect stings, nettles, burns and scalds.

ADMINISTERED AS: expressed juice, poultice, infusion, fresh leaves, fluid extract, decoction, ointment.

Pleurisy root Asclepias tuberose.

COMMON NAME: butterfly-weed, swallow-wort, tuber root, wind root, colic root, orange milkweed, white root, flux root, Canada root.

OCCURRENCE: native to North America.

PARTS USED: the root which contains several resins, volatile oil, fatty matter, glucosides including asclepiadin and cardiac glycosides.

MEDICINAL USES: antispasmodic, diaphoretic, expectorant, tonic, carminative, mildly cathartic. One of the most important indigenous North American herbs which has a specific action on the lungs, reducing inflammation, helping expectoration and delivering a mild tonic effect to the pulmonary system. It is of great benefit in pleurisy, pulmonary catarrh and difficult breathing as it relieves the pain. The root also helps in acute and chronic rheumatism, eczema, flatulent colic, indigestion, dysentery and diarrhoea. It is often combined with other herbs, e.g. ANGELICA to best effect. In large doses, pleurisy root can be emetic and purgative in effect.

ADMINISTERED AS: decoction, fluid extract, infusion.

Poke root Phytolacca decandra.

COMMON NAME: garget, pigeon berry, bear's grape, red-ink plant, American spinach, skoke, crowberry, cancer-root, pocan, coakum, poke berry, herbe de la laque, *Phytolaccae radix*, *Phytolacca vulgaris*, *P. americana*, *Blitun americanum*.

OCCURRENCE: indigenous to North America and is grown in most Mediterranean countries.

PARTS USED: dried root and berries. The root is made up of triterpenoid saponins, phytolaccine (an alkaloid), resins, phytolaccic acid and tannin.

MEDICINAL USES: emetic, cathartic, alterative, narcotic. The root is used for conjunctivitis, chronic rheumatism, skin diseases and paralysis of the bowels. It is said to stimulate the lymphatic system and so is good for tonsillitis, swollen glands and mumps. Herbalists disagree as to whether poke root is effective against cancer. It may be effective, when used both as a poultice and taken internally, against breast cancer and mastitis and has been used in cases of uterine cancer. The berries are thought to have a milder action on the body than the root. The use of the root as an emetic is not recommended and the fresh root is poisonous so this drug should only be prescribed by a qualified herbal practitioner.

ADMINISTERED AS: infusion, ointment, tincture, fluid extract.

Polypody root

Polypody root Polypodium vulgare.
COMMON NAME: rock polypody, polypody of the oak, wall fern, brake root, rock brake, oak fern, rock of polypody.
OCCURRENCE: a common fern growing in sheltered places, hedge-banks, old walls and tree stumps in Great Britain and Europe.
PARTS USED: the root.
MEDICINAL USES: alterative, tonic, expectorant, pectoral. This herb is used as a laxative; as a tonic in dyspepsia and loss of appetite. It is also good for skin diseases, coughs and catarrh, consumption, hepatic complaints and some types of parasitic worm. The action of this drug is such that it may cause the formation of a rash, but these spots should disappear after a short period of time with no after effects. This fern is still used as a cure for whooping cough in many rural areas.
ADMINISTERED AS: fresh root, decoction, powdered root, fluid extract.

Poplar Populus tremuloides.
COMMON NAME: white poplar, American aspen, quaking aspen.
OCCURRENCE: native to North America and commonly grown in Great Britain.
PARTS USED: the bark, which is thought to contain salicin and populin.
MEDICINAL USES: febrifuge, diuretic, stimulant, tonic. This drug is very useful against fevers, particularly those of an intermittent nature. It is often used as a substitute for PERUVIAN BARK or quinine, as it lacks dangerous long-term side effects. Poplar bark is helpful in treating chronic diarrhoea, debility, hysteria, indigestion and faintness as well as acting as a diuretic in gleet, gonorrhoea and urinary complaints. This drug could be considered a 'universal tonic'.
ADMINISTERED AS: infusion, fluid extract.

Poppy, Red Papaver rhoeas.
COMMON NAME: headache, corn poppy, corn rose, flores rhoeados.
OCCURRENCE: a common flowering plant in fields and waste ground across Europe and Great Britain.
PARTS USED: flowers and petals. the fresh petals contain rhoeadic and papaveric acids, which give the flowers their colour, and the alkaloid rhoeadine. The amount and quantity of active ingredients in the plant is uncertain so its action is open to debate.
MEDICINAL USES: very slightly narcotic, anodyne, expectorant. The petals can be made into a syrup which is used to ease pain. It may be used for chest complaints, e.g. pleurisy.
ADMINISTERED AS: syrup, infusion, distilled water.

Poppy, White *Papaver somniferum.*
COMMON NAME: opium poppy, mawseed.
OCCURRENCE: indigenous to Turkey and Asia, cultivated in Europe, Great Britain, Persia, India and China for opium production.
PARTS USED: the capsules and flowers. The white poppy contains twenty one different alkaloids of which morphine, narcotine, codeine, codamine and thebaine are the most important.
MEDICINAL USES: hypnotic, sedative, astringent, expectorant, diaphoretic, antispasmodic, anodyne. The use of this drug dates back to Greek and Roman times. It is the best possible hypnotic and sedative drug, frequently used to relieve pain and calm excitement. It has also been used in diarrhoea, dysentery and some forms of cough. The tincture of opium is commonly called laudanum, and when applied externally with soap liniment it provides quick pain relief.
ADMINISTERED AS: syrup, tincture, decoction and poultice.

Primrose *Primula vulgaris.*
OCCURRENCE: a common wild flower found in woods, hedgerows and pastures throughout Great Britain.
PARTS USED: the root and whole herb. Both parts of the plant contain a fragrant oil called primulin and the active principle saponin.
MEDICINAL USES: astringent, antispasmodic, vermifuge, emetic. It was formerly considered to be an important remedy in muscular rheumatism, paralysis and gout. A tincture of the whole plant has sedative effects and is used successfully in extreme sensitivity, restlessness and insomnia. Nervous headaches can be eased by treatment with an infusion of the root, while the powdered dry root serves as an emetic. An infusion of primrose flowers is excellent in nervous headaches and an ointment can be made out of the leaves to heal and salve wounds and cuts.
ADMINISTERED AS: infusion, tincture, powdered root and ointment.

Puffball *Lycoperdon bovista.*
COMMON NAME: *Lycoperdon giganteum.*
OCCURRENCE: grows wild throughout Great Britain and Europe.
PARTS USED: the lower section of the fungi.
MEDICINAL USES: haemostatic. This fungi grows completely enclosing its spores in fungal tissue (peridium), and then matures so that the colour changes from yellow-white to brown and then the peridium ruptures and the spores are released. When young, the spongy fungal tissue makes an excellent food and is consumed with relish by people in many European

areas, including the Gaelic community in the Highlands of Scotland. Once matured, it is not edible but it can then be used to stop bleeding from wounds. It is a highly effective cure. Puffballs were also used as tinder many years ago and are burnt, producing smoke which stupefies bees so that honey can be collected safely.

ADMINISTERED AS: dried or fresh fungal tissue and spores.

Pumpkin Cucurbita maxima.

COMMON NAME: pumpkin seed, melon pumpkin, pompion.

OCCURRENCE: a plant grown for food and animal fodder in the United States and common in gardens in Great Britain.

PARTS USED: the seeds. They contain a fixed oil, a volatile oil, sugar, starch and an acrid resin which may be the active component.

MEDICINAL USES: taeniacide, diuretic, demulcent. This fruit has long been used as a vermifuge, removing parasitic worms including tapeworm. A mixture of the seeds, sugar, milk or water is mixed up and taken over six hours after which CASTOR OIL is given, a few hours after the final dose of pumpkin. The vermifuge effects are thought to come from the mechanical effects of the seeds. A basic infusion of the seeds in water is used in urinary complaints.

ADMINISTERED AS: infusion.

Purslane, Golden Portulaca sativa.

COMMON NAME: garden purslane, pigweed.

OCCURRENCE: an herbaceous annual plant which is distributed all over the world. It is not indigenous to Great Britain.

PARTS USED: the herb, expressed juice and seeds.

MEDICINAL USES: Purslane is a herb with a great history of use for medical complaints. The expressed juice of the herb was good for strangury, dry coughs, shortness of breath, hot agues, headaches, stopping haemorrhages and as an external application to sores and inflammation. When combined with oil of ROSES, the juice was used for sore mouths, swollen gums and to fasten loose teeth. The bruised seeds were made into a decoction with wine and used to expel worms from children. The bruised herb was used as a poultice to remove heat from the head and temples and to reduce eye inflammation. It was also used on cramps or gouty areas.

ADMINISTERED AS: poultice, decoction, expressed juice.

Pyrethrum, Dalmatian Chrysanthemum cinerariaefolium.

COMMON NAME: insect flowers.

OCCURRENCE: the Dalmatian coast and Japan.

PARTS USED: the closed flowers.

MEDICINAL USES: insecticide, vermin killer. A powder of ground flowers is used in powder, lotions and fumigation materials to kill insects. The active ingredient is pyrethrin. The powder is not toxic to mammals.

ADMINISTERED AS: ground flowers.

Quince *Cydonia oblongata.*

COMMON NAME: quince seed, *Cydonica vulgaris*.

OCCURRENCE: grown in England for its fruit but is native to Persia.

PARTS USED: the fruit and seeds.

MEDICINAL USES: astringent, mucilaginous, demulcent. The fruit is used to prepare a syrup which is added to drinks when ill, as it restrains looseness of the bowels and helps relieve dysentery and diarrhoea. The soaked seeds form a mucilaginous mass similar to that produced by FLAX. A decoction of the seeds is used against gonorrhoea, thrush and in irritable conditions of the mucous membranes. The liquid is also used as a skin lotion or cream and administered in eye diseases as a soothing lotion.

ADMINISTERED AS: syrup, decoction or lotion.

Radish *Raphanus satinus.*

OCCURRENCE: a native plant of China, Japan and Vietnam and widely cultivated in Europe, Great Britain and temperate Asia.

PARTS USED: the root, which has been found to contain a volatile oil, an amylclytic enzyme and a chemical called phenylethyl isothiocyanite.

MEDICINAL USES: antiscorbutic, diuretic. This plant is a very good food remedy for scurvy, gravel and stone. The juice has been beneficial in preventing the formation of gallstones.

ADMINISTERED AS: expressed juice, fresh root, dietary item.

Ragwort *Senecio jacobaea.*

COMMON NAME: St. James's wort, stinking nanny, staggerwort, ragweed, dog standard, cankerwort, stammerwort, fireweed.

OCCURRENCE: an abundant wild plant, widely distributed over Great Britain, Europe, Siberia and north-west India.

PARTS USED: the herb.

MEDICINAL USES: diaphoretic, detergent, emollient, cooling, astringent. The leaves were used as emollient poultices, while the expressed juice of the herb was utilized as a wash in burns, eye inflammation, sores and cancerous ulcers. It has been successful in relieving rheumatism, sciatica, gout and in reducing inflammation and swelling of joints when applied as a poultice. Ragwort makes a good gargle for ulcerated throats and mouths and a decoction of its root is said to help internal bruising and wounds. The herb was previously thought to be able to prevent infection. This plant is poisonous to cattle and should be removed from their pastures. The alkaloids in the ragwort have cumulative effects in the cattle and low doses of the chemical eaten over a period of time can built up to a critical level, where the cattle show obvious symptoms and death then results. It is uncertain if sheep are also susceptible to this chemical.

ADMINISTERED AS: poultice, infusion and decoction.

Raspberry Rubus idaeus.

COMMON NAME: American raspberry, raspbis, hindberry, bramble of Mount Ida, *Rubus strigosus*.

OCCURRENCE: found wild in Great Britain and cultivated in many parts of Europe.

PARTS USED: the leaves and fruit. The fruit contains fruit sugar, a volatile oil, pectin, mineral salts and citric and malic acids.

MEDICINAL USES: astringent and stimulant. Tea made of raspberry leaves is employed as a gargle for sore mouths, canker of the throat and as a wash for wounds and ulcers. It was also reckoned to give strength to pregnant women and encourage fast and safe delivery of the child. The leaves make a good poultice for cleaning wounds and promoting healing. Raspberry vinegar made with fruit juice, sugar and white wine vinegar makes a very good cooling drink when added to water, and is beneficial in fevers and as a gargle for sore throats. The infusion of raspberry leaves is also good in extreme laxity of the bowels and in stomach complaints of children.

ADMINISTERED AS: infusion, poultice, tea and liquid extract.

Red root Ceanothus americanus.

COMMON NAME: New Jersey tea, wild snowball.

OCCURRENCE: a shrub indigenous to the United States.

PARTS USED: the root, which contains tannin, a resin, a bitter extract, gum, lignin, a volatile substance and a principle called ceanothine.

MEDICINAL USES: antispasmodic, astringent, expectorant, sedative, anti-syphilis drug. It is very good in chronic bronchitis, whooping cough, consumption, asthma, dysentery and pulmonary complaints. The decoction is an excellent mouth wash or gargle for sores or ulcers. The herb is also used as an injection for gonorrhoea, gleet and leucorrhoea.

ADMINISTERED AS: fluid extract, decoction, injection.

Rest-harrow *Ononis arvensis*.

COMMON NAME: wild liquorice, cammock, stinking tommy, ground furze, land whin, *Ononis spinosa*.

OCCURRENCE: a weed found on arable and waste land in Britain.

PARTS USED: the root.

MEDICINAL USES: diuretic. This herb was taken internally for dropsy, jaundice, gout, rheumatism and bladder stones. When made into a decoction, it was used as a wash for ulcers, fluid accumulation in tissues and enlarged glands. It was also proposed to subdue delirium. The young shoots were used as a vegetable or pickled, when they were said to refresh the breath and remove the smell of alcohol from the breath.

ADMINISTERED AS: decoction, dietary item.

Rhubarb, English *Rheum rhaponticum*.

COMMON NAME: garden rhubarb, bastard rhubarb, sweet round-leaved dock, *Rheum officinale*.

OCCURRENCE: its cultivation started in England around 1777 and spread throughout Great Britain. It is found growing wild or near dwellings.

PARTS USED: the rhizome and root. The stem and leaves of the plant contain potassium oxalate in quantity and some people are more sensitive to these salts and should avoid eating the plant. People with gout or those subject to urinary irritation should avoid the plant as well.

MEDICINAL USES: stomachic, aperient, astringent, purgative. This plant has a milder action than its relative, Turkey rhubarb (*Rheum palmatum*). It has a milder purgative effect and is particularly useful for stomach troubles in infants and looseness of the bowels. In large doses, rhubarb has a laxative effect. A decoction of the seed is proposed to ease stomach pain and increase the appetite. Rhubarb leaves were formerly used as a vegetable in the nineteenth century, and several fatal cases of poisoning were recorded.

ADMINISTERED AS: decoction and powdered root.

Rice *Oryza sativa*.

COMMON NAME: nivona, dhan, bras, paddy, *Oryza montana*, *O. setegera*, *O. latifolia*.

OCCURRENCE: native to China and India; now cultivated in most subtropical countries.

PARTS USED: the seeds.

MEDICINAL USES: nutritive, demulcent, refrigerant. Boiled rice is good in treating upset digestion, bowel problems and diarrhoea. Rice-water, made from a decoction of the seeds, is an excellent demulcent and refrigerant

drink in febrile and inflammatory diseases of the intestines, painful urination and other related conditions. It may be given as an enema for best results. Finely powdered rice flour can be used for burns, scalds and erysipelas or rice starch can be utilized in the same manner as wheat starch.
ADMINISTERED AS: poultice, decoction, dietary item, enema.

Rose, pale Rosa centifolia.
COMMON NAME: cabbage rose, hundred-leaved rose.
OCCURRENCE: cultivated in southern Europe and grown as a garden plant in many countries.
PARTS USED: the petals, which contain an acid red colouring matter, the glucoside quercitrin, gallic acid, tannic acid, sugar, gum and fat. Also the leaves.
MEDICINAL USES: aperient, laxative, astringent. The petals of this pink rose are rarely taken internally in modern herbal medicine, although they do have aperient properties. These flowers are mainly used for the preparation of rose-water, which is used as an eye lotion and as a carrier medium for other medicines. Cold cream is also made from rose-water and it is used on the skin of the hand and face to soothe abrasions and lesions. Rose leaves are laxative and astringent and were used to heal wounds.
ADMINISTERED AS: distilled water, ointment.

Rose, red Rosa gallica.
COMMON NAME: rose flowers, Provence rose, provins rose.
OCCURRENCE: a native plant of southern Europe and grown in gardens all over the world.
PARTS USED: the petals. Their composition is the same as that of the PALE ROSE, except they do not contain tannic acid.
MEDICINAL USES: tonic, astringent. Today, the petals are not normally taken internally. The petals are prepared in three manners which are then used. A confection is made of petals and sugar and this is utilized in making pills. The fluid extract is prepared using powdered rose petals, glycerine and dilute alcohol while an acid infusion is made with dried rose petals, sulphuric acid, sugar and boiling water. The infusion may be used as a flavouring for other medicines, as a lotion for eye complaints and for the treatment of night sweats relating to depression. Syrup of roses, honey of rose and rose vinegar are also preparations used medicinally in various countries around Europe. The petals are also used as flavour enhancers in two alcoholic liqueurs. *Rosa gallica* petals are used in aromatherapy.
ADMINISTERED AS: pills, lotion, infusion, poultice, syrup, fluid extract.

Rosemary *Rosmarinus officinalis.*

COMMON NAME: polar plant, compass-weed, compass plant, romero, *Rosmarinus coronarium.*

OCCURRENCE: native to the dry hills of the Mediterranean, from Spain westward to Turkey. A common garden plant in Britain, having been cultivated prior to the Norman Conquest.

PARTS USED: the herb and root. Oil of rosemary is distilled from the plant tops and used medicinally. Rosemary contains tannic acid, a bitter principle, resin and a volatile oil.

MEDICINAL USES: tonic, astringent, diaphoretic, stimulant. The essential oil is also stomachic, nervine and carminative and cures many types of headache. It is mainly applied externally as a hair lotion which is said to prevent baldness and the formation of dandruff. The oil is used externally as a rubefacient and is added to liniments for fragrance and stimulant properties. Rosemary tea can remove headache, colic, colds and nervous diseases and may also lift nervous depression.

ADMINISTERED AS: infusion, essential oil and lotion.

Rosinweed *Silphium paciniatum.*

COMMON NAME: compass plant, compass-weed, polar plant.

OCCURRENCE: native to the western United States, especially Ohio. This plant is closely related to *Silphium laciniatum* and is often confused with it.

PARTS USED: the root, which yields a resinous secretion very similar to MASTIC.

MEDICINAL USES: tonic, diaphoretic, alterative, emetic, diuretic, antispasmodic, expectorant. The root is used in dry, stubborn coughs, asthma and other pulmonary diseases. The decoction of the root is said to be emetic and has cured intermittent fevers. A strong infusion is good against enlarged spleen, internal bruising, liver problems and digestive ulcers. The resin has diuretic qualities and taints the urine, giving it a strong odour.

ADMINISTERED AS: fluid extract, decoction, infusion.

Rowan tree *Pyrus aucuparia.*

COMMON NAME: mountain ash, *Sorbus aucuparia, Mespilus aucuparia.*

OCCURRENCE: generally distributed over Great Britain and Europe, especially at high altitudes.

PARTS USED: the bark and fruit. The fruit may contain tartaric, citric or malic acids dependent upon its stage of ripeness. It also contains sorbitol, sorbin, sorbit, parascorbic acid and bitter, acrid colouring matters. The bark contains amygdalin.

MEDICINAL USES: astringent, antiscorbutic. A decoction of Rowan bark is given for diarrhoea and as a vaginal injection for leucorrhoea. The berries are made into an acid gargle to ease sore throats and inflamed tonsils. An infusion of the fruit is administered to ease haemorrhoids. The berries may also be made into jelly, flour, cider, ale or an alcoholic spirit. The rowan tree planted next to a house was said to protect the house against witchcraft.

ADMINISTERED AS: decoction, injection, infusion and dietary item.

Rue *Ruta graveolens.*

COMMON NAME: herb of grace, garden rue, herbygrass, ave-grace.

OCCURRENCE: indigenous to southern Europe and was introduced into Great Britain by the Romans.

PARTS USED: the herb. The herb is covered by glands which contain a volatile oil. The oil is composed of methylnonylketone, limonene, cineole, a crystalline substance called rutin and several acids. The plant also contains several alkaloids including fagarine and arborinine as well as coumarins.

MEDICINAL USES: stimulant, antispasmodic, emmenagogue, irritant, rubefacient. This is a very powerful herb and the dose administered should be kept low. It is useful in treating coughs, croup, colic, flatulence, hysteria and it is particularly good against strained eyes and headaches caused by eyestrain. An infusion of the herb is good for nervous indigestion, heart palpitations, nervous headaches and to expel worms. The chemical, rutin, strengthens weak blood vessels and aids varicose veins. In Chinese medicine, rue is a specific for insect and snake bites. When made into an ointment, rue is effective in gouty and rheumatic pains, sprained and bruised tendons and chilblains. The bruised leaves irritate and blister the skin and so can ease sciatica. This herb should not be used in pregnancy as the volatile oil, alkaloids and coumarins in the plant all stimulate the uterus and strongly promote menstrual bleeding. When a fresh leaf is chewed, it flavours the mouth and relieves headache, giddiness or any hysterical spasms quickly.

ADMINISTERED AS: fresh leaf, volatile oil, ointment, infusion, decoction, tea, expressed juice.

Rupturewort *Herniara glabra.*

COMMON NAME: herniary, breastwort.

OCCURRENCE: found in temperate and southern Europe and Russian Asia. It is a British native plant, particularly in southern and central England.

PARTS USED: the herb, which contains the alkaloid paronychine, and a crystalline principle called herniarne.

MEDICINAL USES: astringent, diuretic. This is a very active drug which has been successful in treating catarrhal infections of the bladder and oedema of cardiac or kidney origins.

ADMINISTERED AS: infusion.

Sabadilla *Veratrum sabadilla* or *Veratrum officinale.*

COMMON NAME: cevadilla, sabadillermer, caustic barley, *Schoenocaulon officinale, Melanthian sabadilla, Helonias officinalis, Sabadilla officinarum, Asagraea officinalis.*

OCCURRENCE: grows in southern North America, guatemala, Venezuela and Mexico.

PARTS USED: the seeds. They contain several alkaloids including veratrine, sabadillie, sabadine, sabadinine and cevadine, which hydrolyzes to cevine. They also contain voatric acid, cevadic acid, resin and fat.

MEDICINAL USES: drastic emetic and cathartic, vermifuge. The powdered seeds have been used to expel parasitic worms and to kill and remove parasitic mites or other vermin from the hair. An extract called veratria is derived from the seeds and despite it being highly poisonous, it is occasionally taken internally in minute doses. When taken internally, it can ease acute rheumatic pain and gout and also help some inflammatory diseases. Veratria is more commonly used as an ointment for neuralgia and rheumatism. This drug has a powerful action on the heart causing it to slow and eventually stop beating entirely.

ADMINISTERED AS: powdered seeds, ointment.

Saffron *Crocus sativus.*

COMMON NAME: crocus, karcom, Alicante saffron, Valencia saffron, krokos, gatinais, saffron, hay saffron, saffron crocus.

OCCURRENCE: grown from Persia and Kurdistan in the east to most European countries including Great Britain.

PARTS USED: the dried flower pistils. These parts contain an essential oil composed of terpenes, terepene alcohols and esters, a coloured glycoside called crocin and a bitter glucoside, called picrocrocin.

MEDICINAL USES: carminative, diaphoretic, emmenagogue. This herb is used as a diaphoretic drug for children and can also benefit female hysteria, absent or painful menstruation and stop chronic haemorrhage of the uterus in adults.

ADMINISTERED AS: tincture, powdered saffron.

Saffron, Meadow *Colchicum autumnale.*

COMMON NAME: colchicum, naked ladies.

OCCURRENCE: grows wild in North Africa and Europe and is found in meadows and limestone areas in the British Isles.

PARTS USED: the root and seeds.

MEDICINAL USES: cathartic, emetic, anti-rheumatic. This herb is very useful for acute rheumatic and gouty ailments, and it is normally taken along with an alkaline diuretic for best results. The active chemical in the plant is colchinine, an alkaline substance which is very poisonous. It has sedative effects and particularly acts on the bowels and kidneys. It acts as an irritant poison in large doses, and can cause undue depression. As such, care should be used when utilizing this herb.

ADMINISTERED AS: fluid extract, powdered root, tincture, solid extract.

Sage, Common *Salvia officinalis.*

COMMON NAME: garden sage, red sage, saurge, broad-leaved white sage, *Salvia salvatrix.*

OCCURRENCE: native to the northern Mediterranean and cultivated through Britain, France and Germany.

PARTS USED: the leaves, whole herb. The herb contains a volatile oil, tannin and resin and is distilled to produce sage oil. This is made up of salvene, pinene, cineol, vorneol, thujone and some esters.

MEDICINAL USES: stimulant, astringent, tonic, carminative, aromatic. Sage makes an excellent gargle for relaxed throat and tonsils, bleeding gums, laryngitis and ulcerated throat. Sage tea is valuable against delirium of fevers, nervous excitement and accompanying brain and nervous diseases; as a stimulant tonic in stomach and nervous system complaints and in weak digestion. It also works as an emmenagogue, in treating typhoid fever, bilious and liver problems, kidney troubles and lung or stomach haemorrhages. The infusion is used in head colds, quinsy, measles, painful joints, lethargy, palsy and nervous headaches. Fresh leaves are rubbed on the teeth to cleanse them and strengthen gums—even today sage is included in toothpowders. The oil of sage was used to remove mucus collections from the respiratory organs and is included in embrocations for rheumatism. The herb is also applied warm as a poultice.

ADMINISTERED AS: infusion, essential oil, tea and poultice.

Salep: *early purple orchid*, Orchis mascula; *spotted orchid*, Orchis maculata; *marsh orchid*, Orchis latifolia.

COMMON NAME: saloop, schlep, satrion, Levant salep.

OCCURRENCE: *Orchis mascula* is found in woods throughout England. *O. maculata* grows wild on heaths and commons; *O. latifolia* is found growing in marshes and damp pastures across Great Britain.

PARTS USED: the tuberous root, which contains mucilage, sugar, starch and volatile oil.

MEDICINAL USES: very nutritive, demulcent. This herb is used as a food item for convalescent people and children, made with milk or water and flavoured. It is prepared in a similar way to arrowroot. A decoction with sugar, spice or wine was given to invalids to build them up. The root is used to stop irritation of the gastro-intestinal canal and for invalids suffering from bilious fevers or chronic diarrhoea. In the old sailing ships, salep was carried and used as an emergency food source. It was sold on street corners in London as a hot drink, before COFFEE replaced its use as a beverage.

ADMINISTERED AS: decoction, dietary item.

Samphire *Crithmum maritimum.*

COMMON NAME: sea fennel, crest marine, sampier, rock fennel, rock samphire.

OCCURRENCE: found on rocks or salt marshes around the west or south of England but rare in the North and Scotland.

PARTS USED: the herb.

MEDICINAL USES: an infusion of samphire has a diuretic effect and acts on the kidneys. It is reputed to be an excellent treatment for obesity. It is eaten as a condiment, as a salad ingredient or pickled.

ADMINISTERED AS: infusion.

Sandalwood *Santalum album.*

COMMON NAME: santalwood, sanders-wood.

OCCURRENCE: a tree native to India and the Malay Archipelago.

PARTS USED: the wood oil.

MEDICINAL USES: aromatic, antiseptic, diuretic. The oil is given internally for chronic mucous conditions, e.g. bronchitis, inflammation of the bladder. It is also used in chronic cystitis, gleet and gonorrhoea. The oil is used in aromatherapy to lessen tension and anxiety and it was also considered a sexual stimulant in folk traditions. The fluid extract of sandalwood may be better tolerated by some people than the oil.

ADMINISTERED AS: wood oil, fluid extract.

Sarsaparilla, Jamaican *Smilax ornata.*

COMMON NAME: red-bearded sarsaparilla, *Smilax medica*, *Smilax officinalis*.

OCCURRENCE: a perennial climbing plant which grows in central America, primarily Costa Rica. It is termed Jamaican sarsaparilla as the plant was exported to Europe through Jamaica.

PARTS USED: the root, which is composed of starch, sarsapic acid, the glucoside sarsaponin and palmitic, stearic, behenic, oleic and linoleic fatty acids. The active principle is a crystalline compound called porillin or smilacin.

MEDICINAL USES: alterative, tonic, diaphoretic, diuretic. This root was introduced into Europe in 1563 as a remedy for syphilis. It is used in other chronic diseases, particularly rheumatism or skin diseases. It is still considered an excellent blood purifier, often given in conjunction with SASSAFRAS or BURDOCK. When smoked, Jamaican sarsaparilla was recommended for asthma.

ADMINISTERED AS: powdered root, fluid extract, solid extract.

Sassafras *Sassafras officinale.*

COMMON NAME: laurus sassafras, sassafrax, *Sassafras radix*, *Sassafras varifolium*.

OCCURRENCE: native to the eastern United States and Canada then south to Mexico.

PARTS USED: the root-bark, root and pith. The root-bark contains a heavy and light volatile oil, resin, wax, tannic acid, lignin, starch and camphorous matter. The pith is made up of mucilage which is used as a demulcent. The bark yields an oil, which is mainly safrol. This is a heavy volatile oil associated with sassafras camphor when cold.

MEDICINAL USES: aromatic, stimulant, diaphoretic, alterative, diuretic. This herb is usually given in combination with other herbs, e.g. SARSAPARILLA, to treat chronic rheumatism, skin diseases or syphilis. The oil relieves pain after childbirth and due to obstructed menstruation and also benefits gonorrhoea and gleet. A decoction of the pith is used as an eye wash in eye complaints and in general inflammations. Safrol, when taken internally, can produce narcotic poisoning, but when used externally it can be used for rheumatic pains and as a dental disinfectant.

ADMINISTERED AS: oil of sassafras, fluid extract, decoction.

Sassy bark *Erythrophloeum guineense.*

COMMON NAME: maneona bark, casca bark, doom bark, ordeal bark, saucy bark, red water bark, nkasa, *Cortex erythrophei*.

OCCURRENCE: a large tree native to the west coast of Africa in Upper Guinea, Senegal, Gambia and Sudan.

PARTS USED: the bark, which contains the poisonous chemical erythrophleine, tannin and resin.

MEDICINAL USES: narcotic, astringent, anodyne, laxative. It has been used successfully in dysentery, diarrhoea and passive haemorrhages. The chemical erythrophleine acts on the pulse rate, peristalsis and the nerve centres to cause relief from pain, purging and vomiting. It needs more research to see if erythrophleine would make a good anaesthetic drug. Since it is very poisonous and has severe effects on the body, it is rarely used in modern herbal medicine. In native West African cultures, this drug is given as an ordeal in trials of witchcraft and sorcery to determine the truth.

ADMINISTERED AS: fluid extract, powdered bark.

Savory, Summer *Satureja hortensis.*

COMMON NAME: garden savory.

OCCURRENCE: a shrub native to the Mediterranean region and introduced into Great Britain.

PARTS USED: the herb.

MEDICINAL USES: aromatic, carminative. This herb is mainly used in cookery, as a pot-herb or flavouring. In medicine, it is added to remedies to flavour and add warmth. It was formerly used for colic, flatulence and was considered a good expectorant. A sprig of summer savory rubbed on a wasp or bee sting relieves the pain quickly.

ADMINISTERED AS: fresh or dried herb.

Savine *Juniperus sabina.*

COMMON NAME: savin, savine tops.

OCCURRENCE: indigenous to the northern states in the USA and middle and southern Europe, e.g. Switzerland, Italy and Austria.

PARTS USED: the tops of the herb. It contains gallic acid, resin, chlorophyll, a volatile oil, lilgnin, calcium salts, gum and a fixed oil.

MEDICINAL USES: emmenagogue, diuretic, anthelmintic. This herb is rarely given internally as it is an irritant herb and also poisonous, whose use can be fatal if not properly managed. It is a powerful emmenagogue which can induce abortion when given in large doses—should never be taken when pregnant. It used to be administered with TANSY, PENNY ROYAL and HEMLOCK. As a vermifuge, it has been used for worms along with PINK ROOT and SENNA. Mainly used externally as an ointment for skin eruptions, blisters and syphilitic warts. It is said to remove warts from the hands.

ADMINISTERED AS: powdered herb, tincture, fluid extract.

Saw palmetto Sarenoa serrulata.

COMMON NAME: sabal, *Sabal serrulata.*

OCCURRENCE: native to the North Atlantic coast of the United States and southern California.

PARTS USED: the ripe fruit, which contains volatile oil, glucose and a fixed oil.

MEDICINAL USES: nutritive, tonic, diuretic, sedative. This herb affects the mucous membranes of the respiratory system to ease many diseases linked to chronic catarrh. Saw palmetto is a tissue-building herb which aids atony of the testicles or breasts. It reduces catarrhal irritation in the body and can ease catarrh of the bladder and urethra.

ADMINISTERED AS: solid extract, powdered fruit, fluid extract.

Saxifrage, Burnet Pimpinella saxifraga.

COMMON NAME: lesser burnet, saxifrage.

OCCURRENCE: found on dry, chalky pastures throughout the British Isles.

PARTS USED: the root and the herb.

MEDICINAL USES: resolvent, diaphoretic, diuretic, stomachic, aromatic, carminative. This herb is prescribed for flatulent indigestion, toothache, paralysis of the tongue, asthma and dropsy. A decoction is used as a gargle in throat infections and hoarseness. The herb was added to casks of beer or wine to impart its aromatic flavour to the drink.

ADMINISTERED AS: fresh root, decoction dried root.

Scullcap, Virginian Scutellaria lateriflora.

COMMON NAME: mad-dog scullcap, helmet flower, madweed, mad-dog weed, skullcap, Quaker bonnet.

OCCURRENCE: native to the United States of America.

PARTS USED: the herb, which contains a volatile oil called scutellonin, flavonoid glucosides including scutellonin and scutellanein, some bitter principle, sugar, cellulose, tannin and fat.

MEDICINAL USES: strong tonic, nervine, antispasmodic, astringent. This herb is an invaluable tonic for the nervous system treating nervous headaches, anxiety, depression, insomnia and neuralgia. It is most beneficial in hysteria, convulsions, rickets, epilepsy and Speakman's chorea where it soothes nervous excitement and induces sleep without any unpleasant side effects. The bitter taste of the herb stimulates and strengthens the digestion. It is said that many cases of hydrophobia have been cured by the use of this herb alone. The European species, *Scutellaria galericulata*, was once used for malaria and it shares the nervine qualities of Virginian scullcap. This herb may be difficult to obtain as most commercial supplies of it are adulterated with wood sage (*Teucrium scorodonia*).

ADMINISTERED AS: fluid extract, infusion, decoction, powdered herb.

Scurvy grass *Cochlearia officinalis.*

COMMON NAME: spoonwort.

OCCURRENCE: native to the coastline of Scotland, Ireland and England; also found in the sea coasts of northern and western Europe, the Arctic Circle and at altitude on the mountain chains of Europe.

PARTS USED: the herb.

MEDICINAL USES: stimulant, aperient, diuretic, antiscorbutic. It was formerly used on sea voyages to prevent scurvy. The essential oil from the herb is beneficial in cases of rheumatism or paralysis. When made into scurvy grass ale it was drunk as a tonic.

ADMINISTERED AS: infusion, essential oil.

Self-heal *Prunella vulgaris.*

COMMON NAME: prunella, all-heal, hook-heal, slough-heal, brunella, heart of the Earth, blue curls, siclewort.

OCCURRENCE: a very abundant wild plant in woods and fields all over Europe and Great Britain.

PARTS USED: the whole herb, containing a volatile oil, a bitter principle, tannin, sugar and cellulose.

MEDICINAL USES: astringent, styptic and tonic. An infusion of the herb is taken internally for sore throats, internal bleeding, leucorrhoea and as a general strengthener.

ADMINISTERED AS: infusion, injection and decoction.

Senega *Polygala senega.*

COMMON NAME: snake root, seneca, milkwort, mountain flax, rattlesnake root, senega snakeroot, seneka, *Senegae radix, Polygala virginiana, Plantula marilandica, Senega officinalis.*

OCCURRENCE: grows wild throughout central and western North America.

PARTS USED: the dried root, which contains polygalic acid, virgineic acid, pectic and tannic acids, fixed oil, albumen, sugar and various mineral salts. The active chemical is called senegin which is almost identical to the saponin chemical found in SOAPWORT (*Saponaria officinale*).

Senna

MEDICINAL USES: stimulant, expectorant, diaphoretic, diuretic, emmena-gogue. It is highly effective in treating acute bronchial catarrh, chronic pneumonia or bronchitis and kidney-related dropsy. senega is also of benefit for croup, whooping cough and rheumatism. The ancient herbalists of Greek or Roman times considered senega of identical action with IPECAC-UANHA (*Cephaelis ipecacuanha*). In large doses senega is an emetic and cathartic drug, and overdoses are possible.

ADMINISTERED AS: powder, fluid extract, syrup, tincture, infusion.

Senna, Alexandrian *Cassia acutifolia*; Senna, East Indian *Cassia angustifolia*.

COMMON NAME: Nubian senna, Egyptian senna, *Cassia senna*, *Cassia lenitiva*, *Cassia officinalis*, *Cassia aethiopica*, *Senna acutifolia*.

OCCURRENCE: *C. acutifolia* is native to the upper and middle Nile in Egypt and Sudan. *C. angustifolia* is indigenous to southern Arabia and is cultivated in southern and eastern India.

PARTS USED: the dried leaflets and pods. The active principles of senna can be extracted using water or dilute alcohol. The drug contains anthraquinone derivatives and their glucosides, as well as cathartic acid as its active chemicals.

MEDICINAL USES: laxative, purgative, cathartic. This drug acts primarily on the lower bowel, acts locally upon the intestinal wall, increasing the peristaltic movements of the colon. The taste is nauseating and prone to cause sickness and griping pains. It is generally combined with aromatics, e.g. GINGER or CINNAMON and stimulants to modify senna's deleterious effects. When the problems are overcome, senna is a very good medicine for children, delicate women and elderly persons. Senna pods have milder effects than the leaves and lack their griping effects.

ADMINISTERED AS: infusion, powdered leaves, syrup, fluid extract, tincture, dried pods.

Sheep's sorrel *Rumex acetosella*.

COMMON NAME: field sorrel.

OCCURRENCE: this grows in pastures and dry places around the globe, except in the tropics and is abundant in the British Isles.

PARTS USED: the herb.

MEDICINAL USES: diaphoretic, diuretic, refrigerant. The fresh juice of the herb is used for kidney and urinary diseases. Less active than SORREL (*Rumex acetosa*).

ADMINISTERED AS: expressed juice.

Shepherd's purse *Capsella bursa-pastoris.*

COMMON NAME: shepherd's bag, shepherd's scrip, lady's purse, witches' pouches, case-weed, pick-pocket, blindweed, pepper and salt, sanguinary, mother's heart, poor man's parmacettie, clappedepouch.

OCCURRENCE: native to Europe and found all over the world outside tropical zones.

PARTS USED: the whole plant which contains various chemicals which have not yet been entirely analyzed but they include an organic acid, a volatile oil, a fixed oil, a tannate, an alkaloid and a resin.

MEDICINAL USES: haemostatic, antiscorbutic, diuretic, stimulant. As an infusion of the dried plant, shepherd's purse is one of the best specifics for arresting bleeding of all kinds, particularly from the kidneys, uterus, stomach or lungs. It is said to be as effective as ERGOT or GOLDEN SEAL. It has been used for diarrhoea, haemorrhoids, dysentery, dropsy and kidney complaints. Shepherd's purse is an important remedy in catarrhal infections of the bladder and ureter and in ulcerated and abscess of the bladder where it increases the flow of urine and provides relief. Externally, the bruised herb is used as a poultice on bruised and strained areas, rheumatic joints and some skin problems. Since the herb tastes slightly unpleasant it is normally taken internally with other herbs to disguise the flavour, e.g. COUCH GRASS, JUNIPER, PELLITORY-OF-THE-WALL.

ADMINISTERED AS: fluid extract, poultice, decoction, infusion.

Silverweed *Potentilla anserina.*

COMMON NAME: trailing tansy, wild tansy, goosewort, silvery cinquefoil, goose grey, goose tansy, wild agrimony, moor grass, prince's feathers.

OCCURRENCE: very abundant in Great Britain and across temperate regions from Lapland to the Azores. It also grows in New Zealand, Chile, Armenia and China.

PARTS USED: the herb, which contains tannin.

MEDICINAL USES: astringent, tonic. An infusion is used as a lotion for bleeding haemorrhoids, as a gargle for sore throats and for cramps in the abdomen, stomach or heart. The infusion may also be used as a compress. A tea of Silverweed has been good for tetanus infections, for malarial infections, in gravel and as a specific in jaundice. A decoction of silverweed is useful for mouth ulcers, spongy gums, fixing loose teeth, toothache and preserving gums from scurvy. A distilled water made from the herb was used as a cosmetic to remove freckles, spots and pimples and to reduce the skin damage after sunburn.

ADMINISTERED AS: decoction, infusion, poultice, distilled water.

Simaruba *Simaruba amara.*

COMMON NAME: dysentery bark, mountain damson, slave wood, maruba, sumaruppa, bitter damson, quassia simaruba.

OCCURRENCE: native to French Guiana, Brazil, Florida and the islands of Dominica, Martinique, St. Lucia, St. Vincent and Barbados.

PARTS USED: the bark, which contains a volatile oil, malic and gallic acids, lignin, resinous matter, various mineral salts and a bitter principle very similar to quassin.

MEDICINAL USES: bitter tonic. It was used successfully against dysentery in France from 1718 onwards. The drug restores lost tone of the intestines and encourages the patient to sleep. It is also useful in loss of appetite, weakened digestion and when convalescing after a fever. In large doses, simaruba can cause sickness and vomiting, so care should be taken when using this drug. It is seldom used in herbal medicine today.

ADMINISTERED AS: infusion, fluid extract.

Skunk cabbage *Symplocarpus foetidus.*

COMMON NAME: dracontium, skunkweed, meadow cabbage, polecat weed, *Dracontium foetidum*, *Spathyema foetida*, *Ictodes foetidus*.

OCCURRENCE: grows in moist places across the middle and northern United States of America.

PARTS USED: the root, which contains resin, silica, iron, manganese, an acrid principle and a volatile oil.

MEDICINAL USES: antispasmodic, diaphoretic, expectorant, narcotic, sedative. This plant is so-named as it has an unpleasant odour when bruised. The root has been used for asthma, chronic rheumatism, chorea, dropsy, hysteria and chronic catarrh. It is good for tightness of the chest, irritant coughs and other spasmodic respiratory disorders. The herb is also believed to be effective against epilepsy and convulsions which can occur during pregnancy or labour. It has a diuretic action and can be used to calm the nervous system. Skunk-cabbage forms an ingredient in well-known herbal ointments and powders.

ADMINISTERED AS: powdered root, tincture, fluid extract.

Slippery elm *Ulmus fulva.*

COMMON NAME: red elm, moose elm, Indian elm.

OCCURRENCE: the United States and Canada.

PARTS USED: the inner bark of the tree, which contains mucilage similar to that of flax, starch and calcium oxalate.

MEDICINAL USES: demulcent, emollient, expectorant, diuretic, nutritive, pectoral. This is one of the most valuable remedies in herbal practice. Finely powdered bark makes very good gruel or food which can be used in all cases of weakness, stomach inflammation, bronchitis, etc. It has a soothing and healing action on all the parts it comes into contact with. A drink of the powder and water called Slippery elm food is excellent in cases of irritation of the mucous membrane of the stomach and intestines, induces sleep and gives very good results in gastritis, colitis and enteritis and gastric catarrh. May also be employed as a heart and lung remedy and is used in typhoid fever.

The coarse powdered bark is the finest available poultice for all inflamed areas, ulcers, wounds, burns, boils, skin diseases, etc. It is utilized by various methods in treating many disorders of the bowel and urinary systems. It is also used to remove worms and is an ingredient in many specialist preparations, e.g. poultices, ointments, etc.

ADMINISTERED AS: infusion, injection, poultice, ointment and dietary item.

Smartweed *Polygonum hydropiper.*

COMMON NAME: water pepper, pepper plant, smartass, ciderage, red knees, culrage, biting persicaria, bloodwort, arsesmart.

OCCURRENCE: a native plant of most parts of Europe and Russian Asia up to the Arctic regions. Also seen in Great Britain and Ireland, although rarer in Scotland. It mainly grows in areas that are under water in the winter period.

PARTS USED: the whole herb and the leaves. The active principle is called polygonic acid but its action is not fully understood. It is destroyed by heat or drying.

MEDICINAL USES: stimulant, diuretic, diaphoretic, emmenagogue. As a cold water infusion, this herb is used for amenorrhoea, gravel, coughs and colds and gout. It is also of benefit in dysentery, sore mouths, bowel complaints, jaundice and dropsy. After simmering with water and vinegar, the herb has been utilized on gangrenous or dead tissue, applied to chronic ulcers and haemorrhoidal tumours. In poultice form, smartweed has been used in chronic erysipelas infections, flatulent colic, cholera and rheumatism. There is a tradition which is mentioned in old herbals, that if a handful of the plant is placed under the saddle of a horse then it will be able to travel for some time before requiring feeding or watering. This belief dates back to the Ancient Greek period.

ADMINISTERED AS: infusion, tincture, fluid extract.

Snapdragon

Snapdragon Antirrhinum magus.
COMMON NAME: calves, snout, lyons snap.
OCCURRENCE: naturalized in Great Britain and is a garden plant.
PARTS USED: the leaves.
MEDICINAL USES: bitter, stimulant. The fresh leaves have been applied as a poultice to tumours and ulcers. In old herbals, it is mentioned that the herb protects against witchcraft and that it makes the wearer 'look gracious in the sight of people.'
ADMINISTERED AS: poultice.

Soap tree Quillaja saponia.
COMMON NAME: quillaia, soap bark, cullay, Panama bark.
OCCURRENCE: native to Chile and Peru in South America.
PARTS USED: the dried inner bark, which contains calcium exalate, can sugar and saponin which is made from a mixture of two glucosides—guillaic acid and guillaia—sapotoxin. The active principles are the same as those found in SENEGA.
MEDICINAL USES: alterative, expectorant, detergent, diuretic, stimulating, sternutatory. This bark can be used in aortic hypertrophy. Since Saponin is a powerful irritant and muscular poison, it can be fatal if used in too large doses and is only occasionally used today. The bark has been used to produce a foam head on beverages and for washing clothes and hair.
ADMINISTERED AS: injection, tincture, powdered bark.

Soapwort Saponaria officinalis.
COMMON NAME: latherwort, soaproot, bruisewort, fuller's herb, crow soap, sweet betty, wild sweet william, bouncing bet.
OCCURRENCE: a common garden plant in Great Britain and it also grows wild in central and southern Europe.
PARTS USED: the dried root and leaves. The root contains gum, resin, woody fibre, mucilage and saponin.
MEDICINAL USES: alterative, detergent, tonic, sternutatory. This herb has been used for scrofula and other skin complaints and in jaundice and other visceral obstructions. It is also good for chronic venereal diseases and in rheumatism or skin eruptions due to infection with syphilis. This drug should be very carefully administered due to the very poisonous nature of saponin. In large doses, soapwort is strongly purgative so should only be given by a qualified herbalist. Soapwort is also used to clean clothes, skin and hair and is an ingredient of most herbal shampoo.
ADMINISTERED AS: decoction, expressed juice from fresh root, fluid extract.

Solomon's seal *Polygonatum multiflorum.*

COMMON NAME: lady's seals, St. Mary's seal, sigillum sanctae Mariae.

OCCURRENCE: a native plant of northern Europe and Siberia. It is found wild in some localities in England but naturalized in Scotland and Ireland.

PARTS USED: the rhizome which contains asparagin, gum, sugar, starch, pectin and convallarin, one of the active chemicals in LILY OF THE VALLEY.

MEDICINAL USES: astringent, demulcent, tonic. When combined with other herbs, it is good for bleeding of the lungs and pulmonary complaints. It is used on its own in female complaints and as a poultice for tumours, inflammations, bruises and haemorrhoids. As it is mucilaginous, it makes a very good healing and restorative tonic for inflammation of the bowels and stomach, haemorrhoids and chronic dysentery. A decoction was used to cure erysipelas and was taken by people with broken bones, as Solomon's Seal was supposed to 'encourage the bones to knit'. A distilled water prepared from the root was used as a cosmetic to remove spots, freckles and marks from the skin.

ADMINISTERED AS: decoction, infusion, poultice, distilled water.

Sorrel *Rumex acetosa.*

COMMON NAME: garden sorrel, green sauce, sour grabs, sour suds, cuckoo sorrow, cuckoo's meate, gowke-meat.

OCCURRENCE: indigenous to Britain and found in moist meadows throughout Europe.

PARTS USED: the leaves, dried and fresh.

MEDICINAL USES: refrigerant, diuretic, antiscorbutic. Sorrel is given as a cooling drink in all febrile conditions and can help correct scrofulous deposits. Its astringent qualities meant it was formerly used to stop haemorrhages and was applied as a poultice on cutaneous tumours. Sorrel juice and vinegar are said to cure ringworm, while a decoction was made to cure jaundice, ulcerated bowel, and gravel and stone in the kidneys.

ADMINISTERED AS: expressed juice, decoction, poultice and dried leaves.

Spearmint *Mentha viridis.*

COMMON NAME: mackerel mint, Our Lady's mint, green mint, spire mint, sage of Bethlehem, fish mint, lamb mint, menthe de Notre Dame, erba Santa Maria, *Mentha spicata*, *Mentha crispa*, yerba buena.

OCCURRENCE: originally a Mediterranean native and was introduced into the British Isles by the Romans.

PARTS USED: the herb and essential oil. The main component of the essential oil is carvone along with phellandrine, limonene and dihydrocarveol acetate. The oil also has the esters of acetic, butyric and caproic acids within it.

MEDICINAL USES: antispasmodic, aromatic, carminative, stimulant. This herb is very similar to peppermint, but it seems to be less powerful. It is more suited to children's remedies. A distilled water from spearmint is used to relieve hiccoughs, flatulence and indigestion while the infusion is good for fevers, inflammatory diseases and all infantile troubles. Spearmint is considered a specific in stopping nausea and vomiting and in easing the pain due to colic. As a homeopathic remedy, spearmint has been used for strangury, gravel and as a local application for painful haemorrhoids.

ADMINISTERED AS: distilled water, infusion, tincture, fluid extract.

Spearwort, Lesser *Ranunculus flammula.*
OCCURRENCE: a very common plant throughout Britain, growing in wet and boggy heaths and commons.

PARTS USED: the whole plant.

MEDICINAL USES: rubefacient, emetic. The bruised leaves have a long history of use on the Isle of Skye and in the Highlands of Scotland in raising blisters. A distilled water from the plant is used as a painless emetic drug while a tincture is good at curing ulcers.

ADMINISTERED AS: distilled water, tincture, poultice.

Speedwell, Common *Veronica officinalis.*
COMMON NAME: bird's-eye, cat's-eye.

OCCURRENCE: a common wild plant in Europe and Great Britain.

PARTS USED: the herb.

MEDICINAL USES: diaphoretic, alterative, expectorant, astringent, diuretic, tonic. Lesser spearwort was formerly used in pectoral and nephritic complaints, haemorrhages, skin diseases and in treating wounds. An infusion of the dried herb is good for catarrh, coughs and most skin problems. May promote menstruation.

ADMINISTERED AS: infusion and dried herb.

Sphagnum moss *Sphagnum cymbifolium.*
COMMON NAME: bog moss.

OCCURRENCE: found in wet and boggy land, normally on peat soils on mountains and moors in Scotland, England, Ireland and parts of western Europe.

PARTS USED: the moss, which is made up of plant cells which are penetrated with a system of tubes and air spaces. This capillary tube system makes the moss resemble a very fine sponge and allows the plant to absorb huge quantities of water.

MEDICINAL USES: wound dressing. The use of sphagnum as a dressing for wounds can be dated back to the Battle of Flodden. There is a long history of use in Lapland where the dried moss is used as a mattress and blankets for infants. The moss has many advantages over other surgical dressings, e.g. cotton wool. Prepared moss can retain twice as much moisture as cotton; a 2oz dressing can absorb up to 2lb of liquid. This means that dressings need to be changed less frequently with less disturbance to the patient. In many times of war sphagnum was prepared in gauze bags, often in association with GARLIC for its antiseptic qualities. Sphagnum moss also has an antibiotic action due to micro-organisms associated with the plant which aids healing. The moss has also been used as bedding in stables and for hanging baskets and other gardening applications.

Spinach *Spinacio oleracea.*

OCCURRENCE: originally native to Persia and Asia and was introduced into Europe in the fifteenth century.

PARTS USED: the leaves, which contain iron, nitrogenous substances, hydrocarbons, chlorophyll and vitamins A and D.

MEDICINAL USES: nutritive, antiscorbutic. Spinach is primarily used as a food source as it is a good source of iron and vitamins. Experiments have shown the benefit of eating spinach on people weakened by illness.

ADMINISTERED AS: expressed juice, dietary item.

Spindle tree *Euonymus atropurpureus. Euonymus europoeus.*

COMMON NAME: Indian arrowroot, burning bush, wahoo, gatten, pigwood, dogwood, skewerwood, prickwood, gadrose, fusanum, fusoria.

OCCURRENCE: *Euonymus europoeus* is found in copses and hedges across Great Britain. *E. atropurpureus* is commonly found in the eastern United States and is the variety normally used in herbal medicine.

PARTS USED: the root, bark and berries. The chief constituents of the plant include an intensely bitter principle called euonymin resin, euonic acid, asparagin, resins, fat, dulcitol and a crystalline glucoside.

MEDICINAL USES: alterative, cholagogue, laxative, hepatic stimulant, tonic. This drug is particularly good in liver complaints which follow or accompany fever, and in stimulating the liver and producing a free flow of bile. Depending on the dose given euonymin has different effects on the digestive system. In large doses it irritates the intestine and has cathartic effects, but in smaller doses it can stimulate the appetite and the flow of gastric juices. The herb is normally administered with other tonic or laxative herbs for best results.

ADMINISTERED AS: pills, powdered root or bark, decoction, fluid extract.

St John's wort *Hypericum perforatum.*

OCCURRENCE: found in woods, hedges, roadsides and meadows across Britain, Europe and Asia.

PARTS USED: the herb and flowers.

MEDICINAL USES: aromatic, astringent, resolvent, expectorant, diuretic and nervine. It is generally utilized in all pulmonary complaints, bladder trouble, suppression of urine, dysentery, diarrhoea and jaundice. It is good against hysteria, nervous depression, haemorrhages, coughing up blood and dispelling worms from the body. If children have a problem with night incontinence, an infusion of St John's wort taken before bed will stop the problem. The herb is used externally to break up hard tissues, e.g. tumours, bruising and swollen, hard breasts when feeding infants.

ADMINISTERED AS: an infusion and poultice.

Stavesacre *Delphinium staphisagria.*

COMMON NAME: starvesacre, staphisagris, lousewort.

OCCURRENCE: indigenous to southern Europe and Asia Minor, and is now cultivated in France and Italy.

PARTS USED: the dried ripe seeds. The main components of the seeds are alkaloid compounds including the poisonous delphinine, delphisine, delphinoidine, staphisagroine and staphisagrine, which may make up twenty five per cent of the seeds.

MEDICINAL USES: vermifuge, vermin-destroying, violent emetic and cathartic. The seeds are so very poisonous that they are rarely taken internally. Occasionally, the powdered seeds may be used as a purge in treating dropsy, with the dose monitored very carefully. The seeds are used externally as a parasiticide to kill lice of the genus *Pediculus*, and as a poultice or decoction compress on some skin eruptions and scrofula. The extracted alkaloid delphinine has been used both internally and externally to ease neuralgia. It resembles ACONITE in its action, slowing the pulse and respiration rates, paralysing the spinal cord and leading to death by asphyxia when taken in large doses. It can be used as an antidote to poisoning by strychnine.

ADMINISTERED AS: ointment, expressed oil, powdered seeds, decoction, poultice, fluid extract.

Stockholm tar *Pinus sylvestris* (and other species).

COMMON NAME: tar, *Pix liquida.*

OCCURRENCE: obtained from various *Pinus* species grown across the northern hemisphere in Sweden, Russia, North America and Switzerland.

PARTS USED: the tar is an impure turpentine obtained from the stems and roots of *Pinus* species by destructive distillation.

MEDICINAL USES: antiseptic, diuretic, diaphoretic, expectorant, stimulant. It may be used for chronic coughs and consumption but is mainly used externally as a cutaneous stimulant and as an ointment for eczema. It is mainly used in veterinary practices.

ADMINISTERED AS: ointment, fluid extract.

Stramonium *Datura stramonium.*

COMMON NAME: thornapple, jimsonweed, Jamestownweed, devil's apple, devil's trumpet, datura, mad apple, stinkweed, apple of Peru.

OCCURRENCE: a plant of unknown origin that is currently found throughout the world except in cold or Arctic areas.

PARTS USED: the whole plant has medicinal qualities but it is the leaves and seeds that are most commonly used today. The leaves contain the same alkaloids as BELLADONNA, but in slightly smaller amounts. The alkaloids include lyoscyamine, atropine, lyoscine along with malic acid, volatile oil, gum, resin and starch. The seeds are made up of fixed oil and the same alkaloids as the leaves, but the fixed oil makes the alkaloids difficult to extract so the leaves are the most extensively utilized.

MEDICINAL USES: antispasmodic, anodyne, narcotic. A herb which acts in a very similar manner to belladonna except it does not cause constipation. An extract of the seeds is given in pill form to stop coughing in spasmodic bronchial asthma, to ease whooping cough and spasm of the bladder. It is considered a better cough remedy than opium, but is used with extreme care as it can act as a narcotic poison in overdoses. When smoked with tobacco, alone or with other herbs, e.g. SAGE and BELLADONNA, stramonium can ease asthma by relaxing spasms of the bronchioles during an attack. Taken in this form, it can also help control the spasms that occur in Parkinson's disease. The herb can relieve the pain of sciatica and rheumatism when used externally in the form of an ointment.. Signs of an overdose of stramonium include dryness of the throat and mouth and an overdose can cause double vision, thirst, palpitations, restlessness, confusion and hallucinations. This drug is highly toxic and should only be used under the guidance of a herbal medicine practitioner or doctor. In India, thieves and assassins used to give their victims Stramonium in order to make them insensible while history states that the herb was taken by the priests of Apollo at Delphi, in Ancient Greece, to assist them in their prophecies.

Stramonium was considered to be a plant which aided witches in their ill-doing, and during the time of the witch and wizard hunt in England, it was exceedingly dangerous to grow stramonium in your garden as it was said to confirm the supernatural powers of the householder. Many people were sentenced to death purely because stramonium was found in their garden.

ADMINISTERED AS: powdered leaves, powdered seeds, fluid extract, tincture and ointment.

Strawberry *Fragaria vesca.*

OCCURRENCE: found through the whole of the northern hemisphere, excluding the tropics.

PARTS USED: the leaves, which contain cissotanic, malic and citric acids, sugar, mucilage and a volatile aromatic chemical which is, as yet, unidentified.

MEDICINAL USES: laxative, diuretic, astringent. The berries are of great benefit for rheumatic gout while the root is good against diarrhoea. The leaves have similar properties and are used to stop dysentery. Fresh strawberries remove discolouration of the teeth if the juice is left on for about five minutes and then the teeth are cleaned with warm water, to which a pinch of bicarbonate of soda has been added. Sunburn could be relieved by rubbing a cut strawberry over a freshly washed face.

ADMINISTERED AS: infusion, fresh berries.

Strophanthus *Strophanthus kombé.*

COMMON NAME: kombe seeds, *Strophanthus hispidus*, *S. semina*.

OCCURRENCE: native to tropical East Africa.

PARTS USED: the seeds. These contain the glucoside strophanthus, the alkaloid inoeine and a fixed oil.

MEDICINAL USES: cardiac tonic. This drug has a large influence on the circulatory system. It is used in chronic heart weakness, muscular debility of the heart and in cardiac pains with difficult or laboured breathing. It acts in the same way as digitalis (FOXGLOVE, *Digitalis purpurea*), but with increased digestive disturbance and strophanthus does not have a cumulative poisoning effect. Strophanthus has diuretic powers and is beneficial in dropsy, particularly when related to heart problems. In urgent cases, the intravenous injection of strophanthus can be used to increase circulation. The strength and power of the seeds are highly variable, and the seeds are so highly poisonous that they should only be used under medical supervision. In Africa, strophanthus is used as an arrow poison.

ADMINISTERED AS: liquid extract, tincture, solid extract.

Sumbul Ferula sumbul.

COMMON NAME: musk root, ouchi, ofnokgi, racine de sumbul, sumbulwurzel, moschuswurzel, jatamarsi, *Sumbul radix.*

OCCURRENCE: thought to be native to Turkestan, northern India and Russia.

PARTS USED: the root and rhizome. They contain two balsamic resins (thought to cause the strong musk-like odour), wax, gum, a bitter substance, a volatile oil, starch and angelic and valeric acids.

MEDICINAL USES: nerve stimulant, antispasmodic, tonic. Sumbul resembles VALERIAN in action and is very good for various hysterical conditions. It is thought to have a specific action on the pelvic organs and is used for dysmenorrhoea and similar female problems. Sumbul acts as a stimulant of the mucous membranes easing chronic diarrhoea and dysentery as well as pneumonia, chronic bronchitis and asthma. The side effects of the drug can occur producing narcotic symptoms, confusion, tingling feelings and a strong odour on the breath which may take two days to disappear.

ADMINISTERED AS: solid extract, tincture, fluid extract.

Sundew Drosera rotundifolia.

COMMON NAME: roundleaved sundew, dew plant, red rot, youthwort, rosa solis, herba rosellae, rosée du soleil.

OCCURRENCE: an insectivorous plant found in bogs, wet places and river edges throughout Britain, Europe, India, China, North and South America and Russian Asia.

PARTS USED: the air-dried flowering plant.

MEDICINAL USES: pectoral, expectorant, demulcent, anti-asthmatic. In small doses sundew is a specific in dry, spasmodic, tickling coughs and is considered very good in whooping cough, for which it may also be used as a prophylactic drug. The fresh juice is used to remove corns and warts. In America, the sundew has been advocated as a cure for old age and has been used with colloidal silicates in cases of thickening of arteries due to old age, or calcium or fat deposition.

ADMINISTERED AS: fluid extract, expressed juice, solid extract.

Sunflower Helicanthus annuus.

COMMON NAME: helianthus, marigold of Peru, *Sola indianus, Chrysanthe-*

mum peruvianum, Corona solis.

OCCURRENCE: native to Peru and Mexico and was introduced into America, Europe and Great Britain as a garden plant.

PARTS USED: the seeds. These contain a vegetable oil, carbonate of potash, tannin and vitamins B1, B3 and B6. The oil is expressed from the crushed seeds and, according to the range of temperature to which the seeds are heated, several grades of oil are obtained.

MEDICINAL USES: diuretic, expectorant. It has been used successfully in treating pulmonary, bronchial and laryngeal afflictions as well as whooping cough, colds and coughs. The leaves are used, in some parts of the world, to treat malaria and the tincture may replace quinine in easing intermittent fevers and the ague. Sunflowers produce the seed cake which is used as cattle food; the fresh leaves are given to poultry; the plants can be used as a vegetable; the stems are used as bedding for ducks; the plant used for silage, fuel, manure, textiles and as a soil improver.

ADMINISTERED AS: sunflower oil, tincture, decoction, poultice.

Tag alder *Alnus semulata.*
COMMON NAME: smooth alder, red alder, common alder, *Alnus rubra.*

OCCURRENCE: a common tree found in Europe, Great Britain and the United States of America.

PARTS USED: the bark and cones.

MEDICINAL USES: tonic, alterative, emetic, astringent. This plant is good for scrofula, diarrhoea, dyspepsia, indigestion, secondary syphilis and debility of the stomach. A decoction of the cones was said to be astringent in effect and of use in all types of haemorrhages. The bark was also of benefit to some cutaneous diseases and intermittent fevers.

ADMINISTERED AS: infusion, decoction, fluid extract.

Tansy *Tanacetum vulgare.*
COMMON NAME: buttons.

OCCURRENCE: a hardy perennial plant, commonly seen in hedges and on waste ground all over Europe and Great Britain.

PARTS USED: the herb. It contains the chemicals tanacetin, tannic acid, a volatile oil, thujone, sugar and a colouring matter.

MEDICINAL USES: anthelmintic, tonic, emmenagogue, stimulant. Tansy is largely used for expelling worms from children. It is good in female disorders, like hysteria and nausea and in kidney weakness. The herb is also used for slight fevers, for allaying spasms and as a nervine drug. In large doses, the herb is violently irritant and induces venous congestion of the abdominal organs. In Scotland, an infusion was administered to cure gout. Tansy essential oil, when given in small doses, has helped in epilepsy and has also been used externally to help some eruptive diseases of the skin. Bruised fresh leaves can reduce swelling and relieve sprains, as can a hot infusion used as a poultice.

ADMINISTERED AS: essential oil, infusion, poultice, fresh leaves, solid extract.

Tarragon *Artemisia dracunculus.*

COMMON NAME: mugwort, little dragon.

OCCURRENCE: cultivated in kitchen gardens across Europe and Great Britain. Tarragon originally arose from both Siberia and southern Europe to form the French and Russian tarragon we know today.

PARTS USED: the leaves, which contain an essential volatile oil which is lost on drying.

MEDICINAL USES: today there are few medicinal uses for tarragon but it has been used previously to stimulate the appetite and to cure toothache. Tarragon is mostly used in cooking—particularly on the European continent. It is used for dressings, salads, vinegar and pickles.

ADMINISTERED AS: fresh root, fresh herb.

Tea *Camellia thea.*

COMMON NAME: *Camellia theifera, Thea sinensis, Thea veridis, Thea bohea, Thea stricta jassamica.*

OCCURRENCE: native to Assam in India, and the plant has spread to Sri Lanka, Java, China and Japan.

PARTS USED: the dried leaves.

MEDICINAL USES: stimulant, astringent. The infusion of the leaves has a stimulating effect on the nervous system, producing a feeling of comfort. It may also act as a nerve sedative where it can relieve headaches. When drunk in excessive quantities, tea can produce unpleasant nervous symptoms, dyspepsia and unnatural wakefulness.

ADMINISTERED AS: infusion.

Thistle, Holy *Carbenia benedicta.*

COMMON NAME: blessed thistle, *Cnicus benedictus, Carduus benedictus.*

OCCURRENCE: a native of southern Europe and has been cultivated in Britain for hundreds of years.

PARTS USED: the whole herb which contains a volatile oil, a bitter crystalline compound called cnicin which is said to be similar to salicin in its properties.

MEDICINAL USES: tonic, stimulant, diaphoretic, emetic and emmenagogue. Very useful as an infusion to weak and debilitating stomach conditions, creating appetite and preventing sickness. It is said to be good in all fevers, as a purifier of the blood and circulation and its main modern day use is for bringing on a proper supply of milk in nursing mothers. In large doses, however, holy thistle is a strong emetic, producing vomiting. It may be used as a vermifuge. ADMINISTERED AS: infusion and fluid extract.

Thistle, Scotch *Onopordon acanthium.*
COMMON NAME: woolly thistle, cotton thistle.
OCCURRENCE: a common plant in all of Great Britain, found in waste ground and roadsides.
PARTS USED: the leaves and root.
MEDICINAL USES: ancient herbalists believed that the Scotch thistle was a specific against cancer and even today the expressed juice of the plant has been used to good effect on cancers and ulcers. A decoction of thistles was thought to restore a healthy, growing head of hair when applied to a bald head, while a root decoction has astringent effects and reduces production from mucous membranes. Thistles were also supposed to be effective against rickets in children, a crick in the neck and nervous complaints.
ADMINISTERED AS: expressed juice, decoction.

Thyme *Thymus vulgaris.*
COMMON NAME: garden or common thyme, tomillo.
OCCURRENCE: cultivated in temperate countries in northern Europe.
PARTS USED: the herb. Thyme gives rise to oil of thyme after distillation of the fresh leaves. This oil contains the phenols, thymol and carvacrol, as well as cymene, pinene and borneol.
MEDICINAL USES: antiseptic, antispasmodic, tonic, carminative. The fresh herb, in syrup, forms a safe cure for whooping cough, as is an infusion of the dried herb. The infusion or tea is beneficial for catarrh, sore throat, wind spasms, colic and in allaying fevers and colds. Thyme is generally used in conjunction with other remedies in herbal medicine.
ADMINISTERED AS: fluid extract, essential oil and infusion.

Tobacco *Nicotiana tabacum, N. acuminata, N. rustica* and other varieties.
COMMON NAME: leaf tobacco, tabacca.
OCCURRENCE: native to America and cultivated in many sub-tropical countries including China, Greece, France and Turkey.
PARTS USED: the cured and dried leaves, which contain five alkaloids including nicotine. Upon smoking, nicotine decomposes into

various chemicals—the very poisonous carbon monoxide, pyridine and hydrogen cyanide.

MEDICINAL USES: narcotic, sedative, diuretic, expectorant, emetic. Medicinally, tobacco has been used internally for hernias, constipation, tetanus, retention of urine, worms and hysterical convulsions. It is best utilized externally as a plaster or poultice to ease cutaneous diseases, haemorrhoids and facial neuralgia. A combination of tobacco leaves along with the leaves of STRAMONIUM or BELLADONNA make a very good treatment for spasmodic afflictions, painful tumours and obstinate ulcers. Tobacco is a local irritant and the nicotine within it is very poisonous, causing heart palpitations and irregularity and disturbing the digestive and circulatory organs. The use of tobacco as a medicine is unusual in today's western herbal medicine, although it is still used in some native societies. The poisonous nature of the alkaloids within the plant have discouraged its use as use of tobacco, even within small doses, can cause depression, convulsions and even death.

ADMINISTERED AS: poultice, ointment, suppositories, smoking herb.

Tree of heaven Ailanthus glandulosa.

COMMON NAME: ailanto, vernis de Japan, Chinese sumach.

OCCURRENCE: indigenous to China and India, and is now cultivated through Europe and the United State.

PARTS USED: the root and the inner bark of the tree. The bark contains chlorophyll, pectin, lignin, volatile oil, resin, quassin, tannin and various mineral salts.

MEDICINAL USES: astringent, antispasmodic, cardiac depressant. Despite this herb's unpleasant and nauseating action on patients, it has been successful against diarrhoea, dysentery, leucorrhoea, prolapse of the rectum and for tapeworms. A tincture prepared from the root bark of the tree has been good for epilepsy, asthma and cardiac palpitations.

ADMINISTERED AS: infusion, tincture.

Turpentine oil distilled from *Pinus palustris, Pinus maritima* and other species.

MEDICINAL USES: rubefacient, irritant, diuretic. When taken internally, turpentine forms a valuable remedy in bladder, kidney, and rheumatic problems and diseases of the mucous membranes. The oil is also used for respiratory complaints and externally as a liniment, an embrocation and an inhalant for rheumatism and chest problems. Turpentine may be combined with other aromatic oils as a remedy.

ADMINISTERED AS: essential oil.

Valerian

Valerian Valeriana officinalis.

COMMON NAME: all-heal, great wild valerian, amantilla, setwall, sete-wale, capon's tail.

OCCURRENCE: found throughout Europe and northern Asia. It is common in England in marshy thickets, riverbanks and ditches.

PARTS USED: the root, which contains a volatile oil, two alkaloids called chatarine and valerianine as well as several unidentified compounds.

MEDICINAL USES: powerful nervine, stimulant, carminative anodyne and antispasmodic herb. It may be given in all cases of nervous debility and irritation as it is not narcotic. The expressed juice of the fresh root has been used as a narcotic in insomnia and as an anticonvulsant in epilepsy. The oil of valerian is of use against cholera and in strengthening the eyesight. A herbal compound containing valerian was given to civilians during the Second World War, to reduce the effects of stress caused by repeated air raids and to minimize damage to health.

ADMINISTERED AS: fluid and solid extract, tincture, oil, expressed juice.

Verbena, Lemon Lippia citriodora.

COMMON NAME: herb Louisa, lemon-scented verbena, *Verveine citronelle* or *odorante*, *Verbena triphylla*, *Lippia triphylla*, *Aloysia citriodora*.

OCCURRENCE: originally from Peru and Chile, it was introduced into England in 1784 and is now a common garden plant.

PARTS USED: the leaves and flowering tops.

MEDICINAL USES: febrifuge, sedative. This herb has similar uses to BALM, PEPPERMINT, ORANGE flowers and SPEARMINT in relieving flatulence, indigestion and dyspepsia through its antispasmodic and stomachic actions. It is commonly made into a refreshing tisane. The leaves of lemon verbena were once used in finger bowls at banquets and the essential oil distilled from the herb was used to impart a strong lemon scent to cosmetics and soaps.

ADMINISTERED AS: tea.

Vervain Verbena officinalis.

COMMON NAME: herb of grace, herbe sacrée, herba veneris, *Verbena hastrata*.

OCCURRENCE: grows across Europe, China, Japan and Barbary. Also found in England by roadsides and in sunny pastures.

PARTS USED: the herb. Vervain contains a peculiar tannin, which has not yet been fully investigated.

MEDICINAL USES: nervine, tonic, emetic, sudorific, astringent, diaphoretic,

antispasmodic. This herb is recommended in many complaints including intermittent fevers, ulcers, pleurisy, ophthalmic disorders and is said to be a good galactogogue. May also be administered as a poultice to ease headache, ear neuralgia, rheumatism and taken as a decoction to ease bowel pain during purging. Vervain is often applied externally for piles.
ADMINISTERED AS: fluid extract, decoction.

Vine *Vitis vinifera.*

COMMON NAME: grape vine.

OCCURRENCE: a very ancient plant, frequently mentioned in the Bible after the Great Flood. It now grows in Asia, central and southern Europe, Africa, Australia, Greece, California and South America.

PARTS USED: the fruit, leaves and juice. The wine sold commercially is made from fermented fruit juice. This juice, which is called 'must', contains malic acid, gum, sugar, inorganic salts and potassium bicarbonate. The leaves contain tartaric acid, tannin, malic acid, gum, quercetine, quercitrin, potassium bitartrate, cane sugar and glucose.

MEDICINAL USES: the leaves and seeds have an astringent action, with the leaves previously used to stop haemorrhages and bleeding. Ripe grapes, when eaten in some quantity, increase the flow of urine and can be of great benefit in exhaustion, anaemia, smallpox, sleeplessness and neuralgia. They are also eaten for poor biliary function and torpid liver. Grape sugar is chemically different to other sugars, as the saliva has no enzymatic effect on it. Thus it acts faster to warm up the body and build tissues, to increase strength and repair the body after illness. Raisins have demulcent, nutritive and slightly laxative effects on the body.

ADMINISTERED AS: fermented fruit juice, fresh or dried leaves, fresh or dried fruits.

Violet *Viola adorata.*

COMMON NAME: blue violet, sweet violet, sweet-scented violet.

OCCURRENCE: native to Great Britain and found widely over Europe, northern Asia and North America.

PARTS USED: the dried flowers and leaves and whole plant when fresh.

MEDICINAL USES: antiseptic, expectorant, laxative. The herb is mainly taken as syrup of violets which has been used to cure the ague, epilepsy, eye inflammation, pleurisy, jaundice and sleeplessness which are some of the many other complaints that benefit from treatment with this herb. The flowers possess expectorant properties and have long been used to treat coughs. The flowers may also be crystallized as a sweetmeat or added to salads. The rhizome is strongly emetic and purgative and has violent effects when administered. The seeds also have purgative and diuretic effects and are beneficial in treating urinary complaints and gravel. In the early part of this century, violet preparations were used to great effect against cancer. Fresh violet leaves are made into an infusion which was drunk regularly, and a poultice of the leaves was applied to the affected area. The herb has been used successfully to both allay pain and perhaps cure the cancer. It is said to be particularly good against throat cancer.

ADMINISTERED AS: infusion, poultice, injection, ointment, syrup and powdered root.

Walnut *Juglans nigra.*
COMMON NAME: carya, Jupiter's nuts, *Juglans regia.*
OCCURRENCE: cultivated throughout Europe and was probably native to Persia.
PARTS USED: the bark and leaves. The active principle of the walnut tree is nucin or juglon, while the kernels also contain oil, mucilage, albumin, cellulose, mineral matter and water.
MEDICINAL USES: alterative, laxative, detergent, astringent. The bark and leaves are used in skin problems, e.g. scrofulous diseases, herpes, eczema and for healing indolent ulcers. A strong infusion of the powdered bark has purgative effects, while the walnut has various properties dependent upon its stage of ripeness. Green walnuts are anthelminthic and vermifuge in action and are pickled in vinegar, which is then used as a gargle for sore and ulcerated throats. The wood is used for furniture, gun-stocks and for cabinets. Walnut oil expressed from the kernels is used in wood polishing, painting and is used as butter or frying oil.
ADMINISTERED AS: fluid extract, infusion, expressed oil, whole fruit.

Water betony *Scrophularia aquatica.*
COMMON NAME: water figwort, brownwort, bishop's leaves, crowdy kit, fiddlewood, fiddler, *Betonica aquatica.*
OCCURRENCE: found growing wild in damp places, on the banks of rivers and ponds throughout Great Britain and Europe.
PARTS USED: the leaves, fresh and dried.
MEDICINAL USES: detergent, vulnerary. The leaves are used as a poultice, or as an ointment for wounds, sores, haemorrhoids, ulcers and scrofulous glands in the neck. It was also used to expel nightmares, cure toothache and as a cosmetic for blemished or sunburnt skin.
ADMINISTERED AS: decoction, poultice, ointment.

Watercress Nasturtium officinale
OCCURRENCE: a perennial creeping plant often growing near springs and running water across Great Britain and Europe.
PARTS USED: the stem and leaves, which contain nicotinamide, volatile oil, a glucoside, gluconasturtin and vitamins A, C and E.
MEDICINAL USES: stimulant, expectorant, nutritive, antiscorbutic, diuretic. Watercress was proposed as a specific in tuberculosis and has a very long history of medical use. It is used to treat bronchitis and coughs as well as boosting digestion, lowering blood sugar and helping the body to remove toxic wastes from the blood and tissues. The herb is of value nutritionally as it contains many vitamins and mineral salts which help during convalescence and general debility. It can be bruised and made into a poultice for arthritis and gout, and is chewed raw to strengthen gums.
ADMINISTERED AS: expressed juice, poultice, dietary item.

Water dock Rumex aquaticus.
COMMON NAME: red dock, bloodwort.
OCCURRENCE: found in fields, meadows and ditches throughout Europe and Great Britain and is particularly common in the northern latitudes.
PARTS USED: the root.
MEDICINAL USES: alterative, deobstruent, detergent. It has a powerful tonic action and is used externally to clean ulcers in afflictions of the mouth. It is applied to eruptive and scorbutic diseases, skin ulcers and sores. As a powder, Water dock has a cleansing and detergent effect upon the teeth.
ADMINISTERED AS: fluid extract and infusion.

Willow, White Salix alba.
COMMON NAME: European willow.
OCCURRENCE: a large tree growing in moist places and running streams around Great Britain and Europe.
PARTS USED: the bark and leaves. The bark contains tannin and salicin.
MEDICINAL USES: tonic, antiperiodic, astringent. The bark has been used in febrile diseases of rheumatic or gouty origin, diarrhoea and dysentery. It has been used in dyspepsia connected with digestive organ disorders. The bark has also been of benefit in convalescence after acute diseases and against parasitic worms.
ADMINISTERED AS: decoction, powdered root.

Wintergreen Gaultheria procumbens.

COMMON NAME: mountain tea, teaberry, boxberry, thé du Canada, aromatic wintergreen, partridge berry, deerberry, checkerberry.

OCCURRENCE: native to the northern United States and Canada from Georgia northwards.

PARTS USED: the leaves, which produce a volatile oil upon distillation. The oil is made up of methyl salicylate, gaultherilene, an aldehyde, a secondary alcohol and an ester. The aromatic odour of the plant is due to the alcohol and the ester.

MEDICINAL USES: aromatic, tonic, stimulant, diuretic, emmenagogue, astringent, galactogogue. The oil is of great benefit in acute rheumatism, but must be given in the form of capsules so stomach inflammation does not occur. The true distilled oil when applied to the skin can give rise to an eruption and so the synthetic oil of wintergreen is recommended for external use as it still contains methyl salicylate, but with no deleterious effects. The synthetic oil is exceedingly valuable for all chronic joint and muscular troubles, lumbago, sciatica and rheumatism. The oil is also used as a flavouring for toothpowders and mouth washes, particularly when combined with menthol and EUCALYPTUS. The berries are a winter food for many animals and also produce a bitter tonic, after being steeped in brandy. The leaves are either used to flavour tea or as a substitute for tea itself.

ADMINISTERED AS: capsules, synthetic oil, infusion, tincture.

Witch hazel Hamamelis virginiana.

COMMON NAME: spotted alder, winterbloom, snapping hazelnut.

OCCURRENCE: native to the United States of America and Canada.

PARTS USED: the dried bark, both fresh and dried leaves. The leaves contain tannic and gallic acids, volatile oil and an unknown bitter principle. The bark contains tannin, gallic acid, a physterol, resin, fat and other bitter and odorous bodies.

MEDICINAL USES: astringent, tonic, sedative. Valuable in stopping internal and external haemorrhages and in treating piles. Mainly used for bruises, swelling, inflammation and tumours as a poultice. It may also be utilized for diarrhoea, dysentery and mucous discharges. A decoction is used against tuberculosis, gonorrhoea, menorrhagia and the debilitated state resulting from abortion. Tea made from the bark or leaves aids bleeding of the stomach, bowel complaints and may be given as an injection for bleeding piles. Witch hazel is used to treat varicose veins as a moist poultice, as an extract to ease burns, scalds and insect and mosquito bites, and to help inflammation of the eyelids.

ADMINISTERED AS: liquid extract, injection, tincture, lotion, ointment, suppositories, poultice, infusion and decoction.

Woodruff *Asperula odorata.*
COMMON NAME: wuderove, wood-rova, sweet woodruff, woodroof, waldmeister tea.
OCCURRENCE: grows in woods or shaded hedges in England.
PARTS USED: the herb, which contains coumarin, a fragrant crystalline chemical, citric, malic and rubichloric acids and tannic acid.
MEDICINAL USES: diuretic, tonic. The fresh leaves, when applied to wounds, were said to have a strong healing effect. A strong decoction of the fresh herb was used as a cordial and stomachic and is said to be useful in removing biliary obstructions of the liver.
ADMINISTERED AS: a poultice and decoction.

Wormseed, American *Chenopodium anthelminticum.*
COMMON NAME: Mexican tea, Jesuit's tea, herba Sancti Mariae, *Chenopodium ambrosioides*.
OCCURRENCE: indigenous to Mexico and South America, and naturalized in almost all areas of the eastern United States.
PARTS USED: the fruits and seeds. An oil is distilled from the crushed fruits called chenopodium oil. It is made up of ascaridole, an unstable substance, choline, betzine, sylvestrene and several other compounds.
MEDICINAL USES: anthelmintic, vermifuge. The herb is used to expel roundworms and hookworms, particularly in children. The drug should be given in one full dose, then fasting until an active purgative drug e.g. CASTOR OIL is given two hours later. The treatment should be repeated ten days later. The drug may be given as volatile oil, expressed juice of the fresh plant, the fluid extract, or the bruised fruit. Chenopodium oil has been of benefit in chorea, malaria, hysteria and similar nervous diseases and has been used as a pectoral drug in asthma and catarrh. Unfortunately the chenopodium oil on the market varies as to the quantity of ascaridole within it and care must be taken to prevent overdoses occurring. Toxic symptoms caused by this drug include temporary dizziness and vomiting.
ADMINISTERED AS: distilled oil, expressed juice, bruised fruit, fluid extract.

Wormwood *Artemisia absinthium.*
COMMON NAME: green ginger, old women, ajenjo.
OCCURRENCE: a plant found wild in many parts of the world including Siberia, Europe and the United States of America.

Woundwort

PARTS USED: the whole herb. The herb contains a volatile oil made up of thujone, pinene, cadinene and chamazulene, a bitter principle called absinthum, carotene, tannins and vitamin C.

MEDICINAL USES: bitter tonic, anthelmintic, febrifuge, stomachic. The liqueur, absinthe, was made using this plant as flavouring and it was banned in France in 1915 as excess intake caused irreversible damage to the nervous system. In modern herbal medicine, it is used as a bitter tonic to stimulate the appetite, the liver and gall bladder, production of digestive juices and peristalsis. Wormwood also expels parasitic worms, particularly roundworms and threadworms. The plant contains chemicals which have anti-inflammatory effects and help reduce fevers. Since ancient times this herb has been used by women to encourage menstruation, and it is applied as an external compress during labour to speed up the birth process. After labour, wormwood was taken both internally and externally to expel the afterbirth. This herb should not be used during pregnancy and should only be administered for short time periods.

ADMINISTERED AS: infusion, essential oil, fluid extract.

Woundwort *Stachys palustris.*

COMMON NAME: all-heal, panay, opopanewort, clown's woundwort, rusticum vulna herba, downy woundwort, stinking marsh stachys.

OCCURRENCE: common to marshy meadows, riversides and ditches in most parts of Great Britain.

PARTS USED: the herb.

MEDICINAL USES: antiseptic, antispasmodic. The herb relieves cramp, gout, painful joints and vertigo, while bruised leaves will stop bleeding and encourage healing when applied to a wound. Woundwort had an excellent reputation as a vulnerary among all of the early herbalists. A syrup made of the fresh juice will stop haemorrhages and dysentery when taken internally. The tuberous roots are edible as are the young shoot which resemble ASPARAGUS.

ADMINISTERED AS: poultice or syrup.

Yam, wild *dioscorea villosa.*

COMMON NAME: dioscorea, colic root, rheumatism root, wilde yamwurzel.

OCCURRENCE: native to the southern United States and Canada.

PARTS USED: the roots and rhizome, which contain steroidal saponins, phytosterols, tannins, starch and various alkaloids including dioscorine.

MEDICINAL USES: antispasmodic, diuretic. This plant has a history of traditional use in relieving menstrual cramps and in stopping threatened miscarriage. It brings quick relief for bilious colic and flatulence, particularly in pregnant women. It is prescribed for the inflammatory stage of rheumatoid arthritis and in painful disorders of the urinary tract. Wild Yam is also beneficial for poor circulation, spasmodic hiccoughs, neuralgic complaints and spasmodic asthma. Prior to 1970, the wild yam was the only source of diosgenin, one of the starting materials used in commercial manufacturing of steroid hormones for the contraceptive pill.

ADMINISTERED AS: fluid extract, powdered bark, infusion.

Yerba santa *Eriodictyon glutinosum.*

COMMON NAME: mountain balm, gum bush, bear's weed, holy or sacred herb, consumptive's weed, *Eriodictyon californicum.*

OCCURRENCE: native to California and northern Mexico.

PARTS USED: the dried leaves which contain five phenolic chemicals, free acids including free formic acids, volatile oil, phytosterol, glucose, a resin and some glycerides of fatty acids.

MEDICINAL USES: bitter tonic, stimulant, expectorant, aromatic. This herb is recommended in laryngeal and bronchial problems, catarrh, hay fever, asthma and chronic lung afflictions. It is also used for catarrh of the bladder and haemorrhoids. Yerba santa is used as a bitter tonic upon the digestion and is highly effective in masking the unpleasant taste of quinine, when given as an aromatic syrup. The dried leaves are smoked to ease asthma.

ADMINISTERED AS: powdered leaves, fluid extract, syrup.

Yew *Taxus baccata.*

OCCURRENCE: found in Europe, North Africa and Western Asia. The tree has been closely associated with the history and legends of Europe.

PARTS USED: the leaves, seeds and fruit. The seeds and fruit are the most poisonous parts of the plant and contain an alkaloid toxine and another principle milrossin.

MEDICINAL USES: it has few medicinal uses due to its poisonous nature but the leaves were once used effectively in treating epilepsy. The wood was used for making longbows.

ADMINISTERED AS: powdered leaves.

Homeopathy:
An Introduction

The aim of homeopathy is to cure an illness or disorder by treating the whole person rather than merely concentrating on a set of symptoms. Hence, in homeopathy the approach is holistic, and the overall state of health of the patient, especially his or her emotional and psychological wellbeing, is regarded as being significant. A homeopath notes the symptoms that the person wishes to have cured but also takes time to discover other signs or indications of disorder that the patient may regard as being less important. The reasoning behind this is that illness is a sign of disorder or imbalance within the body. It is believed that the whole 'make-up' of a person determines, to a great extent, the type of disorders to which that individual is prone and the symptoms likely to occur. A homeopathic remedy must be suitable both for the symptoms and the characteristics and temperament of the patient. Hence, two patients with the same illness may be offered different remedies according to their individual natures. One remedy may also be used to treat different groups of symptoms or ailments.

Homeopathic remedies are based on the concept that 'like cures like', an ancient philosophy that can be traced back to the 5th century BC, when it was formulated by Hippocrates. In the early 1800s, this idea awakened the interest of a German doctor, Samuel Hahnemann, who believed that the medical practices at the time were too harsh and tended to hinder rather than aid healing. Hahnemann observed that a treatment for malaria, based on an extract of cinchona bark (quinine), actually produced symptoms of this disease when taken in a small dose by a healthy person. Further extensive studies convinced him that the production of symptoms was the body's way of combating illness. Hence, to give a minute dose of a substance that stimulated the symptoms of an illness in a healthy person could be used to fight that illness in someone who was sick. Hahnemann conducted numerous trials (called 'provings'), giving minute doses of substances to healthy people and recording the symptoms produced. Eventually, these very dilute remedies were given to people with illnesses, often with encouraging results.

Modern homeopathy is based on the work of Hahnemann, and the medicines derived from plant, mineral and animal sources are used in extremely dilute amounts. Indeed, it is believed that the curative properties are enhanced by each dilution because impurities that might cause unwanted side effects are lost. Substances used in homeopathy are first soaked in alcohol to extract their essential ingredients. This initial solution, called the 'mother tincture', is diluted successively either by factors of ten (called the 'decimal scale' and designated X) or 100 (the 'centesimal scale' and designated C). Each dilution is shaken vigorously before further ones are made, and this is thought to make the properties more powerful by adding energy at each stage while impurities are removed. The thorough shakings of each dilution are said to energize, or 'potentiate', the medicine. The remedies are made into tablets or may be used in the form of ointment, solutions, powders, suppositories, etc. High potency (i.e. more dilute) remedies are used for severe symptoms and lower potency (less dilute) for milder ones.

The homeopathic view is that during the process of healing, symptoms are redirected from more important to less important body systems. It is also held that healing is from innermost to outermost parts of the body and that more recent symptoms disappear first, this being known as the 'law of direction of cure'. Occasionally, symptoms may worsen initially when a homeopathic remedy is taken, but this is usually short-lived and is known as a 'healing crisis'. It is taken to indicate a change and that improvement is likely to follow. Usually, with a homeopathic remedy, an improvement is noticed fairly quickly although this depends upon the nature of the ailment, health, age and wellbeing of the patient and potency of the remedy.

A first homeopathic consultation is likely to last about one hour so that the specialist can obtain a full picture of the patient's medical history and personal circumstances. On the basis of this information, the homeopathic doctor decides on an appropriate remedy and potency (which is usually 6C). Subsequent consultations are generally shorter, and full advice is given on how to store and take the medicine. It is widely accepted that homeopathic remedies are safe and non-addictive, but they are covered by the legal requirements governing all medicines and should be obtained from a recognized source.

Potency table for homeopathic medicines
The centesimal scale

1C =	1/100	$(1/100^1)$	of mother tincture
2C =	1/10 000	$(1/100^2)$	of mother tincture
3C =	1/1 000 000	$(1/100^3)$	of mother tincture
6C =	1/1 000 000 000 000	$(1/100^6)$	of mother tincture

Homeopathy: An Introduction

The decimal scale

1X =	1/10	$(1/10^1)$	of mother tincture
2X =	1/100	$(1/10^2)$	of mother tincture
6X =	1/1 000 000	$(1/10^6)$	of mother tincture

The development of homeopathy

The Greek physician Hippocrates, who lived several hundred years before the birth of Christ (460-370 BC), is regarded as the founding father of all medicine. The Hippocratic Oath taken by newly qualified doctors in orthodox medicine binds them to an ethical code of medical practice in honour of Hippocrates. Hippocrates believed that disease resulted from natural elements in the world in which people lived. This contrasted with the view that held sway for centuries that disease was some form of punishment from the gods or God. He believed that it was essential to observe and take account of the course and progress of a disease in each individual, and that any cure should encourage that person's own innate healing power. Hippocrates embraced the idea of 'like being able to cure like' and had many remedies that were based on this principle. Hence, in his practice and study of medicine he laid the foundations of the homeopathic approach although this was not to be appreciated and developed for many centuries.

During the period of Roman civilization a greater knowledge and insight into the nature of the human body was developed. Many herbs and plants were used for healing by people throughout the world, and much knowledge was gained and handed down from generation to generation. The belief persisted, however, that diseases were caused by supernatural or divine forces. It was not until the early 1500s that a Swiss doctor, Paracelsus (1493–1541), put forward the view that disease resulted from external environmental forces. He also believed that plants and natural substances held the key to healing and embraced the 'like can cure like' principle. One of his ideas, known as the 'doctrine of signatures', was that the appearance of a plant, or the substances it contained, gave an idea of the disorders it could cure.

In the succeeding centuries, increased knowledge was gained about the healing properties of plants and the way the human body worked. In spite of this, the methods of medical practice were extremely harsh, and there is no doubt that many people suffered needlessly and died because of the treatment they received. It was against this background that Samuel Hahnemann (1755-1843), the founding father of modern homeopathy, began his work as a doctor in the late 1700s. In his early writings,

Hahnemann criticized the severe practices of medicine and advocated a healthy diet, clean living conditions and high standards of hygiene as a means of improving health and warding off disease. In 1790, he became interested in quinine, extracted from the bark of the cinchona tree, which was known to be an effective treatment for malaria. He tested the substance first on himself, and later on friends and close family members, and recorded the results. These early experiments were called 'provings'. The results led him to conduct many further investigations and provings of other natural substances, during the course of which he rediscovered and established the principle of like being able to cure like.

By 1812, the principle and practice of homeopathy, based on the work of Hahnemann, had become established, and many other doctors adopted the homeopathic approach. Hahnemann himself became a teacher in homeopathy at the University of Leipzig and published many important writings—the results of his years of research. He continued to practise, teach and conduct research throughout his life, especially in producing more dilute remedies that were succussed, or shaken, at each stage and were found to be more potent. Although his work was not without its detractors, Hahnemann had attracted a considerable following by the 1830s. In 1831 there was a widespread cholera epidemic in central Europe for which Hahnemann recommended treatment with camphor. Many people were cured, including Dr Frederick Quin (1799–1878), a medical practitioner at that time. He went on to establish the first homeopathic hospital in London in 1849. A later resurgence of cholera in Britain enabled the effectiveness of camphor to be established beyond doubt, as the numbers of people cured at the homeopathic hospital were far greater than those treated at other hospitals.

In the United States of America, homeopathy became firmly established in the early part of the 19th century, and there were several eminent practitioners who further enhanced knowledge and practice. These included Dr Constantine Hering (1800–80), who formulated the 'laws of cure', explaining how symptoms affect organ systems and move from one part of the body to another as a cure occurs. Dr James Tyler Kent (1849–1916) introduced the idea of constitutional types, which is now the basis of classical homeopathy, and advocated the use of high potency remedies.

In the later years of the 19th century, a fundamental split occurred in the practice of homeopathy, which was brought about by Dr Richard Hughes (1836–1902), who worked in London and Brighton. He insisted that physical symptoms and the nature of the disease itself was the important factor rather than the holistic approach based on the make-up of the whole individual person. Hughes rejected the concept of constitutional types and advocated the use of low potency remedies. Although he worked as a homeopath, his approach was to attempt to make homeopathy more scientific and to bring it closer to the practices of conventional medicine. Some other homeopathic doctors followed the approach of Hughes, and the split led to a collapse in faith in the whole practice of homeopathy during the earlier part of the 20th century. As the 20th century advanced, however, homeopathy regained its following and respect. Conventional medicine and homeopathy have continued to advance, and there is now a greater sympathy and understanding between the practitioners in both these important disciplines.

Homeopathic Remedies in Common Use

Aconitum napellus

Aconite, monkshood, wolfsbane, friar's cap, mousebane

Aconitum is a native plant of Switzerland and other mountainous regions of Europe, where it grows in the damp conditions of alpine meadows. Attractive purple/dark blue flowers are borne on tall, upright stems produced from tubers developed from the root system. Aconite is highly poisonous, and its sap was used by ancient hunters on the ends of their arrows. 'Wolfsbane' refers to this use, and *Aconitum* is derived from the Latin word *acon*, meaning 'dart'. This was one of the homeopathic remedies extensively tested and proved by Hahnemann. He used it for the acute infections and fevers, accompanied by severe pain, that were usually treated by blood-letting by the physicians of his day. This remains its main use in modern homeopathy, and the whole plant is used to produce the remedy.

Aconite is a valuable treatment for acute illnesses of rapid onset in people who have previously been healthy and well. These often occur after the person has been out in cold wet weather. It is used especially at the start of feverish respiratory infections, such as colds and influenza and those affecting the eyes and ears. The person usually experiences restlessness, a hot, flushed face and pains and disturbed sleep but may be pale when first getting up. It is also used to treat the menopausal symptoms of hot flushes. It is an effective remedy for some mental symptoms, including extreme anxiety and fear, palpitations and attacks of panic, especially the belief that death is imminent during illness. The remedy encourages sweating and is sometimes used in conjunction with BELLADONNA. Symptoms are made worse by cold, draughts, tobacco smoke, stuffy, airless, warm rooms, listening to music, at midnight and by lying on the painful part. They improve out in the fresh air and with warmth. The people who benefit from Aconite are typically strong, solid or well-built, high-coloured and usually enjoy good health but have a poor opinion of themselves. Because of this, they tend to have a constant need to prove their own worth, to the point of insensitivity or unkindness to others. When in good health, Aconite people have a need for the company of others. However, they also have fears that they keep concealed and may be frightened of going out or of being in a crowd. When ill, they are inclined to be morbid and to believe that death is imminent, and they cope badly with any kind of shock.

Actea racemosa

Actea rac.; cimic, *Cimifuga racemosa*, black snakeroot, rattleroot, bugbane, rattleweed, squawroot.

This plant is a native of woodlands in North America and was used by the American Indian peoples as a remedy for the bite of the rattlesnake. It was also used as a tranquillizer and for pain relief in labour and menstruation. An infusion made from the plant was sprinkled in the home to protect against supernatural forces and evil spirits. The plant has a dark, woody underground stem (rhizome) and roots, and produces feathery, tall stems of white flowers. The fresh rhizomes and roots are used in homeopathy, being collected, cut and dried in the autumn after the stems and leaves have died down and the fruit has been formed. The rhizome has a faint, unpleasant smell and the taste is acrid and bitter. The remedy was extensively tested and proved by the English homeopath Dr Richard Hughes, who used it in the treatment of a stiff neck and associated headache. It is used for this purpose in modern homeopathy and also to treat pain in the lower back and between the shoulder blades. Also for rheumatic pain and swelling of joints or muscles and other sudden, sharp pains. Actea rac. is considered to be of great value in the treatment of menstrual problems with cramps, bloatedness, and pain and symptoms of pregnancy, e.g. morning sickness and abdominal discomfort. It is also of value for postnatal depression and menopausal symptoms. Emotional symptoms that accompany these periods of hormonal change, such as weepiness, anxiety and irritability, are also eased by this remedy. Symptoms are made worse by exposure to cold, wet, draughty conditions, by any sudden change in the weather, on drinking alcohol and with excitement. They improve with keeping warm, with gentle exercise and in the fresh, open air. A person suitable for this remedy is often a woman. She may be a bubbly, extrovert, talkative person or withdrawn, depressed and sad, heaving great sighs. The woman is usually emotionally intense with a fear of dying and madness. These fears are at their height in a woman going through the menopause.

Allium

Allium cepa; Spanish onion

The onion has been cultivated and used for many centuries, both for culinary and medicinal purposes, and was important in the ancient Egyptian civilization. The volatile oil released when an onion is sliced stimulates the tear glands of the eyes and mucous membranes of the nose, throat and air passages. Hence, in homeopathy the onion is used to treat ailments with symptoms of a streaming nose and watering eyes. The red Spanish onion, which is cultivated throughout the world, is used to make the homeopathic remedy. It is used to treat allergic conditions, such as hay fever, colds and pains or symptoms that go from one side to the other. It is useful for shooting, stabbing or burning pains associated with neuralgia, which may alternate from side to side, frontal headaches, painful molar teeth and earache in children. The symptoms are made worse by cold, damp conditions and improve in fresh air and cool, dry surroundings.

Apis mellifica
Apis; *Apis mellifera*, the honey bee
The source of the medicine is the entire body of the honey bee, which is crushed or ground to prepare the remedy. It is used particularly to treat inflammation, redness, swelling and itching of the skin, which is sensitive to touch, and with stinging hot pains. There is usually feverishness and thirst and the pains are worsened by heat and relieved by cold. The remedy is used for insect stings, nettle rash, allergic conditions, blisters, whitlow (an abscess on the fingertip) and infections of the urinary tract, including cystitis, with stabbing hot pains. Also for urinary incontinence in elderly persons, fluid retention causing swelling of the eyelids or other areas, allergic conditions that cause sore throat and swallowing difficulty, and tonsillitis. The person often experiences hot, stabbing headaches and has dry skin. Apis is additionally valued as a remedy for swollen, painful inflammation of the joints as in arthritic conditions and for peritonitis and pleurisy. The symptoms are made worse by heat and touch, stuffy airless rooms following sleep and in the early evening. They improve in the fresh, cool open air, after taking a cold bath, or any cold application. A person suitable for the Apis remedy tends to expect high standards and may be rather irritable and hard to please. He (or she) likes to organize others and is jealous of his own domain, tending to be resentful of anyone new. Apis types may seem to be rushing around and working hard but may achieve very little as a result.

Argenticum nitricum
Argent. nit; silver nitrate, devil's stone, lunar caustic, hellstone
Silver nitrate is obtained from the mineral acanthite, which is a natural ore of silver. White silver nitrate crystals are derived from a chemical

solution of the mineral ore and these are used to make the homeopathic remedy. Silver nitrate is poisonous in large doses and has antiseptic and caustic properties. In the past it was used to clean out wounds and prevent infection. In homeopathy, it is used to treat states of great anxiety, panic, fear or apprehension about a forthcoming event, e.g. taking an examination, having to perform a public role (speech-making, chairing a public meeting, acting, singing), going for an interview, or any activity involving scrutiny and criticism by others. It was also used as a remedy for digestive complaints including indigestion, abdominal pain, wind, nausea and headache. Often, there is a longing for sweet 'comfort' or other types of food. Argent. nit. may be given for laryngitis, sore throat and hoarseness, eye inflammation such as conjunctivitis, and period pains. Other types of pain, asthma and warts may benefit from Argent. nit.

Often, a person experiences symptoms mainly on the left side, and these are worse with heat and at night. Also, they are made worse by anxiety and overwork, emotional tension and resting on the left side. Pains are made worse with talking and movement. Symptoms improve in cold or cool fresh air and are relieved by belching. Pains are helped by applying pressure to the painful part. People suitable for Argent nit. are quick-witted and rapid in thought and action. They may appear outgoing and happy but are prey to worry, anxiety and ungrounded fears that make them tense. All the emotions are quick to surface, and Argent nit. people are able to put on an impressive performance. They enjoy a wide variety of foods, particularly salty and sweet things although these may upset the digestion. They have a fear of heights, crowds, of being burgled and of failure and arriving late for an appointment. Also, of serious illness, dying and madness. Argent. nit. people are generally slim and full of restless energy and tension. They may have deeply etched features and lines on the skin that make them appear older than their real age.

Arnica montana
Arnica; leopard's bane, sneezewort, mountain tobacco

Arnica is a native plant of woodland and mountainous regions of central Europe and Siberia. It has a dark brown root system from which a central stem arises, producing pairs of elongated green leaves and bright yellow flowers. If the flowers are crushed or bruised and a person then inhales the scent, this causes sneezing. All the fresh parts of the flowering plant are used to prepare the homeopathic remedy. It is a commonly used first aid remedy for symptoms relating to injury or trauma of any kind, e.g. bruising, swelling, pain and bleeding. It is also used to treat physical and mental shock. It is helpful following surgery, childbirth or tooth extraction, promoting healing, and also for gout, rheumatic joints with pain, heat and inflammation, sore sprained or strained muscles, concussion, and osteoarthritis. Taken internally, it is a remedy for black eyes, eye strain, skin conditions such as eczema and boils. Arnica is helpful in the treatment of whooping cough in children and also wetting the bed when the cause is nightmares. Symptoms are made worse with heat, touch and continued movement, and also with heat and resting for a long period. The symptoms improve when the person first begins to move and with lying down with the head at a lower level than the feet. A person suitable for this remedy tends to be solemn, fatalistic and subject to morbid fears. Arnica types usually deny the existence of any illness, even when obviously not well, and do not seek medical help, preferring to manage on their own.

Arsenicum album
Arsen. alb.; white arsenic trioxide

This is a widely used homeopathic remedy, the source being white arsenic trioxide derived from arsenopyrite, a metallic mineral ore of arsenic. Arsenic has been known for centuries as a poison and was once used as a treatment for syphilis. White arsenic trioxide used to be given to improve muscles and skin in animals such as horses. It is used to treat acute conditions of the digestive system and chest and mental symptoms of anxiety and fear. Hence it is a remedy for diarrhoea and vomiting caused by eating the wrong kinds of food, or food poisoning or overindulgence in alcohol. Also, for dehydration in children following gastroenteritis or feverish illness. It is a remedy for asthma and breathing difficulty, mouth ulcers, carbuncle (a collection of boils), dry, cracked lips, burning skin, inflamed, watering stinging eyes and psoriasis. Also, for sciatica, shingles, sore throat and painful swallowing, candidiasis (fungal infection) of the mouth and motion sickness. There may be oedema (retention of fluid) showing as a puffiness around the ankles.

An ill person who benefits from Arsen. alb. experiences burning pains but also feels cold. The skin may be either hot or cold to the touch. The symptoms are worse with cold in any form, including cold food and drink, and between midnight and 3 a.m. They are worse on the right side and if the person is near the coast. Symptoms improve with warmth, including warm drinks, gentle movement and lying down with the head raised. People suitable for Arsen. alb. are precise, meticulous and ambitious and loathe any form of disorder. They are always immaculately dressed and everything in their life is neat and tidy. However, they tend to have great worries, especially about their financial security and their own health and that of their family. They fear illness and dying, loss of financial and personal status, being burgled, darkness and the supernatural. Arsen. alb. people have strongly held views and do not readily tolerate contrary opinions or those with a more relaxed or disordered lifestyle. They enjoy a variety of different foods, coffee and alcoholic drinks. They are usually thin, with delicate, fine features and pale skin that may show worry lines. Their movements tend to be rapid and their manner serious and somewhat restless, although always polite.

Atropa belladonna

Belladonna, deadly nightshade, black cherry, devil's cherries, naughty man's cherries, devil's herb

Belladonna is a native plant of most of Europe although it is uncommon in Scotland. The plant is extremely poisonous, and many children have died as a result of being tempted to eat the shiny black berries of deadly nightshade. It is a stout, stocky plant with light brown roots, growing to about four feet high, with green oval leaves and pale purple, bell-shaped flowers. In medieval times, the plant had its place in the potions of witchcraft. Italian women used extracts of the plant as eye drops to widen the pupils of the eye and make them more beautiful (hence *bella donna*, which means 'beautiful woman'). The plant contains atropine, an alkaloid substance that induces paralysis of nerves and is used in orthodox medicine to relieve painful spasms and in ophthalmic (eye) procedures.

In homeopathy, the remedy is obtained from the pulped leaves and flowers. It was investigated and proved by Hahnemann as a treatment for scarlet fever. Belladonna is used to treat acute conditions that arise suddenly in which there is a throbbing, pulsing headache and red, flushed skin, high fever and staring wide eyes. The skin around the mouth and lips may be pale, but the tongue is a fiery red and the hands and feet are cold. It is used as a remedy for infectious diseases such as influenza, scarlet fever, measles, whooping cough, chicken pox, mumps and the early stages of pneumonia. Also for boils, earache (particularly on the right side and worse when the head is cold or wet), cystitis, boils, conjunctivitis, tonsillitis, inflammation of the kidneys, neuralgia (sharp pain along the course of a nerve) and sore throat. Other conditions that benefit from this remedy include labour pains, soreness of the breasts in breast-feeding, fever and teething in children, with broken sleep and whitlow (an infection of a fingernail). The symptoms are worse at night and with lying down, and occur more intensely on the right side. Also, they are exacerbated by loud noises, bright lights, jarring of the body, touch or pressure and with cool surroundings.

They improve with sitting upright or standing and keeping warm or warm applications to the painful area. People suitable for belladonna usually enjoy good health, being fit, energetic and ready to tackle any task. They are amusing, sociable and popular when in good health. However, if they become ill the reverse is often true and they may be restless, irritable and possibly even violent.

Aurum metallicum
Aurum met.; gold

Gold was highly prized by Arabian physicians in the early Middle Ages who used it to treat heart disorders. In the early part of this century, it was used in the treatment of tuberculosis. Gold is now used in conventional medicine for some cancer treatments and for rheumatic and arthritic complaints. In homeopathy, pure gold is ground down to produce a fine powder, and it is used to treat both physical and mental symptoms. It is used as a remedy for congestive circulatory disorders and heart diseases including angina pectoris. The symptoms include a throbbing, pulsing headache, chest pain, breathlessness and palpitations. It is also used to treat liver disorders with symptoms of jaundice, painful conditions of bones and joints (especially the hip and knee), inflammation of the testes and an undescended testicle in small boys (especially if the right side is affected). It is a remedy for sinusitis and severe mental symptoms of despair, depression and thoughts of suicide. The person who is suitable for this remedy tends to drive himself very hard to the point of being a workaholic. He (or she) is excessively conscientious but usually feels that he has not done enough and is oversensitive to the criticism of other people. The person may come to regard himself as a failure and become severely clinically depressed or even suicidal. Symptoms are made worse by mental effort and concentration, or physical exercise, especially in the evening or night and by emotional upheaval. They improve with cold bathing, walking in the fresh air and with rest and quiet.

Bryonia alba
Bryonia, European white bryony, black-berried white bryony, wild hops

Bryony is a native plant of many parts of Europe and grows in England, although it is rarely found in Scotland. It has large, white, branched roots with swollen, expanded portions that are highly poisonous. The smell given off is unpleasant and, if eaten, the taste is very bitter and death soon follows. The tall stems of the plant climb up supports by means of corkscrew tendrils and round black berries are produced in the autumn. Bryony was used by the physicians of ancient Greece and Rome and was described by Hippocrates. The homeopathic remedy is made from the fresh pulped root of the plant, and is mainly used for conditions producing acute stitch-like pains, which are made worse by even slight movement and relieved by rest. These ailments usually develop slowly and accompanying symptoms include dry skin, mouth and eyes with great thirst. It is used as a remedy for inflammation of the lining of joints in arthritic and rheumatic disorders with swelling, heat and pains. Also, for chest inflammation, pleurisy, chesty bronchitis and pneumonia with severe pain and dry, hacking cough. Digestive problems that are eased by Bryonia include indigestion, colic, constipation, nausea, vomiting and diarrhoea. Breast inflammation because of breast-feeding, colic in babies, gout and lumbago may be helped by Bryonia. The symptoms are made worse by movement and bending and improve with rest and pressure applied to the painful area. People suitable for Bryonia are hard-working, conscientious and reliable but have a dread of poverty. They tend to measure success in life in financial or materialistic terms. They cope badly with any threat to their security or lifestyle, becoming extremely worried, fretful and depressed.

Calcerea carbonica
Calc. carb.; calcium carbonate
This important homeopathic remedy is made from powdered mother-of-pearl, the beautiful, translucent inner layer of oyster shells. Calcium is an essential mineral in the body, being especially important for the healthy development of bones and teeth. The Calc. carb. remedy is used to treat a number of different disorders, especially those relating to bones and teeth, and also certain skin conditions and symptoms relating to the female reproductive system. It is a remedy for weak or slow growth of bones and teeth and fractures that take a long time to heal. Also, for teething problems in children, pains in bones, teeth and joints, headaches and eye inflammations affecting the right side, and ear infections with an unpleasant-smelling discharge. Premenstrual syndrome, heavy periods and menopausal disorders are helped by Calc. carb., and also chapped skin and eczema.

Calc. carb. may be used as a remedy for verruca (a type of wart) and thrush infections. People who benefit from Calc. carb. are very sensitive to the cold, particularly in the hands and feet and tend to sweat profusely. They suffer from fatigue and anxiety, and body secretions (sweat and urine) smell unpleasant. Children who benefit from Calc. carb. have recurrent ear, nose and throat infections, especially tonsillitis and glue ear. Symptoms are made worse by draughts and cold, damp weather and also at night. They are worse when the person first wakens up in the morning and for physical exercise and sweating. In women, symptoms are worse premenstrually. They improve in warm, dry weather and are better later on in the morning and after the person has eaten breakfast. People suitable for Calc. carb. are often overweight or even obese with a pale complexion. They are shy and very sensitive, quiet in company and always worried about what other people think of them. Calc. carb. people are hard-working, conscientious and reliable and easily upset by the suffering of others. They need constant reassurance from friends and family and tend to feel that they are a failure. Usually, Calc. carb. people enjoy good health but have a tendency for skeletal weakness. They enjoy a wide variety of different foods and tend to overeat, but are upset by coffee and milk. They are afraid of dying and serious illness, the supernatural, madness, being a failure and becoming poor, and they tend to be claustrophobic.

Calcarea fluorica

Calc. fluor.; fluorite, calcium fluoride, fluoride of lime

This homeopathic remedy is one of the Schussler tissue salts (*see* GLOSSARY). Calcium fluoride occurs naturally in the body in the enamel of the teeth, bones, skin and connective tissue. It is used to treat disorders of these body tissues or to maintain their elasticity. It is used to treat chronic lumbago, scars, and to prevent the formation of adhesions after operations, gout and arthritic nodules. Also, for rickets, slow growth of bones in children, enlarged adenoids that become stony because of persistent, recurrent respiratory tract infections and cataracts. It is used to strengthen weak tooth enamel and strained and stretched ligaments and muscles, e.g. around a joint. People suitable for Calc. fluor. are intelligent and punctual but tend to make mistakes through lack of planning. They benefit from the guidance of others to work efficiently and fear poverty and illness. They are often prone to piles, varicose veins, swollen glands and muscle and ligament strain. The manner of walking may be rapid with jerking of the limbs. Symptoms are made worse on beginning movement and in cold, damp, draughty conditions. They improve with warmth and heat and for continual gentle movement.

Calcarea phosphorica

Calc. phos., phosphate of lime, calcium phosphate

This homeopathic remedy is a SCHUSSLER TISSUE SALT (*see* Glossary) and

Calendula officinalis

calcium phosphate is the mineral that gives hardness to bones and teeth. It is obtained by a chemical reaction between dilute phosphoric acid and calcium hydroxide, when a white precipitate of calcium phosphate is formed. Since calcium phosphate is an essential mineral in the normal, healthy development of bones and teeth, it is used to treat disorders in these tissues. It is particularly helpful as a remedy for painful bones, difficult fractures that are slow to heal, teeth prone to decay, problems of bone growth and teething in children and 'growing pains'. Also, it is beneficial during convalescence when a person is weakened and tired after an illness, and for digestive problems including diarrhoea, stomach pains and indigestion. It may be used as a remedy for tonsillitis, sore throats and swollen glands. Children who benefit from this remedy tend to be thin, pale, miserable and fail to thrive, and are prone to sickness and headaches. They are often fretful and demanding. Adults are also unhappy and discontented with their circumstances, although endeavour to be friendly towards others. They are restless and need plenty of different activities and stimulation, hating routine and needing a good reason to get out of bed in the morning. Symptoms are made worse by any change in the weather, and in cold, wet conditions, e.g. thawing snow. Also for worry or grief and too much physical activity. Symptoms improve when the weather is warm and dry, in summer, and from taking a hot bath.

Calendula officinalis
Calendula, marigold, garden marigold, marygold
This is a familiar garden plant that grows well in all parts of the United Kingdom, having light green leaves and bright orange flowers. The plant has been known for centuries for its healing properties and was used in the treatment of various ailments. The parts used in homeopathy are the leaves and flowers, and the remedy is of value in first aid for its antiseptic and anti-inflammatory activity. It is used in the treatment of boils, stings, cuts and wounds, and to stem bleeding, often in the form of an ointment that can be applied to broken skin. It is helpful when applied to skin tears following childbirth. It is used in the form of an antiseptic tincture as a mouth wash and gargle after tooth extraction, for mouth ulcers or a septic sore throat. When taken internally it prevents suppuration (pus formation) and may be used for persistent chronic ulcers and varicose ulcers, fever and jaundice. It is a useful remedy in the treatment of children's ailments. The symptoms are made worse in damp, draughty conditions and cloudy weather and after eating. They improve with walking about and lying absolutely still.

Cantharis vesicatoria
Cantharis, Spanish fly

This remedy is derived from the body and wings of a bright green iridescent beetle that is found mainly in the southern parts of Spain and France. The beetle, *Cantharis vesicatoria*, secretes a substance called canthardin, which has irritant properties, is also poisonous and is an ancient remedy to cure warts. It was also used as an aphrodisiac, reputedly by the notorious Maquis de Sade. The beetles are dried and ground to produce a powder that is then used in homeopathy. It is an irritant, blistering agent acting externally on the part of the body to which it is applied and internally on the bladder, urinary tract and genital organs. Hence it is used to treat conditions in which there are stinging and burning pains. An accompanying symptom is often a great thirst but a reluctance to drink. It is used to treat cystitis with cutting hot pains on passing urine, urinary frequency with pain and other urinary infections. Also, certain inflammations of the digestive system in which there is abdominal distension and burning pains and diarrhoea. In general it is used as a remedy for conditions that worsen rapidly. It is a remedy for burns and scalds of the skin, including sunburn, insect stings, and rashes with spots that contain pus. Some mental symptoms are eased by Cantharis, including angry and irritable or violent behaviour, extreme anxiety and excessive sexual appetite. Symptoms are made worse with movement, touch and after drinking coffee or chilled water. They improve when gastro-intestinal wind is eliminated and with warmth, at night time and with very light massage.

Carbo vegetabilis
Carbo veg., vegetable charcoal

The homeopathic remedy Carbo veg. is made from charcoal, which itself is obtained from heating or partially burning wood without oxygen. The charcoal is hard and black or dark grey, and is a form of carbon that is present in all living things. Charcoal has been made for centuries, and usually silver birch, beech or poplar trees are the source of wood that is used. The homeopathic remedy is used to treat a person who is run down, weak or exhausted, especially after a debilitating illness or operation. It is also used for postoperative shock, when there is a clammy, cold, pale skin but the person feels a sensation of heat or burning inside. It is helpful as a remedy for ailments of poor circulation such as varicose veins. Again, the skin tends to be pale, clammy and chilly with a bluish colour and the extremities feel cold. The legs may be puffy, and additional symptoms include hoarseness and laryngitis and lack of energy. Carbo veg. is a useful remedy for digestive problems, and carbon is also used for this purpose in orthodox medicine. Symptoms are those of indigestion, heartburn and flatulence with a sour taste in the mouth. Morning headaches with accompanying symptoms of nausea and giddiness or fainting may be relieved by Carbo veg., particularly if the cause is a large, heavy meal the night before. People suitable for this remedy often complain of a lack of energy and may indeed be physically and mentally exhausted, with poor powers of concentration and lapses of memory. They usually have fixed attitudes, with a lack of interest in news of the wider world. They do not like the night and are fearful of the supernatural. Symptoms are made worse by warm, moist weather, in the evening and night, and with lying down. They are also exacerbated after eating meals of fatty foods, coffee and milk and drinks of wine. They improve with burping and with circulating cool, fresh air.

Chamomilla
Chamomile, common chamomile, double chamomile

A creeping and trailing plant that produces daisy-like flowers in summer and prefers dry, sandy soils. Chamomiles are native to Britain and others part of northern Europe and have been used in medicine since ancient times, being described by Hippocrates. When walked on, it gives off an aromatic perfume and was gathered and strewn on the floor in medieval dwellings to counter unpleasant odours. It is prized for its many medicinal uses, the flowers and leaves both being used for a number of different ailments. Herbalists use chamomile to treat skin conditions such as eczema, and for asthma and disturbed sleep. In homeopathy, it is used for its soothing and sedative effect on all conditions producing restlessness, irritability and pains. It is a useful remedy for children's complaints such as teething where the child is fretful and cries if put down, colicky pains and disturbed sleep. Also, for toothache, when one cheek is red and the other white, that is exacerbated by heat and relieved by cold. It is used to treat a blocked ear and earache, painful, heavy periods and soreness and inflammation associated with breast-feeding. People suitable for this remedy are very sensitive to pain, which causes sweating or fainting, especially in children and women. They are irritable and fretful when ill. Symptoms are made worse if the person becomes angry or in cold winds and the open air. They improve if the person fasts for a time and if the weather is wet and warm. People who are suitable for chamomile are noisy sleepers, in that they frequently cry out or talk while dreaming. If woken suddenly from sleep they are extremely irritable and they like to poke their feet out from the bed covers to keep them cool.

Chincona officinalis
Cinchona succirubra; china, Peruvian bark, Jesuit's bark

This homeopathic remedy, known as china, is obtained from the dried bark of the cinchona tree and contains quinine. The attractive evergreen cinchona, with its red bark, is a native of the hot tropical forests of South America, but it is also cultivated in India, Sri Lanka and southeast Asia. A preparation of powdered bark was used to treat a feverish illness suffered by the Countess of Cinchon, wife of the viceroy of Peru in 1638. After her recovery she publicized the remedy, and the tree was called cinchona from this time. The value of the bark as a cure for malaria had long been known and used by Jesuit priests. This was the first homeopathic substance tested and proved by Hahnemann on himself.

In modern homeopathy it is used mainly as a remedy for nervous and physical exhaustion resulting from chronic debilitating illnesses. It is used for weakness because of dehydration, sweating, chills and fever, and headaches that are relieved if firm pressure is applied. The person wants drinks during periods of chills and shivering rather than when feverish and hot. He or she usually has a washed-out unhealthy complexion with very sensitive skin. China is also used as a remedy for neuralgia, muscles that twitch because of extreme fatigue, bleeding, including nosebleeds, and tinnitus (noises in the ears). It has a helpful effect on the digestion and is used to treat gastro-intestinal upset and gall bladder. Some mental symptoms are helped by this remedy, including irritability and tetchy behaviour that is out of character, apathy and loss of concentration and sleeplessness.

People who are suitable for this remedy tend to be artistic, imaginative and highly strung. They find it easier to empathize with the natural world rather than with the people around them. They are intense and dislike trivial conversation and fatty foods such as butter, but have a liking for alcoholic drinks. Their nature makes them prone to irritability and depression, and they tend to draw up grand schemes at night that are later abandoned. Symptoms are made better by warmth and plenty of sleep and by the application of steady continuous pressure to a painful area. They are made worse by cold, draughty weather, particularly in the autumn, and in the evening and night.

Citrullus colocynthis
Colocynth; bitter cucumber, bitter apple

The plant *Citrullus colocynthis* is a native of Turkey and is also found in parts of Asia and Africa, flourishing in dry, arid conditions. It produces yellow flowers and then yellow-orange smooth fruits, about the size of a large apple, which contain many seeds embedded in a whitish pulp. The homeopathic remedy colocynth is obtained from the dried fruits from which the seeds have been removed. This is then ground down to produce a powder. The fruit itself is poisonous, having a violent irritant effect on the digestive tract, causing severe, cramp-like pains, inflammation and bleeding. This is caused by the presence of a substance called colocynthin. According to tradition, Elisha, the Old Testament prophet, is said to have performed a miraculous transformation of the fruit during the famine in Gilgal, making it fit for the people to eat. In homeopathy, colocynth is used to treat colicky abdominal pains that may be accompanied by sickness and diarrhoea (including colic in young babies). Also, for neuralgia, especially of the face, sciatica, ovarian or kidney pain because of nerves, rheumatic disorders and headache.

People who are helped by colocynth are often reserved, with a tendency to bottle up anger. They have strong opinions about what is right and wrong, and may become quite agitated if someone else has a contrary viewpoint. Physical symptoms of colicky pains or neuralgia and upset stomach may follow on from becoming upset or angry. The symptoms are made worse when the person becomes irritated or angry and in cold, damp weather conditions. Also, eating meals and drinking exacerbate the symptoms. They are relieved by warmth and pressure on the painful part and drinking coffee. Abdominal flatulence also relieves the symptoms.

Cuprum metallicum
Cuprum met.; copper

Copper ore, which is found in rocks in many parts of the world, has been mined and used for many centuries in the manufacture of weapons, utensils and jewellery, etc. In earlier times, physicians made an ointment from the ground metal and this was applied to raw wounds to aid healing. Copper is poisonous in large doses affecting the nervous system and causing convulsions, paralysis and possibly death because of its effects upon respiratory muscles. Toxic effects were recognized in those who worked with the metal and who developed wasting because of poor absorption of food, coughs and respiratory symptoms, and colicky pains. The ruddy, gold-coloured metal is ground to produce a fine red powder that is used in homeopathy to treat cramping, colicky pains in the abdomen, and muscular spasms in the calves of the legs, feet and ankles. It is also used as a remedy for epilepsy and problems of breathing and respiration such as asthma, croup and whooping cough in which there are spasms. The person may turn blue because of the effort of breathing.

The symptoms are made worse by touch, hot, sunny weather and for keeping emotions bottled up. They improve with sweating and drinking cold fluids. People who benefit from Cuprum met. have mood swings that alternate from stubbornness to passivity, weepiness and depression. They tend to be serious people who judge themselves severely and keep their emotions very much suppressed. As babies or toddlers, they may be breath-holders who turn blue with anger or as a result of a tantrum. As children, some are destructive and others are loners who dislike the company of others.

Daphne mezereum
Daphne, spurge laurel, wild pepper, spurge olive, flowering spurge, dwarf bay

This poisonous plant is native to upland areas of Europe and is cultivated in the United Kingdom. It produces cheerful bright-red flowers and dark green leaves, and the bark is the part used in homeopathy. It is used to treat skin conditions characterized by blistering, especially erysipelas, shingles and varicose ulcers. Also, for any condition in which there is a persistent, dry cough and tightness around the chest and a mucus discharge from the nose. There may be burning pains that are worse at night.

Drosera rotundifolia
Drosera, sundew, youthwort, red rot, moor grass

This small, carnivorous (insect-eating) plant is found widely throughout Europe and in Britain, where it grows in the poor, acidic soils of bogs, damp uplands, moorlands and woodlands. It is a small plant growing close to the ground, and needs to trap insects for extra nutrients as the soil in which it grows is so poor. It is remarkable for its leaves, which are covered with long red hairs, each with a small, fluid-containing gland at the top. When the sun shines on the leaves it resembles dew, hence the name sundew. An insect landing on the leaf is trapped because this curls over and inwards, and the sticky fluid secreted by the hairs holds it fast. The secretion contains enzymes that digest the body and the nutrients are absorbed by the plant. The small, white flowers of sundew are fully open in the early morning but close up when the sun is shining strongly. In medieval times, the plant was used to treat tuberculosis and the plague, and it was employed as a remedy for skin disorders in early Asian medicine. It was noticed that sheep who inadvertently cropped sundew developed a paroxysmal type of cough like whooping cough. It was investigated and proved as a remedy for this illness in homeopathy, and the whole plant is used to prepare the medicine. Any condition in which there is a violent, dry, persistent barking cough of a spasmodic nature, as in whooping cough, benefits from the use of sundew, which has a particular action on the upper respiratory tract. Accompanying symptoms are gagging, sickness, sweating and nosebleeds. It is also used to treat bronchitis, asthma, corns and warts, growing pains and pains in the bones.

People who benefit from this remedy are restless and fearful of being alone when they are ill, and they tend to be stubborn and lack concentration. They are suspicious and may feel that others are talking about them or concealing bad news. They are sensitive to the supernatural and are afraid of ghosts. The symptoms are worse for being too warm in bed, after midnight, with crying, lying down, laughing, singing and talking. Also, for meals of cold food and drinks. Symptoms improve out in the fresh air, with walking or gentle exercise, sitting propped up in bed, with pressure applied to the painful part and in quiet surroundings.

Euphrasia officinalis
Euphrasia, eyebright

Eyebright is an attractive wild flower that is variable in size and grows widely throughout Europe, including Britain, and in North America. It has been known since medieval times as a remedy for inflammation of the eyes, and this remains its main use in homeopathy. The plant flourishes on well-drained, chalky soils and may be between two and eight inches in height, depending upon conditions. It is partly parasitic, deriving some nourishment from the roots of grass, and produces pretty white, purple-veined flowers with yellow centres. The whole plant and flowers are used in homeopathy, and the remedy is used to treat eye disorders characterized by redness, inflammation, watering, burning, stinging or itching. These include conjunctivitis, blepharitis (inflammation of eyelids), injuries to the eye and dry eyes. It is also used as a remedy for allergic conditions such as hay fever, in which the eyes are very much affected, and colds producing eye symptoms. It is a remedy for the early stages of measles, headaches, some menstrual problems and inflammation of the prostate gland in men. Symptoms are worse in the evening, in windy and warm weather and for being inside. They improve in subdued light, with drinking a cup of coffee and with cold applications.

Ferrum phosphoricum
Ferrum phos.; ferric phosphate of iron, iron phosphate

Ferrum phos. is one of the SCHUSSLER TISSUE SALTS (*see* GLOSSARY), and the iron phosphate powder is obtained by chemical reaction between sodium phosphate, sodium acetate and iron sulphate. Iron is a very important substance in the body, being found in the haemoglobin pigment of red blood cells that transports oxygen to all the tissues and organs. The homeopathic remedy is used to treat the early stages of infections, inflammations and feverish conditions, before any other particular symptoms occur. It is used to treat colds and coughs in which there may be a slowly developing fever, headache, nosebleeds, bronchitis, hoarseness and loss of the voice, earache and rheumatic pains. Digestive symptoms such as sour indigestion, inflammation of the stomach (gastritis), and vomiting and some disorders of menstruation are helped by this remedy. It is also used to treat the early symptoms of dysentery. The person tends to be pale but is prone to flushing, and feels cold in the early afternoon. There may be a rapid weak pulse. Symptoms are worse at night and in the early morning between 4 a.m. and 6 a.m. Also, they are worse for heat and hot sun, movement and jarring of the body, pressure and touch and resting on the right side and suppressing sweating by the use of deodorants, etc. Symptoms improve for cold applications and with gentle movements. People who are suitable for Ferrum phos. tend to be thin and pale but may be liable to flush easily. They are intelligent and quick to absorb new concepts, having plenty of original ideas of their own. They may be prone to digestive and respiratory complaints, stomach upsets and coughs and colds.

Gelsemium sempervirens
Gelsemium, yellow jasmine, false jasmine, Carolina jasmine, wild woodbine
This attractive climbing plant is a native of the southern United States and parts of Mexico. It has a woody stem that twists around any available tree trunk, and grows on stream banks and on the sea coast. It produces attractive, large, bell-shaped, perfumed yellow flowers in the early spring, which belie the poisonous nature of the plant. It has an underground stem, or rhizome, from which arise a tangle of yellow roots that have an aromatic smell. The root is the part used in homeopathy and, if eaten in significant amounts, it affects the central nervous system, causing paralysis and possible death through failure of the nerves and muscles of the respiratory system. In homeopathy it is used to treat both physical and mental symptoms. The physical ailments treated mainly involve the nervous and respiratory systems. These include headaches that are worsened with bright light and movement, multiple sclerosis, eye pain, especially on the right side, sore throat and influenza-like symptoms, earache and feverish muscular pains. Accompanying symptoms include chills and shivering,

Graphites

flushed face and malaise. It is used to treat some menstrual problems including pain. Mental symptoms that are helped by Gelsemium include fears and phobias with symptoms of fatigue, weakness, trembling and apprehension. These fears may arise before an examination, interview or public performance (stage fright). Excitement or fear that causes the heart to skip a beat and extreme anxiety causing sleeplessness are helped by Gelsemium. Symptoms are made worse in the sun and in warm, moist, humid weather or damp and fog. They are also worse with smoking and for excitement, anticipation, stress or bad news. Symptoms improve with movement in the fresh air and after sweating and drinking alcohol or a stimulant drink. They improve after urinating—a large quantity of pale urine is usually passed. People suitable for Gelsemium tend to be well-built with a blue-tinged skin and often complain of feeling weak and tired. They are beset by fears, and may be cowardly and too fearful to lead or enjoy a normal active life.

Graphites
Graphite; black pencil lead

Graphite is a form of carbon that is the basis of all life. It is found in older igneous or metamorphic rocks, such as granite and marble, and is mined for its industrial uses, e.g. in batteries, motors, pencil leads, cleaning and lubricating fluids. It was investigated and proved by Hahnemann after he learned that it was being used by some factory workers to heal cold sores. The powder used in homeopathy is ground graphite, and it is mainly used for skin disorders that may be caused by metabolic imbalances and stomach ulcers. It is a remedy for eczema, psoriasis, acne, rough, dry skin conditions with pustules or blisters, scarring and thickened cracked nails and cold sores. Also, for stomach ulcers caused by a thinning or weakness in the lining of the stomach wall, problems caused by excessive catarrh, loss of hair, and cramping pains or numbing of the feet and hands. In women it is used to treat some menstrual problems. The symptoms are worse in draughty, cold and damp conditions and for eating sweet meals or sea foods. Also, the use of steroids for skin complaints and, in women, during menstruation. Symptoms are often worse on the left side. They improve with warmth as long as the air is fresh and it is not stuffy, when it is dark and for eating and sleep. People suitable for Graphites are usually well-built and may be overweight, often having dark hair. They like to eat well but lack physical fitness, and sweat or flush with slight exertion. They are prone to dry, flaky skin conditions that may affect the scalp. Graphites people are usually lethargic and may be irritable, lacking in concentration for intellectual activities. They are prone to mood swings and subject to bouts of weeping, especially when listening to music. A Graphites person feels that he or she is unlucky and is inclined to self-pity, often feeling fearful and timid.

Guaiacum officinale
Guaiac, resin of lignum vitae
This attractive evergreen tree is a native of the West Indies and the northern coastal regions of South America. The tree grows to a height of 40-60 feet and produces striking, deep blue flowers. The part used in homeopathy is a resin obtained from the wood. The wood is unusual in being very dense, which means that it sinks in water, and this property caused much interest when it was first discovered in the Middle Ages. The resin is obtained by firing the cut log, and the melted resin then flows out of a hole made in the wood and is collected. This is allowed to cool and harden, and it is usually exported in large blocks that split readily into glassy fragments. The remedy is used to treat inflammation of the pharynx (pharyngitis) and tonsillitis, being very helpful in relieving painful soreness of the throat. It is particularly indicated where there is foul-smelling sputum and sweating. It is also a remedy for gout and rheumatic conditions with severe and stabbing joint pains. The symptoms are made worse by extremes of heat and cold and damp weather, and also with movement. They may be relieved by rest and keeping warm.

Hamamelis virginiana
Hamamelis, witch hazel, spotted alder, snapping hazelnut, winterbloom
This plant is a native of the eastern United States and Canada but it is also grown in Europe. It is a shrub with grey-green leaves and yellow flowers that appear in the autumn. The part used in homeopathy is the bark of stems and twigs and the outer part of the fresh root. This has the effect of causing body tissues, especially blood vessels, to contract, and it is used to arrest bleeding. Its curative properties were known to the native North American Indians, and it was first investigated and proved in homeopathy by Dr Hering. Its main effect is on the blood circulation of the veins, particularly when the walls of the vessels are inflamed and weakened, and bleeding does not stop easily. It is used as a remedy for haemorrhoids, or piles with bleeding, varicose veins and ulcers, phlebitis (inflamed veins), nosebleeds, heavy periods, internal bleeding and pain associated with bruising or bleeding. Some headaches are helped by Hamamelis and, also, mental symptoms of depression, irritability and impatience. The symptoms

are made worse by warmth and moisture and with physical activity. They improve out in the fresh air and for concentrating on a particular task or event and for conversation, thinking and reading.

Hepar sulphuris calcareum
Hepar sulph.; sulphide of calcium

This remedy is impure calcium sulphide, which is obtained by heating crushed and powdered oyster shells with flowers of sulphur. This is an old remedy that was, at one time, applied externally to treat swellings caused by tuberculosis, gout, rheumatism and thyroid disorders (goitre) and also itching skin. It was investigated and proved by Hahnemann as a remedy for the toxic effects of mercury, which was widely used by contemporary physicians. It is now used to treat infections and any condition where there is a discharge of foul-smelling pus. It is used to treat skin conditions where the skin is highly sensitive to touch, such as boils and acne, and also, tonsillitis, sinusitis, earache, sore throat, hoarseness and laryngitis, mouth ulcers and cold sores. A wheezing, croup-like type of cough or chesty cough that may develop into a cold or influenza is helped by Hepar sulph. This remedy helps those who, when ill, tend to produce bodily secretions that have an unpleasant sour smell. During illness, those who benefit from this remedy are irritable, difficult to please and easily offended. They are difficult patients who make unreasonable demands and hate noise or disturbance, being touched or cold air. Symptoms are worse for cold and for getting chilled when undressing during winter and for touch. They improve with warmth and warm applications and for covering the head and for eating a meal. People suitable for Hepar sulph. tend to be overweight, lethargic, with pale skin and often depressed. They feel that life has dealt with them harshly and feel the symptoms of illness and pain acutely. They may appear to be calm but tend to be anxious and restless.

Hypericum perforatum
Hypericum, St John's wort

A perennial herbaceous plant that is a native of Britain, Europe and Asia, but is cultivated throughout the world. It grows between one and three feet in height, producing elongated, oval dark green leaves that appear to be covered in minute spots or holes (hence *perforatum*, or perforate). In fact, these are minute oil-secreting glands that secrete a bright red solution. The large, bright yellow flowers appear in June, July and August and have small black dots around the edges of the petals. The crushed flowers produce a blood-coloured juice that was used, in early times, to treat raw wounds. It was also believed that the plant could be hung up to ward off evil spirits (the name *Hypericum* being derived from the Greek, meaning 'over an apparition'). There are two traditions associated with the common name, St John's wort. One links the plant with 29 August, believed to be the anniversary of the execution of St John the Baptist. The other is that the plant is named after an ancient order of knights going back to the time of the Crusades, the knights of St John of Jerusalem.

The whole fresh green plant and flowers are used in homeopathy to produce the mother tincture. It is mainly used to treat damage to nerves and nerve pain following accidental injury. Typically, there are shooting, stabbing pains that radiate upwards, and it is indicated especially where there are many nerve endings concentrated in a particular part of the body, e.g. the fingers and toes. It is very effective in pains associated with the spinal nerves and spinal cord, concussion, head or eye injuries. It is also a remedy for wounds and lacerations producing stabbing pains indicating nerve damage, and accidental crushing injuries. It is useful for bites, stings, splinters and puncture wounds, toothache and pain following dental extractions. In addition, it is a treatment for asthma and some digestive complaints of indigestion, sickness and diarrhoea. It is sometimes helpful in the treatment of piles, or haemorrhoids, and some menstrual problems with accompanying headache. The symptoms are made worse by cold, damp or foggy weather, before a storm and getting chilled when undressing. Also for touch and for a close, stuffy atmosphere. Symptoms improve when the person remains still and tilts the head backwards.

Ignatia amara
Agnate; *Strychnos ignatii*, St Ignatius' bean

Ignatia amara is a large tree that is native to the Philippine Islands, China and the East Indies. The tree has many branches and twining stems and produces stalked white flowers. Later, seed pods are produced, each containing ten to twenty large, oval seeds, that are about one inch long and are embedded in pulp. The seeds are highly poisonous and contain strychnine, which affects the central nervous system. Similar active constituents and properties are found in nux vomica. The tree is named after the founder of the Jesuits, Ignatius Loyola (1491-1556), and Spanish priests belonging to this order brought the seeds to Europe during the 1600s. The homeopathic remedy is made from the powdered seeds and is used especially for emotional symptoms. It is used for grief, bereavement, shock and loss, particularly when a person is having difficulty coming to terms with his or her feelings and is inclined to suppress the natural responses.

Ipecacuanha

Accompanying symptoms include sleeplessness, anger and hysteria. Similar emotional and psychological problems are helped by this remedy, including anxiety and fear, especially of appearing too forward to others, a tendency to burst into fits of crying, self-doubt, pity and blame, and depression. Nervous tension headaches and digestive upsets, feverish symptoms, chills and pains in the abdomen may be helped by Ignatia. Some problems associated with menstruation, especially sharp pains or absence of periods are relieved by this remedy, as are conditions with changeable symptoms. These are worse in cold weather or conditions, with emotional trauma, being touched, for smoking and drinking coffee. They improve with warmth, moving about, eating, lying on the side or area that is painful and after passing urine.

The person for whom Ignatia is suitable is usually female and with a tendency towards harsh, self criticism and blame; she is usually a creative artistic person, highly sensitive but with a tendency to suppress the emotions. She is perceptive and intelligent but inclined to be hysterical and subject to erratic swings of mood. Typically, the person expects a high standard in those she loves. The person enjoys dairy products, bread and sour foods but sweets, alcoholic drinks and fruit upset her system. She is afraid of crowds, tends to be claustrophobic, and fears being burgled. Also, she is afraid of being hurt emotionally, and is very sensitive to pain. The person is usually dark-haired and of slim build with a worried expression and prone to sighing, yawning and excessive blinking.

Ipecacuanha

Ipecac.; *Cephaelis ipecacuanha*, *Psychotria ipecacuanha*, the ipecac plant

This plant is a native of South America, particularly Brazil, Bolivia and New Grenada. The plant contains the alkaloids emetine and cephaeline, and different varieties contain differing proportions of these alkaloids. The root is the part used in homeopathy, and the preparations may be in a number of different forms. It is used to treat conditions where the main symptoms are nausea and vomiting, which are intractable and persistent, e.g. motion sickness and morning sickness. It is also used as a remedy for bronchitis, breathlessness because of the presence of fluid in the lung, whooping cough and heart failure. The symptoms are made worse by cold weather and lying down, and after a meal of pork or veal. They improve in the fresh open air and while resting with the eyes shut.

Kalium bichromicum

Kali bich.; potassium dichromate, potassium bichromate

This substance has several uses in industry (e.g. in the preparations of dyes and in batteries) as well as its medicinal purposes. The crystals of potassium dichromate are bright orange and are prepared from a chemical reaction involving the addition of a solution of potassium chromate to an acid. It is used for discharges of mucus and disorders of the mucous membranes, particularly involving the vagina and genital and urinary tracts, throat, nose and stomach. The remedy is useful for catarrhal colds and sinusitis, feelings of fullness and pressure, headache, migraine and glue ear. Also, for joint and rheumatic disorders with pains that may move about or even disappear. People who benefit from this remedy are highly sensitive to cold and chills when ill, but also experience a worsening of symptoms in hot, sunny conditions. They tend to be people who adhere very closely to a regular routine and may be somewhat rigid and inflexible. They like everything to be done properly down to the smallest detail and are law-abiding, moral and conformist. Symptoms are worse during the summer and also in wet and chilly conditions. They are at their height in the early hours of the morning between 3 and 5 a.m., and also on first waking up. Drinking alcohol and becoming chilled while taking off clothes exacerbates the symptoms. They improve with moving around and after eating a meal. Also, symptoms improve with warmth and heat (but not hot sun) and after vomiting.

Kalium iodatum

Kali iod.; *Kali hydriodicum*, potassium iodide

This is prepared by chemical reaction from potassium hydroxide and iodine and is an old remedy for syphilis. It is recommended that potassium iodide should be added to animal feed concentrates and table salt to prevent deficiency in iodine. The homeopathic remedy is used to relieve catarrh in those who are prone to chesty conditions. It is also used to treat swollen glands, sore throats, sinusitis, hay fever and influenza-type infections. It is used to treat male prostate gland disorders. The symptoms tend to improve with movement and from being out in the fresh air. They are made worse by heat and touch and are at their most severe between two and five in the early morning. People who suit this remedy tend to be dogmatic, knowing exactly what they think about a particular subject. They may be irritable or bad-tempered and not easy to get along with. They have a preference for cool rather than warm or hot weather.

Kalium phosphoricum

Kali phos.; potassium phosphate, phosphate of potash

This remedy is one of the Schussler tissue salts (*see* Glossary), and it is obtained from a chemical reaction between dilute phosphoric acid and solution of potassium carbonate. Potassium carbonate is derived from potash, the white powder that is left when wood is burnt completely. Potassium is an essential element in the body, vital for the healthy functioning of nerve tissue. Kali phos. is used to treat mental and physical exhaustion and depression, particularly in young persons in whom it may have been caused by too much work or studying. Accompanying symptoms include jumping at noise or interruption and a desire to be alone. Also, there may be a pus-containing discharge from the bladder, vagina, bowels or lungs and extreme muscular fatigue. They may suffer from gnawing hunger pains, anxiety, insomnia, tremor and have a tendency to perspire on the face when excited or after a meal. People who are suitable for Kali phos. are usually extrovert, hold clearly formed ideas and are easily exhausted. They become distressed by bad news, including that which does not affect them directly, such as a disaster in another country. They tend to crave sweet foods and dislike bread. Symptoms are made worse by any anxiety, in cold, dry weather and in winter and on drinking cold drinks. Also, they are exacerbated by noise, conversation, touch and physical activity. Symptoms improve with heat, gentle exercise, in cloudy conditions and after eating.

Lachesis
Trigonocephalus lachesis, *Lachesis muta*, venom of the bushmaster or surukuku snake

This South African snake produces a deadly venom that may prove instantly fatal because of its effects upon the heart. The venom causes the blood to thin and flow more freely, hence increasing the likelihood of haemorrhage. Even a slight bite bleeds copiously with a risk of blood poisoning or septicaemia. The snake is a ferocious hunter, and its African name, surukuku, describes the sound it makes while in pursuit of prey. The properties of the venom were investigated by the eminent American homeopathic doctor Constantine Hering during the 1800s. He tested and proved the remedy on himself. It is effective in treating a variety of disorders, particularly those relating to the blood circulation and where there is a risk of blood poisoning, or septicaemia. It is used to treat varicose veins and problems of the circulation indicated by a bluish tinge to the skin. The remedy is useful for those suffering from a weak heart or angina, palpitations and an irregular, fast or weak pulse. There may be symptoms of chest pain and breathing difficulty. It is of great benefit in treating uterine problems, particularly premenstrual congestion and pain that is relieved once the period starts. It is also an excellent remedy for menopausal symptoms, especially hot flushes, and for infections of the bladder and rectum. It is used to treat conditions and infections where symptoms are mainly on the left side, such as headache or stroke. Also, as a treatment for sore throats and throat infections, tonsillitis, lung abscess, boils, ulcers, wounds that heal slowly, vomiting because of appendicitis and digestive disorders, fevers with chills and shivering, nosebleeds and bleeding piles.

It is used to treat severe symptoms of measles and serious infections including scarlet fever and smallpox. Symptoms are made worse by touch and after sleep and by tight clothing. They are worse for hot drinks and baths, exposure to hot sun or direct heat in any form. For women, symptoms are worse during the menopause. They improve for being out in the fresh air and drinking cold drinks and for release of normal bodily discharges. People suitable for Lachesis tend to be intelligent, creative, intense and ambitious. They have strong views about politics and world affairs and may be impatient of the views of others. They may be somewhat self-centred, possessive and jealous, which can cause problems in close relationships with others. They dislike being tied down and so may be reluctant to commit themselves to a relationship. Lachesis people have a liking for sour pickled foods, bread, rice and oysters and alcoholic drinks. They like coffee, but hot drinks and wheat-based food tends to upset them. They have a fear of water, people they do not know, being burgled and of dying or being suffocated. Lachesis people may be somewhat overweight and are sometimes red-haired and freckled. Alternatively, they may be thin and dark-haired, pale and with a lot of energy. Children tend to be somewhat jealous of others and possessive of their friends, which can lead to naughty or trying behaviour.

Ledum palustre
Ledum; marsh tea, wild rosemary

Wild rosemary is an evergreen shrub that grows in the bogs and cold upland conditions of the northern United States, Canada and northern Europe, especially Scandinavia, Ireland and parts of Asia. The bush produces elongated, dark green leaves, about one or two inches long, that are smooth and shiny on the upper surface but underneath are covered with brown woolly hairs. ('Ledum' is derived from the Greek word *ledos*, meaning 'woolly robe'). The leaves contain a volatile, aromatic oil like camphor, and the plant has been used for centuries by Scandinavian people to repel insects, moths and mice. The plant produces attractive white flowers and is valued for its antiseptic properties. The fresh parts of the plant are gathered, dried and ground to make a powder used in homeopathy, and it is a valuable first aid remedy. It is taken internally for animal bites, insect stings, lacerations and wounds in which there is bruising and sharp stabbing pains. There is usually inflammation, redness, swelling and throbbing accompanied by feverish symptoms of chills and shivering. It is additionally used as a remedy for gout in the big toe, rheumatic pains in the feet that radiate upwards, hot, painful, stiff joints and tendons but with cold skin. People who benefit from this remedy tend to get hot and sweaty at night when ill, and usually throw off the bed coverings. They often have itchy skin on the feet and ankles and have a tendency to sprain their ankles. When ill, they are irritable and hard to please or may be withdrawn, and do not want the company of others. The symptoms are made worse by warmth or heat, touch and at night. They improve with cold applications to the painful part and for cool conditions.

Lycopodium clavatum
Lycopodium; club moss, wolf's claw, vegetable sulphur, stag's-horn moss, running pine

This plant is found throughout the northern hemisphere, in high moorlands, forests and mountains. The plant produces spore cases on the end of upright forked stalks, which contain the spores. These produce yellow dust or powder that is resistant to water and was once used as a coating on pills and tablets to keep them separate from one another. The powder was also used as a constituent of fireworks. It has been used medicinally for many centuries, as a remedy for digestive disorders and kidney stones in Arabian countries and in the treatment of gout. The powder and spores are collected by shaking the fresh, flowering stalks of the plant, and its main use in homeopathy is for digestive and kidney disorders. It is used to treat indigestion, heartburn, the effects of eating a large meal late at night, sickness, nausea, wind, bloatedness and constipation. Also, in men, for kidney stones, with the production of a red-coloured urine containing a sand-like sediment and enlarged prostate gland. It is used in the treatment of some problems of male impotence and bleeding haemorrhoids, or piles. Symptoms that occur on the right side are helped by Lycopodium, and the patient additionally tends to crave sweet, comfort foods. Nettle rash, psoriasis affecting the hands, fatigue because of illness and ME (myalgic encephalomyelitis), some types of headache, cough and sore throat are relieved by this remedy. It is used to relieve emotional states of anxiety, fear and apprehension caused by chronic insecurity or relating to forthcoming events, such as taking an examination or appearing in public (stage fright). Also, night terrors, sleeplessness, shouting or talking in the sleep and being frightened on first waking up can all benefit from this treatment.

The symptoms are worse between 4 p.m. and 8 p.m. and in warm, stuffy rooms and with wearing clothes that are too tight. They are also worse in the early morning between 4 a.m. and 8 a.m., for eating too much and during the spring. They improve outside in cool fresh air, after a hot meal or drink and with loosening tight clothing, with light exercise and at night. People suitable for Lycopodium tend to be serious, hard-working and intelligent, often in professional positions. They seem to be self-possessed and confident but are in reality rather insecure with a low self-opinion. They are impatient of what they perceive as being weakness and are not tolerant or sympathetic of illness. Lycopodium people are sociable but may keep their distance and not get involved; they may be sexually promiscuous. They have a great liking for sweet foods of all kinds and enjoy hot meals and drinks. They are easily filled but may carry on eating regardless of this and usually complain of symptoms on the right side. Lycopodium people are afraid of being left on their own, of failure in life, of crowds, darkness and the supernatural, and tend to be claustrophobic. They are often tall, thin and pale with receding hair or hair that turns grey early in life. They may be bald, with a forehead lined with worry lines and a serious appearance. They tend to have weak muscles and are easily tired after physical exercise. They may have a tendency to unconsciously twitch the muscles of the face and to flare the nostrils.

Mercurius solubilis
Merc. sol.; quicksilver

The mineral cinnabar, which is found in volcanic crystalline rocks, is an important ore of mercury and is extracted for a variety of uses, including dental fillings and in thermometers. Mercury is toxic in large doses, and an affected person produces great quantities of saliva and suffers repeated bouts of vomiting. Mercury has been used since ancient times and was once given as a remedy for syphilis. A powder of precipitate of mercury is obtained from dissolving liquid mercury in a dilute solution of nitric acid, and this is the source of the remedy used in homeopathy. It is used as a remedy for conditions that produce copious bodily secretions that often smell unpleasant, with accompanying symptoms of heat or burning and a great sensitivity to temperature. It is used as a remedy for fevers with profuse, unpleasant sweating, bad breath, inflammation of the gums, mouth ulcers, candidiasis (fungal infection) of the mouth, infected painful teeth and gums, and excessive production of saliva. Also, for a sore infected throat, tonsillitis, mumps, discharging infected ear, and a congested severe headache and pains in the joints. It is good for eye complaints, including severe conjunctivitis, allergic conditions with a running nose, skin complaints that produce pus-filled pustules, spots, and ulcers, including varicose ulcers. The symptoms are made worse by extremes of heat and cold and also by wet and rapidly changing weather. They are worse at night and for sweating and being too hot in bed.

Symptoms improve with rest and in comfortable temperatures where the person is neither too hot nor too cold. People suitable for Merc. sol. tend to be very insecure although they have an outwardly calm appearance. They are cautious and reserved with other people and consider what they are about to say before speaking so that conversation may seem laboured. Merc. sol. types do not like criticism of any kind and may suddenly become angry if someone disagrees with their point of view. They tend to be introverted, but their innermost thoughts may be in turmoil. They tend to be hungry and enjoy bread and butter, milk and other cold drinks but dislike alcohol with the exception of beer. They usually do not eat meat and do not have a sweet tooth. They dislike coffee and salt. Merc. sol. people often have fair hair with fine, unlined skin and an air of detachment. They are afraid of dying and of mental illness leading to insanity, and worry about the wellbeing of their family. They fear being burgled and are afraid or fearful during a thunderstorm.

Natrum muriaticum

Natrum mur.; common salt, sodium chloride

Salt has long been prized for its seasoning and preservative qualities, and Roman soldiers were once paid in salt, such was its value (the word 'salary' comes from the Latin word *salarium*, which refers to this practice). Sodium and chlorine are essential chemicals in the body, being needed for many metabolic processes, particularly the functioning of nerve tissue. In fact, there is seldom a need to add salt to food as usually enough is present naturally in a healthy, well-balanced diet. (An exception is when people are working very hard physically in a hot climate and losing a lot of salt in sweat). However, people and many other mammals frequently have a great liking for salt. If the salt/water balance in the body is disturbed, a person soon becomes very ill and may even die.

In ancient times, salt was usually obtained by boiling sea water, but natural evaporation around the shallow edges of salt lakes results in deposits of rock salt being formed. Rock salt is the usual source of table salt and also of the remedy used in homeopathy. This remedy has an effect on the functioning of the kidneys and the salt/water balance of body fluids, and is used to treat both mental and physical symptoms. Emotional symptoms that benefit from Natrum mur. include sensitivity and irritability, tearfulness and depression, suppressed grief and premenstrual tension. Physical ailments that respond to this remedy are often those in which there is a thin, watery discharge of mucus and in which symptoms are made worse by heat. Hence Natrum mur. is used in the treatment of colds with a runny nose or other catarrhal problems. Also, for some menstrual and vaginal problems, headaches and migraines, cold sores, candidiasis (fungal infection) of the mouth, mouth ulcers, inflamed and infected gums and bad breath. Some skin disorders are helped by Natrum mur., including verruca (a wart on the foot), warts, spots and boils, and cracked, dry lips. It may be used in the treatment of fluid retention with puffiness around the face, eyelids and abdomen, etc, urine retention, constipation, anal fissure, indigestion, anaemia and thyroid disorders (goitre). When ill, people who benefit from this remedy feel cold and shivery, but their symptoms are made worse, or even brought on, by heat. Heat, whether from hot sun and fire or a warm, stuffy room, exacerbate the symptoms, which also are made worse by cold and thundery weather. They are worse on the coast from the sea breeze, and in the morning between 9 and 11 o'clock. Too much physical activity and the sympathy of others exacerbate the symptoms. They improve in the fresh, open air and for cold applications or a cold bath or swim. Also, sleeping on a hard bed and sweating and fasting make the symptoms better. People suitable for Natrum mur. are often women who are highly sensitive, serious-minded, intelligent and reliable. They have high ideals and feel things very deeply, being easily hurt and stung by slights and criticism. They need the company of other people but, being so sensitive, can actually shun them for fear of being hurt. They are afraid of mental illness leading to loss of self-control and insanity, and of dying. Also, they fear the dark, failure in work, crowds, being burgled and have a tendency to be claustrophobic. They worry about being late and are fearful during a thunderstorm. Merc. sol. people tend to become introverted and react badly to the criticism of others. They are highly sensitive to the influence of music, which easily moves them to tears. Natrum mur. people are usually of squat or solid build with dark or fairish hair. They are prone to reddened, watery eyes as though they have been crying, and a cracked lower lip. The face may appear puffy and shiny with an air of stoicism.

Nux vomica

Strychnos nux vomica; poison nut, Quaker buttons

The *Strychnos nux vomica* tree is a native of India but also grows in Burma, Thailand, China and Australia. It produces small, greenish-white flowers and, later, apple-sized fruits, containing small, flat, circular pale seeds covered in fine hair. The seeds, bark and leaves are highly poisonous, containing strychnine, and have been used in medicine for many centuries. In medieval times, the seeds were used as a treatment for the plague. Strychnine has severe effects upon the nervous system but in minute amounts can help increase urination and aid digestion. The seeds are cleaned and dried and used to produce the homeopathic remedy. Nux vomica is used in the treatment of a variety of digestive complaints, including cramping, colicky abdominal pains, indigestion, nausea and vomiting, diarrhoea and constipation. Also, indigestion or stomach upset caused by overindulgence in alcohol or rich food and piles, which cause painful contractions of the rectum. Sometimes these complaints are brought on by a tendency to keep emotions, particularly anger, suppressed and not allowing it to show or be expressed outwardly. Nux vomica is a remedy for irritability, headache and migraine, colds, coughs and influenza-like symptoms of fever, aching bones and muscles and chills and shivering. It is a useful remedy for women who experience heavy, painful periods that may cause fainting, morning sickness during pregnancy and pain in labour. It is also used to treat urinary frequency and cystitis.

The type of person who benefits from this remedy is frequently under stress and experiences a periodic flare-up of symptoms. The person may be prone to indigestion and heartburn, gastritis and stomach ulcer, and piles, or haemorrhoids. The person usually has a tendency to keep everything bottled up but has a passionate nature and is liable to outbursts of anger. Nux vomica people are very ambitious and competitive, demanding a high standard of themselves and others and intolerant of anything less than perfection. They enjoy challenges and using their wits to keep one step ahead. Often they are to be found as managers, company directors, scientists, etc, at the cutting edge of their particular occupation. They are ungracious and irritable when ill and cannot abide the criticism of others. This type of person is afraid of being a failure at work and fears or dislikes crowded public places. He or she is afraid of dying. The person enjoys rich, fattening foods containing cholesterol and spicy meals, alcohol and coffee, although these upset the digestive system. Symptoms are worse in cold, windy, dry weather and in winter and in the early morning between 3 and 4 a.m. They are aggravated by certain noises, music, bright lights and touch, eating (especially spicy meals) and overwork of mental faculties. Nux vomica people usually look serious, tense and are thin with a worried expression. They have sallow skin and tend to have dark shadows beneath the eyes.

Phosphorus
Phos; white phosphorus

Phosphorus is an essential mineral in the body found in the genetic material (DNA), bones and teeth. White phosphorus is extremely flammable and poisonous and was once used in the manufacture of matches and fireworks. As it tends to catch fire spontaneously when exposed to air, it is stored under water. In the past it has been used to treat a number of disorders and infectious diseases such as measles. In homeopathy, the remedy is used to treat nervous tension caused by stress and worry, with symptoms of sleeplessness, exhaustion and digestive upset. Often there are pains of a burning nature in the chest or abdomen. It is a remedy for vomiting and nausea, heartburn, acid indigestion, stomach ulcer and gastroenteritis. It is also used to treat bleeding, e.g. from minor wounds, the gums, nosebleeds, gastric and profuse menstrual bleeding.

Severe coughs, which may be accompanied by retching, vomiting and production of a blood-tinged phlegm, are treated with Phos. as well as some other severe respiratory complaints. These include pneumonia, bronchitis, asthma and laryngitis. Styes that tend to recur and poor circulation may be helped by Phos. Symptoms are worse in the evening and morning and before or during a thunderstorm. They are also made worse for too much physical activity, hot food and drink and lying on the left side. Symptoms improve in the fresh open air and with lying on the back or right side. They are better after sleep or when the person is touched or stroked. People who need Phos. do not like to be alone when ill and improve with the sympathy and attention of others. They are warm, kind, affectionate people who are highly creative, imaginative and artistic. They enjoy the company of other people and need stimulation to give impetus to their ideas. Phos. people have an optimistic outlook, are full of enthusiasm but sometimes promise much and deliver little. They are very tactile and like to be touched or stroked and offered sympathy when unhappy or unwell. They enjoy a variety of different foods but tend to suffer from digestive upsets. Phos. people are usually tall, slim and may be dark or fair-haired, with an attractive, open appearance. They like to wear brightly coloured clothes and are usually popular. They have a fear of illness, especially cancer, and of dying and also of the dark and supernatural forces. They are apprehensive of water and fear being a failure in their work. Thunderstorms make them nervous.

Pulsatilla nigricans
Pulsatilla, *Anemone pratensis*, meadow anemone

This attractive plant closely resembles *Anemone pulsatilla*, the pasqueflower, which is used in herbal medicine but has smaller flowers. *Anemone pratensis* is a native of Germany, Denmark and Scandinavia and has been used medicinally for hundreds of years. The plant produces beautiful deep purple flowers with orange centres and both leaves and flowers are covered with fine, silky hairs. The whole fresh plant is gathered and made into a pulp, and liquid is extracted to make the homeopathic remedy. It is used to treat a wide variety of disorders with both physical and mental symptoms. It is useful for ailments in which there is a greenish, yellowish discharge. Hence it is used for colds and coughs and sinusitis with the production of profuse catarrh or phlegm. Also, eye infections with discharge such as styes and conjunctivitis. Digestive disorders are helped by it, particularly indigestion, heartburn, nausea and sickness caused by eating too much fatty or rich food. The remedy is helpful for female disorders in which there are a variety of physical and emotional symptoms. These include premenstrual tension, menstrual problems, menopausal symptoms and cystitis, with accompanying symptoms of mood swings, depression and tearfulness. It is a remedy for headaches and migraine, swollen glands, inflammation and pain in the bones and joints as in rheumatic and arthritic disorders, nosebleeds, varicose veins, mumps, measles, toothache, acne, frequent urination and incontinence.

Symptoms are worse at night or when it is hot, and after eating heavy, rich food. Symptoms improve out in the cool fresh air and for gentle exercise such as walking. The person feels better after crying and being treated sympathetically by others. Pulsatilla people are usually women who have a mild, passive nature and are kind, gentle and loving. They are easily moved to tears by the plight of others and love animals and people alike. The person yields easily to the requests and demands of others and is a peacemaker who likes to avoid a scene. An outburst of anger is very much out of character, and a Pulsatilla person usually has many friends. The person likes rich and sweet foods, although these may upset the digestion, and dislikes spicy meals. Pulsatilla people may fear darkness, being left alone, dying and any illness leading to insanity. They are fearful of crowds, the supernatural and tend to be claustrophobic. Usually, they are fair and blue-eyed with clear, delicate skin that blushes readily. They are attractive and slightly overweight or plump.

Rhus toxicodendron

Rhus tox.; *Rhus radicaris*, American poison ivy, poison oak, poison vine.
This large bush or small tree is a native species of the United States and
Canada. Its leaves are extremely irritant to the touch, causing an inflamed
and painful rash, swelling and ulceration. Often the person experiences
malaise, swollen glands, headache, feverishness and a lack of appetite.
The plant produces white flowers with a green or yellow tinge in June,
followed later by clusters of berries. The fresh leaves are gathered and
pulped to make the remedy used in homeopathy. It is used especially as a
treatment for skin rashes and lesions with hot, burning sensations and
also for inflammation of muscles and joints. Hence it is used to treat eczema, chilblains, cold sores, shingles, nappy rash and other conditions in
which there is a dry, scaling or blistered skin. Also, for rheumatism, sciatica, lumbago, gout, synovitis (inflammation of the synovial membranes
surrounding joints), osteoarthritis, ligament and tendon strains. Feverish
symptoms caused by viral infections, such as high temperature, chills and
shivering, swollen, watering eyes, aching joints, nausea and vomiting,
may be helped by Rhus tox. Some menstrual problems, including heavy
bleeding and abdominal pains that are relieved by lying down, benefit
from this remedy. People who are helped by Rhus tox tend to be depressed
and miserable when ill, with a tendency to burst into tears, and are highly
susceptible to cold, damp weather. Usually they have a dry, irritating cough
and thirst and are irritable, anxious and restless. The symptoms are made
worse in stormy, wet, windy weather and at night, and when the person
moves after a period of rest. Also, for becoming chilled when undressing.
Warm, dry conditions and gentle exercise improve and lessen the symptoms. Rhus tox people may be initially shy in company, but when they
lose this are charming, entertaining and lively and make friends easily.
They are usually conscientious and highly motivated and serious about
their work to the extent of being somewhat workaholic. Rhus tox people
often have an inner restlessness and become depressed and moody when
affected by illness. They may be prone to carry out small compulsive
rituals in order to function.

Ruta graveolens

Ruta grav.; rue, garden rue, herbygrass, ave-grace, herb-of-grace, bitter herb
This hardy, evergreen plant is a native of southern Europe but has been
cultivated in Britain for centuries, having been first brought here by the
Romans. It thrives in poor soil in a dry and partially shaded situation,
producing yellow-green flowers. The whole plant has a distinctive, pun-

Sepia officinalis

gent, unpleasant smell and was once used to repel insects, pestilence and infections. It has been used medicinally throughout history to treat ailments in both animals and people, and was used to guard against the plague. It was believed to be effective in guarding against witchcraft, and Hippocrates recommended it as an antidote to poisoning. Rue was believed to have beneficial effects on sight and was used by the great artists, such as Michelangelo, to keep vision sharp. In the Catholic High Mass, brushes made from rue were once used to sprinkle the holy water, hence the name herb-of-grace. Taken internally in large doses, rue has toxic effects causing vomiting, a swollen tongue, fits and delirium.

The homeopathic remedy is prepared from the sap of the green parts of the plant before the flowers open. It is indicated especially for bone and joint injuries and disorders, and those affecting tendons, ligaments and muscles where there is severe, deep, tearing pain. Hence it is used for synovitis (inflammation of the synovial membranes lining joints), rheumatism, sprains, strains, bruising, fractures and dislocations and also sciatica. Also, it is a useful remedy for eyestrain with tired, aching eyes, redness and inflammation and headache. Chest problems may be relieved by Ruta grav., particularly painful deep coughs, and some problems affecting the rectum, such as prolapse. Pain and infection in the socket of a tooth after dental extraction may be helped by this remedy. A person who is ill and who benefits from Ruta grav. tends to feel low, anxious, depressed and dissatisfied both with himself (or herself) and others. The symptoms are usually worse in cold, damp weather, for resting and lying down and for exercise out of doors. They improve with heat and gentle movement indoors.

Sepia officinalis
Sepia; ink of the cuttlefish
Cuttlefish ink has been used since ancient times, both for medicinal purposes and as a colour in artists' paint. The cuttlefish has the ability to change colour to blend in with its surroundings and squirts out the dark brown-black ink when threatened by predators. Sepia was known to Roman physicians who used it as a cure for baldness. In homeopathy it is mainly used as an excellent remedy for women experiencing menstrual and menopausal problems. It was investigated and proved by Hahnemann in 1834. It is used to treat premenstrual tension, menstrual pain and heavy bleeding, infrequent or suppressed periods, menopausal symptoms such as hot flushes, and postnatal depression. Physical and emotional symptoms caused by an imbalance of hormones are helped by Sepia. Also,

conditions in which there is extreme fatigue or exhaustion with muscular aches and pains. Digestive complaints, including nausea and sickness, abdominal pain and wind, caused by eating dairy products, and headaches with giddiness and nausea are relieved by Sepia. Also, it is a remedy for incontinence, hot, sweaty feet and verruca (a wart on the foot). A woman often experiences pelvic, dragging pains frequently associated with prolapse of the womb. Disorders of the circulation, especially varicose veins and cold extremities, benefit from sepia.

Symptoms are worse in cold weather and before a thunderstorm, and in the late afternoon, evening and early in the morning. Also, before a period in women and if the person receives sympathy from others. The symptoms are better with heat and warmth, quick vigorous movements, having plenty to do and out in the fresh open air. People suitable for Sepia are usually, but not exclusively, women. They tend to be tall, thin and with a yellowish complexion, and are rather self-contained and indifferent to others. Sepia people may become easily cross, especially with family and close friends, and harbour resentment. In company, they make a great effort to appear outgoing and love to dance. A woman may be either an externally hard, successful career person or someone who constantly feels unable to cope, especially with looking after the home and family. Sepia people have strongly held beliefs and cannot stand others taking a contrary opinion. When ill, they hate to be fussed over or have the sympathy of others. They like both sour and sweet foods and alcoholic drinks but are upset by milk products and fatty meals. They harbour deep insecurity and fear being left alone, illness resulting in madness, and loss of their material possessions and wealth. One physical attribute is that they often have a brown mark in the shape of a saddle across the bridge of the nose.

Silicea terra
Silicea; silica

Silica is one of the main rock-forming minerals and is also found in living things, where its main function is to confer strength and resilience. In homeopathy, it is used to treat disorders of the skin, nails and bones and recurring inflammations and infections, especially those that occur because the person is somewhat rundown or has an inadequate diet. Also, some disorders of the nervous system are relieved by Silicea. The homeopathic remedy used to be derived from ground flint or quartz but is now prepared by chemical reaction. The remedy is used for catarrhal infections such as colds, influenza, sinusitis, ear infections including glue ear. Also, for inflammations producing pus, such as a boil, carbuncle, abscess, stye, whitlow (infection of the fingernail) and peritonsillar abscess. It is beneficial in helping the natural expulsion of a foreign body, such as a splinter in the skin. It is a remedy for a headache beginning at the back of the head and radiating forwards over the right eye, and for stress-related conditions of overwork and sleeplessness.

Symptoms are worse for cold, wet weather, especially when clothing is inadequate, draughts, swimming and bathing, becoming chilled after removing clothes and in the morning. They are better for warmth and heat, summer weather, warm clothing, particularly a hat or head covering, and not lying on the left side. People who are suitable for Silicea tend to be thin with a fine build and pale skin. They often have thin straight hair. They are prone to dry, cracked skin and nails and may suffer from skin infections. Silicea people are usually unassuming, and lacking in confidence and physical stamina. They are conscientious and hard-working to the point of working too hard once a task has been undertaken. However, they may hesitate to commit themselves through lack of confidence and fear of responsibility. Silicea people are tidy and obsessive about small details. They may feel 'put upon' but lack the courage to speak out, and may take this out on others who are not responsible for the situation. They fear failure and dislike exercise because of physical weakness, often feeling mentally and physically exhausted. They enjoy cold foods and drinks.

Sulphur
Sulphur, flowers of sulphur, brimstone
Sulphur has a long history of use in medicine going back to very ancient times. Sulphur gives off sulphur dioxide when burnt, which smells unpleasant ('rotten eggs' odour) but acts as a disinfectant. This was used in mediaeval times to limit the spread of infectious diseases. Sulphur is deposited around the edges of hot springs and geysers and where there is volcanic activity. Flowers of sulphur, which is a bright yellow powder, is obtained from the natural mineral deposit and is used to make the homeopathic remedy. Sulphur is found naturally in all body tissues, and in both orthodox medicine and homeopathy is used to treat skin disorders. It is a useful remedy for dermatitis, eczema, psoriasis and a dry, flaky, itchy skin or scalp. Some digestive disorders benefit from it, especially a tendency for food to rise back up to the mouth and indigestion caused by drinking milk. Sulphur is helpful in the treatment of haemorrhoids, or piles, premenstrual and menopausal symptoms, eye inflamma-tions such as conjunctivitis, pain in the lower part of the back, catarrhal colds and

coughs, migraine headaches and feverish symptoms. Some mental symptoms are helped by this remedy, particularly those brought about by stress or worry, including depression, irritability, insomnia and lethargy. When ill, people who benefit from sulphur feel thirsty rather than hungry and are upset by unpleasant smells. The person soon becomes exhausted and usually sleeps poorly at night and is tired through the day. The symptoms are worse in cold, damp conditions, in the middle of the morning around 11 a.m., and in stuffy, hot, airless rooms. Also, for becoming too hot at night in bed and for wearing too many layers of clothes. Long periods of standing and sitting aggravate the symptoms, and they are worse if the person drinks alcohol or has a wash. Symptoms improve in dry, clear, warm weather and for taking exercise. They are better if the person lies on the right side.

Sulphur people tend to look rather untidy and have dry, flaky skin and coarse, rough hair. They may be thin, round-shouldered and inclined to slouch or be overweight, round and red-faced. Sulphur people have lively, intelligent minds full of schemes and inventions, but are often useless on a practical level. They may be somewhat self-centred with a need to be praised, and fussy over small unimportant details. They enjoy intellectual discussion on subjects that they find interesting and may become quite heated although the anger soon subsides. Sulphur people are often warm and generous with their time and money. They enjoy a wide range of foods but are upset by milk and eggs. They have a fear of being a failure in their work, of heights and the supernatural.

Tarentula cubensis
Tarentula cub.; Cuban tarantula

The bite of the Cuban tarantula spider produces a delayed response in the victim. About 24 hours after a bite, the site becomes inflamed and red, and swelling, fever and abscess follow. The homeopathic remedy, made from the poison of the spider, is used to treat similar septic conditions, such as an abscess, boil, carbuncle or whitlow (an infection of the fingernail) and genital itching. Also, it is a remedy for anthrax and shock, and is of value as a last-resort treatment in severe conditions. The infected areas are often tinged blue, and there may be burning sensations of pain that are especially severe at night. It is of particular value in the treatment of recurring boils or carbuncles. The symptoms tend to improve with smoking and are made worse by physical activity and consuming cold drinks.

Thuja occidentalis

Thuja; tree of life, yellow cedar, arbor vitae, false white cedar

This coniferous, evergreen tree is a native species of the northern United States and Canada and grows to a height of about 30 feet. It has feathery green leaves with a strong, aromatic smell resembling that of camphor. The leaves and twigs were used by the Indian peoples to treat a variety of infections and disorders, and the plant has long been used in herbal medicine. It is an important remedy in aromatherapy. The fresh green leaves and twigs are used to prepare the homeopathic remedy, which is especially valuable in the treatment of warts and wartlike tumours on any part of the body. It is a useful remedy for shingles and also has an effect on the genital and urinary tracts. Hence it is used to treat inflammations and infections such as cystitis and urethritis and also pain on ovulation. It may be given as a remedy for infections of the mouth, teeth and gums, catarrh and for tension headaches.

People who benefit from Thuja tend to sweat profusely, and it helps to alleviate this symptom. They tend to suffer from insomnia and when they do manage to sleep, may talk or cry out. They are prone to severe left-sided frontal headaches that may be present on waking in the morning. Symptoms are worse at night, from being too hot in bed and after breakfast. Also, at 3 a.m. and 3 p.m. and in weather that is cold and wet. Symptoms are felt more severely on the left side. Symptoms improve for movement and stretching of the limbs, massage and after sweating. People suitable for Thuja tend to be insecure and unsure about themselves. They try hard to please others but are very sensitive to criticism and soon become depressed. This may lead them to neglect their appearance. Thuja people are often thin and pale and tend to have greasy skin and perspire easily.

Urtica urens

Urtica; stinging nettle

One of the few plants that is familiar to all and that, for hundreds of years, has been valued for its medicinal and culinary uses. Nettles have always been used as a source of food both for people and animals, the young leaves being a nutritious vegetable with a high content of vitamin C. Nettles were thought to purify the blood, and an ancient cure for rheumatism and muscular weakness was the practice of 'urtication', or lashing the body with stinging nettles. The hairs covering the leaves of the nettle release a volatile liquid when touched, which causes the familiar skin reaction of painful, white bumps to appear. The fresh, green parts of the plant are used to prepare the homeopathic remedy, which is used as a treatment for burning and stinging of the skin. Hence it is used to treat allergic reactions of the skin, urticaria, or nettle rash, insect bites and stings and skin lesions caused by burns and scalds. Also, for eczema, chicken pox, nerve inflammation and pain (neuritis and neuralgia), shingles, rheumatism, gout and cystitis in which there are burning, stinging pains. The person who benefits from this remedy is prone to inflamed, itching and irritated skin complaints and may be fretful, impatient and restless. Symptoms are made worse by touch and in cold, wet weather, snow and for contact with water. Allergic skin reactions may occur if the person eats shellfish such as prawns. The symptoms improve if the affected skin is rubbed and also if the person rests and lies down.

Minor Homeopathic Remedies

Aethusa cynapium
Aethusa; fool's parsley, dog parsley, dog poison, lesser hemlock
This plant is a common weed that grows throughout most of Europe, including Great Britain. It resembles hemlock but is smaller and has three to five long, thin, leaflike bands that hang down beneath each flower head of small, white flowers. The leaves have an unpleasant smell although this is less strong than that of hemlock and is quite different from that of garden parsley. The plant is poisonous, although less potent than hemlock, and has effects on the digestive organs and nervous system. The green parts of the flowering plant are used in homeopathy, and it is used especially to treat bouts of violent vomiting, particularly in babies with an allergy to milk. Accompanying symptoms include abdominal pains and diarrhoea. It is used to treat summer diarrhoea in children and also severe mental symptoms of confusion, fits and delirium. (These symptoms are produced in cases of poisoning with fool's parsley). It is used to help alleviate mental weakness and fatigue and inability to concentrate. Symptoms are made worse by heat, summer weather, in the evening and between 3 and 4 a.m. in the early morning. They improve out in the fresh open air and when the person has the company of others.

Agaricus muscarius
Agaricus; *Amanita muscaria*, common toadstool, fly agaric, bug agaric
This striking toadstool, with its bright red-orange cap studded with small white flakes, grows in damp, boggy, upland woods in Scotland, northern Europe, North America and Asia. It is deadly poisonous, and juice obtained from the fungus used to be extracted and used as a fly killer. It has effects on the mind and has been exploited for its hallucinogenic properties. These attributes mean that it must be handled with very great care and its use is banned in some countries. The whole fresh fungus is used to prepare the homeopathic remedy, which is given for chilblains and itching, burning hot, swollen fingers and toes. Also, it is a remedy for epilepsy and disorders in which there are twitching, jerking spasms of muscles (chorea). It is given as a remedy for dizziness and unsteadiness, confusion, delirium tremens

(alcoholism) and senile dementia. People who benefit from it feel the cold at all times but particularly acutely when not well. Symptoms are made worse by cold conditions or weather, thunderstorms and after a meal. They improve with gentle, slow movements.

Ailanthus olandulosa
Ailanthus; *Ailanthus altissima*, shade tree, Chinese sumach, copal tree, tree of heaven, tree of the gods, ailanto

A large, attractive tree that produces yellow-green flowers with a highly unpleasant smell. When inhaled, the scent causes digestive upset, and the fresh flowers are used to make the homeopathic remedy. The tree is a native of China but was introduced into Britain during the 18th century as an ornamental species. It is used as a remedy for glandular fever in which there is a highly painful sore throat and swollen glands. The tonsils are red and inflamed and it is difficult to swallow. The person may have a severe headache and pains in the muscles. The symptoms are made worse by swallowing and bending the body forwards. Also, for lying down and during the morning, and for being exposed to light.

Aloe socotrina
Aloe; *Aloe ferox*, the common aloe

Aloes are succulent plants, and there are a number of species flourishing in the hotter climates of the world. Juice drained from the cut leaves is dried and made into a resin that is powdered to make the homeopathic remedy. Aloe has been used in medicine for many centuries and was given by Greek and Roman physicians for digestive and abdominal disorders. In more recent times, it has been used as a medicine to purge the bowels.

Aloe was investigated and proved by Dr Constantine Hering in the mid-1800s, and the remedy is used in homeopathy for various congestive problems. These include headache, enlarged prostate gland in men, prolapsed uterus, haemorrhoids, or piles, diarrhoea and constipation and overindulgence in alcoholic drinks. Symptoms are made worse by heat and hot, dry summer weather. They are at their most severe in the very early morning and following meals and drinks. Symptoms improve in cold weather and for cold applications, and also for abdominal flatulence. People who are suitable for Aloe tend to be short-tempered and cross, feeling generally displeased with themselves and those around them. They frequently feel tired and unable to face up to their daily work, and symptoms are at their most severe when the person is constipated. Aloe types enjoy beer but it upsets their digestion.

Aluminum oxide

Aluminium oxide
Alumina; oxide of aluminium

Aluminium is obtained from bauxite, a type of rock containing hydrated aluminium oxide. In conventional medicine, aluminium is used in indigestion remedies where there is an excess of stomach acid. The brain tissue of people suffering from Alzheimer's disease has been found to contain elevated levels of aluminium, and there is some concern that the metal may leach out from cooking utensils, especially when acid fruits are stewed. One of the main uses of the homeopathic remedy is for the treatment of confusional states. It is also used to treat all ailments where there is a slowness or sluggishness in the system. The remedy is given for senile dementia, confusion and memory loss, constipation, poor co-ordination, and heaviness and deadness of the limbs, poor flow of urine, and giddiness when the eyes are closed. Symptoms are worse in the morning and for being out in the cold and also following meals that are high in carbohydrate and salt.

People suitable for alumina are usually pale and thin with dry skin. They are pessimistic and gloomy, beset with feelings of impending disaster, and have a phobia about sharp, pointed objects such as knives. Alumina types may experience strange cravings for inappropriate substances to eat, but they do not like meat or beer.

Ammonium carbonicum
Ammon. carb.; ammonium carbonate, sal volatile

Ammonium carbonate was long in use in medicine in the treatment of scarlet fever and as a constituent of smelling salts. The remedy was investigated and proved by Hahnemann in the 1800s and was found to be an effective treatment for a number of different disorders. The remedy is obtained from a chemical reaction between ammonium chloride and sodium carbonate. It is of particular value if the circulation is slow and if the heart is weak. It can be used to treat post-viral tiredness and ME (myalgic encephalomyelitis). The symptoms are made worse by prolonged exertion and cloudy, overcast weather. They improve in warm, dry weather and surroundings, by lying down with the feet higher than the head and by the application of pressure. People suitable for Ammon. carb. are usually of large build and soon feel tired. They tend to be short-tempered, irritable and are prone to forgetfulness and bouts of crying. They are especially sensitive to the effects of overcast, dull weather.

Ammonium muriaticum

Ammon. mur.; sal ammoniac, ammonium chloride

Ammonium chloride has been used since ancient times and was especially prized by alchemists. There used to be only one source of the substance, which was the Fire Mountain in central Asia, but it is now prepared by chemical reaction. Ammonium chloride is used in conventional medicine in remedies for colds and coughs, and it has several important industrial uses. It is a remedy for conditions in which there is a feeling of tightness and constriction. Ailments include coughs, bronchitis and pneumonia in which it feels as though there is a tight band around the chest, and with a sticky, thick mucus. Also for disorders affecting joints and tendons, backache, lumbago and sciatica with symptoms especially affecting the left side and being worse in the morning. Often the person experiences a frontal headache at the base of the nose and may have an irritated dry scalp and dandruff. Symptoms are worse in the early hours of the morning between 2 and 4 a.m. and also during the afternoon. They are better in the evening and night and improve for brisk exercise, especially out in the fresh air. The person who benefits from Ammon. mur. tends to be obese, although the limbs may appear to be thin, and has a puffy skin because of fluid retention. The metabolism is slow, and the circulation is sluggish and erratic, which may cause pains of a throbbing nature. Ammon. mur. people have a somewhat pessimistic outlook on life and cry easily, and tend to have a painful heel that may be caused by an ulcer. They may take an unreasonable dislike of some people and are afraid of the dark.

Amyl nitrosum

Amyl nitrate

This remedy is used for irregularities of heartbeat and anxiety. Symptoms include a racing heart (tachycardia), throbbing in the head and awareness of the heart rate with the sensation of the heart missing a beat and palpitations. There may be pain and numbness in the chest, which can spread to involve the arm and may be severe, as in angina. The person may experience hot flushes and sweats, especially if a woman going through the menopause. There is a feeling of fullness in the head and the person may flush easily.

Anacardium orientale

Anacard. or.; *Semecarpus anacardium*, cashew nut, marking nut

There are several products of the cashew nut tree that are useful to humans, and these have long been used for culinary and medicinal purposes.

Antimonium tartaricum

The nuts are gathered and eaten and used in cookery, and the fruits also are edible. The nut is surrounded by an inner and outer shell, and in between the two there is a thick, caustic, dark fluid that is the substance used in homeopathy. This fluid causes blistering of the skin and has been used to treat warts, ulcers, corns, bunions and other lesions of the skin. The fluid was also used to make an indelible ink by mixing it with chalk, and this was employed to mark cloth (hence 'marking nut'). Arabian physicians used the juice for treating psychiatric and nervous system disorders, including convulsions, paralysis and dementia. The cashew nut tree has an attractive appearance, produces perfumed pink flowers, and is a native species of the East Indies and Asia. In homeopathy, the remedy is used to treat symptoms of constriction, as though there are tight belts around the body. The person feels as though the digestive system is blocked by a plug, and there is pain, indigestion and constipation. Also, Anacard. or. is given for rheumatism and ulcers, and while symptoms are initially relieved by eating, they are worse once digestion is completed. Symptoms are worse late at night around midnight and for pressure and hot baths. They are relieved by fasting. People suitable for this remedy tend to be totally lacking in self-confidence, feeling constantly inferior. They often have a poor memory and may be prone to mental disorders, particularly an inability to distinguish between reality and fantasy.

Antimonium tartaricum
Antim. tart.; tartar emetic, antimony potassium tartrate
This substance is important in the manufacture of textiles, being used to fix dyes used to colour materials. In orthodox medicine it has been used in cough remedies and as an emetic to cause vomiting. The homeopathic remedy is obtained by means of a chemical reaction between potassium tartrate and antimony oxide. It is used in the treatment of bronchitis and conditions in which there is an accumulation of phlegm. Breathing is difficult and laboured, and the person has a wheezing cough that is ineffective in bringing up the accumulated fluid. It is useful for young children and elderly persons who are in a weakened condition and are not able to cough effectively. Also, it may be used as a remedy for a tension headache with a feeling of tight constriction around the head. The person generally does not feel thirsty and may have some puffiness of the skin because of fluid retention. The tongue appears to be thickly furred. Symptoms are made worse by exercise, lying flat, wet, cold conditions and in warm, stuffy, airless rooms. They are relieved by cold, dry air and resting by sitting propped up.

Apomorphia
Alkaloid of morphine

This is a remedy for severe and persistent vomiting accompanied by weakness, dizziness, fainting and sweating. Nausea may or may not be present. The vomiting may be the result of a number of different causes, such as the morning sickness of pregnancy. Additionally, it may be caused by overindulgence in alcohol or too much rich food or misuse of drugs.

Aranea diadema
Aranea diad.; *Aranea diadematus*, papal cross spider

This spider is widely found in many countries throughout the northern hemisphere. It has a spherical brown body marked with white spots on its back that form the shape of a crucifix. It is a web-spinning spider that paralyses its prey by biting and injecting a venom. The whole spider is used to prepare the homeopathic remedy, which was first investigated and proved by von Grauvogl, a German doctor during the mid 1800s. He used it as a remedy for symptoms of cutting and burning neuralgic pains that are made worse by damp, cold conditions. It is used to treat any kind of neuralgic pains but especially those affecting the face. The pains usually arise suddenly and are intermittent and severe in nature, being hot and searing. There may also be sensations of numbness and symptoms are worsened by exposure to cold, damp conditions and any cold applications. They improve in warm, summer weather and with warm applications. Also, and most unusually, they are relieved by smoking.

Argentum metallicum
Argent. met.; silver

Silver is usually found in association with other metallic minerals in ore deposits in ancient rocks. It has been prized throughout human history and used to make jewellery, utensils, artistic ornamentation and has modern industrial uses, e.g. in photographic film. It is widely used in dentistry in fillings and is valued in conventional medicine for its antiseptic and astringent properties. The homeopathic remedy is used for arthritic and rheumatic disorders, particularly those affecting the joints of the toes, ankles, fingers and wrists. The joints are painful, but usually the pain is intermittent in character and may disappear altogether for a time. Other types of pain from deep within the body may also be relieved by Argent. met. and also asthmatic and bronchitic symptoms and laryngitis. Symptoms are made worse for movement of the affected joints and also late in the morning towards midday. They improve with resting the affected part and being out in fresh clean air. Symptoms are better at night and for the application of gentle pressure.

Arsenicum iodatum
Arsen. iod.; iodide of arsenic

This homeopathic remedy is obtained from a chemical reaction between iodine and metallic arsenic and was formerly used in the treatment of tuberculosis. It is used as a remedy for allergic conditions such as hay fever in which there is a copious watery discharge from the nose. Also, for bronchitis, psoriasis and eczema and hyperactivity in children. The symptoms are worse at night around midnight and are better if the person is out in the fresh, cool air.

Arum triphyllum
Arum triph.; jack-in-the-pulpit, Indian turnip, wild turnip, pepper turnip, dragon root, memory root

This is a common wild plant of North America and Canada, which has unusually shaped leaves that are borne on long stalks. It has a broad, flattened root that is highly irritant if eaten, causing severe symptoms of vomiting, nausea and diarrhoea and burning inflammation of the mucous membranes of the mouth and digestive tract. ('Arum' is derived from the Arabic word for 'fire', ar). The fresh root is used to make the homeopathic remedy, which is used as a remedy for colds and hay fever with symptoms mainly on the left side. There may be cracking and bleeding of the skin around the nose and mouth and dry, sore lips. It is also given for hoarseness and laryngitis. Typically, there is a burning and profuse nasal discharge, and the person may feel hot and unwell. The symptoms may be caused by overuse of the voice, for instance if the person is a singer, or be brought on by exposure to the cold. Symptoms are made worse by cold weather, especially if exposed to biting winds, and also by lying down. They improve for drinking coffee and are also better in the morning.

Asafoetida
Ferula foetida, food of the gods, devil's dung

Ferula foetida is a large plant that is a native of eastern Iran and Afghanistan, and grows to a height of several feet. It has a thick and fleshy root, and when this is cut, a white, gumlike, milky fluid is exuded that hardens into resin. The sap of the plant smells rank and unpleasant and has an effect upon the digestive system. The hardened gum is made into a powder for use in homeopathy, and it is used for digestive disorders and hysteria. It is a remedy for indigestion, abdominal pains and flatulence, bloatedness and hysterical symptoms.

Astacus fluviatilis
Crawfish
This homeopathic remedy is used to treat allergic skin reactions that may have arisen as a result of eating shellfish. There is a raised, itchy skin rash (urticaria) and there may be a high temperature, malaise, chills and swollen glands. Symptoms are made worse by exposure to cold and draughts.

Avena sativa
Avena; wild oats
Oats have been cultivated for centuries as a nutritious source of food for both people and livestock. Oats are the only known food to reduce the level of cholesterol in the blood. The fresh green parts of the plant are used to make the homeopathic remedy, and in both homeopathy and herbal medicine the preparations are used to treat nervous complaints. The homeopathic remedy is given as a treatment for nervous exhaustion, stress, sleeplessness and anxiety. It helps to relieve the nervous symptoms of those suffering from alcohol abuse and may be used to treat impotence. Symptoms are made worse by consumption of alcohol and relieved by a good night's sleep.

Baptisia tinctoria
Baptisia; wild indigo, indigo weed, horsefly weed, rattlebush
This is an herbaceous, perennial plant that grows throughout Canada and most of the United States in dry, upland, wooded habitats. It has a dark woody root that is pale on the inside with many small roots arising from it, and this is the part used in homeopathy. The root was ground down and used by the Indian peoples both as a medicine and as a dye. ('Baptisia' is derived from the Greek word *bapto*, meaning 'to dye'). The plant grows to about three feet in height, producing yellow flowers in August and September. It is poisonous if eaten in large quantities but preparations of the root are valued for their antibacterial, antiseptic, astringent properties. In homeopathy it is used to treat acute, severe infections and fevers. These include influenza, whooping cough, scarlet fever and typhoid fever. The person feels unwell and may be exhausted, confused and delirious with a discoloured tongue and bad breath. There may be diarrhoea with an offensive smell. Symptoms are made worse by hot, humid airless conditions and improve with gentle exercise in the fresh, open air, once the person is convalescent.

Baryta carbonica

Baryta carb., witherite, barium carbonate

The barium carbonate that is used to make the homeopathic remedy is found as white crystals of witherite and barite in ancient rocks. Barium, which is derived from these minerals, is used in radiology and also in the manufacture of glassware. Witherite was once used medicinally to treat swollen glands and tuberculosis. In homeopathy it is a useful remedy for children and elderly persons suffering from intellectual and, possibly, physical impairment. Children may have Down's syndrome or similar disorders, and often have a disproportionately large head and impairment of growth. They tend to suffer from recurrent respiratory infections such as tonsillitis. Elderly persons who benefit from Baryta carb. may suffer from dementia or be physically and intellectually impaired because of an event such as a stroke. People suitable for this remedy are shy and unsure of themselves and they need a great deal of reassurance. They tend to be childlike, and need to be guided into making the right decisions. Symptoms are made worse by cold in any form, especially damp and chilly weather and biting cold winds. They improve with warmth in any form and with exercise in the open air. The person feels better if warm clothing is worn.

Bellis perennis

Bellis; the daisy, bruisewort, garden or common daisy

This little plant with its dark green leaves and white flowers with yellow centres, is so common as to be familiar to all. The leaves contain an acrid liquid that protects the plant from being eaten by insects or grazing animals. The daisy has a long history of medicinal use, having been used since mediaeval times to relieve bruising (hence bruisewort). The whole fresh flowering plant is used to make the homeopathic remedy, which is mainly used to treat bruising, pain and inflammation following accidental injury, trauma or surgery. It is useful for the prevention of infection and in the treatment of boils and abscesses. Symptoms are more severe if the person becomes chilled when already too hot, and glands may be swollen. Arms and legs may feel cold or numb. Bellis may be given during pregnancy to relieve pains and cramps. Symptoms are made worse by chilling, becoming wet and for sweating and being too hot at night in bed. They improve with massage or rubbing of the painful area and for gentle exercise and movement.

Benzoicum acidum
Benz. ac.; benzoic acid

Benzoic acid is found naturally in a resinous substance, benzoin gum, that occurs in some plants. A combination of sodium and benzoic acid forms sodium benzoate, which is used in the preservation of food. The homeopathic remedy is used for arthritic conditions and gout and also for urinary disorders, particularly kidney stones. There is a characteristic clicking of the joints in arthritic conditions and severe, searing pain. Urinary complaints are accompanied by the production of a dark urine that smells offensive and associated pain. The person is very sensitive to cold and often feels chilled. Benz. ac. may also be given as a treatment for menstrual disorders and a prolapsed uterus. Symptoms are made worse for getting cold while undressing or chilling because of winter weather or draughts. They improve with heat and hot applications to the painful part.

Berberis vulgaris
Berberis, barberry, pipperidge bush

Berberis is a common bushy shrub that grows throughout Europe, producing pale green leaves, yellow flowers and glossy red berries. The berries have always been valued for culinary purposes, and the plant also has a long history of medicinal use. The physicians of ancient Greece and Arabia used Berberis to treat feverish conditions, haemorrhage, gastroenteritis, dysentery and jaundice. In herbal medicine it is still used to treat jaundice, liver disorders, gallstones and digestive disorders. The fresh root of the plant is used to prepare the homeopathic remedy, which is used in the treatment of kidney complaints accompanied by severe pain, such as renal colic and kidney stones. These complaints may be accompanied by the production of dark-coloured abnormal urine with an offensive odour. Also, it is used for gallstones, jaundice and biliary colic accompanied by the passing of pale faeces. People suitable for this remedy tend to have an unhealthy appearance, being pale with sunken features and dark shadows beneath the eyes. Symptoms may show rapid fluctuations and are made worse by prolonged standing. They are relieved for stretching exercise and gentle movements.

Borax
Borate of sodium

This homeopathic remedy acts on the gastro-intestinal tract and is used in the treatment of digestive disorders. It is particularly helpful as a remedy for pains, diarrhoea, nausea and vomiting. These may be accompanied by sweating, fever and giddiness. Symptoms are made worse by downward movements such as sitting or lying down.

Bothrops lanceolatus
Bothrops; *Lachesis lanceolatus*, fer-de-lance, yellow pit viper
This greyish-brown snake, marked with a diamond pattern, is a native animal of the Caribbean island of Martinique. It produces a deadly venom, and if a person receives a bite, the affected part swells and eventually becomes affected by gangrene. The venom of the snake is harvested and used to make the homeopathic remedy, which is given for conditions of the blood such as haemorrhage and thrombosis. It is also used for strokes that affect the left side of the brain, producing symptoms of weakness and paralysis on the right side of the body and speech difficulty. People who need Bothrops are frequently exhausted, with slow, weary movements, and may be subject to tremor (involuntary trembling).

Bovista
Lycoperdon bovista; warted puffball, *Lycoperdon giganteum*
This fungus can be found in countries throughout Europe and has the shape of a round, white ball, varying in diameter from four inches to one foot. When the fungus is ripe, an irregular gash forms in its surface and dark browny/green spores are released. Young puffballs are eaten in some countries and they have a long history of use among country dwellers. The puffball was cut and applied to wounds to staunch bleeding and also burnt to produce a smoke that would stupefy bees so that honey could be collected from a hive. In homeopathy, the remedy is used for speech disorders such as stammering and also for skin lesions, including eczema, blisters, warts, bunions, corns and nettle rash. These skin eruptions tend to weep and crust over and produce severe itching. Symptoms are made worse by heat and relieved by cold applications.

Bufo rana
Bufo, the common toad
This toad is found in many countries throughout the world and has a mottled brown and pale warty skin. When the toad is disturbed and feels threatened, it secretes a toxic irritant substance from pores in its skin, especially from the raised pouches above its eyes. This poisonous substance is noxious and prevents the toad from being eaten. It affects the mucous membranes of the mouth, throat, eyes, etc, and can produce quite severe symptoms, even in larger predators that might be tempted to attack the

toad. The poison has a long history of use in Chinese medicine and is collected and prepared to make the homeopathic remedy, which was first investigated and proved by the American homeopath Dr James Tyler Kent. It is used to treat epilepsy, in which the person is disturbed by bright lights or music before the onset of a fit and moves the tongue rapidly (lapping). After the fit, the sufferer is left with a severe headache. Symptoms are made worse at night and for sleep and during menstruation in women. They are much better in the morning and after resting lying down. People who benefit from this remedy have a puffy appearance because of fluid retention. They are apt to lose their temper if unable to make their views understood.

Cactus grandiflorus
Cactus grand; *Selinecereus grandiflorus*, night-blooming cereus, sweet-scented cactus, vanilla cactus, large-flowered cactus
This plant grows in the parched, arid desert regions of South America, Mexico and the United States. It is a shrubby plant with thick fleshy stems and large white flowers with yellow centres. The flowers are about eight to twelve inches across and have a pleasant perfume resembling vanilla. They open in the evening and are closed during the day. The homeopathic remedy is made from the fresh flowers and young stems, and it was investigated and proved in 1862 by Dr Rubins. He discovered that it produced effects on the heart with feelings of constriction and pain. Hence, the remedy is used to treat the unpleasant and frightening symptoms of angina. These include severe, gripping pain that is worse for physical exertion and stress, and a feeling of the chest being held and compressed by tight, constricting bands. There may be numbness, coldness and tingling in the left hand and arm and palpitations. The person feels extremely anxious and fears that death is imminent, and the pain is worse if he or she lies on the left side. Symptoms are worse from late morning until late evening and improve for lying on the right side with the head raised. A person with these symptoms needs reassurance and should not be left alone.

Calcarea hypophosphorosa
Hypophosphate of lime
This is a remedy for persons with the Calcarea constitutional type. The remedy is used for arthritic and rheumatic disorders, especially of the hands and wrists. The hands feel clammy and cold, and the symptoms are made worse by cold, damp weather. The person is very susceptible to cold and has a pale, chilly skin.

Calcarea iodata
Iodide of lime
A remedy for glandular swellings and infections in the neck, including tonsillitis, swollen adenoids and enlarged thyroid (goitre). It is also given for fibroids in the uterus and similar benign breast lumps of a fibrous nature.

Calcarea sulphurica
Calc. sulph.; calcium sulphate, plaster of Paris, gypsum
The source of calcium sulphate is the mineral deposit gypsum, which was formed as a precipitate when salt water evaporated. It is one of the SCHUSSLER TISSUE SALTS (*see* Glossary) and is used to make plaster casts for immobilizing fractured bones. It is a remedy for infected conditions of the skin in which pus is produced. Ailments include boils, carbuncles, skin ulcers and abscesses and infected eczema. The skin looks grey and unhealthy and feels cold and clammy although the soles of the feet may be hot. There may be yellow fur on the tongue, and the person may suffer from malaise and weakness. Symptoms are worse in weather that is wet and cold and improve in dry, fresh open air. They are also better for eating and for drinks of tea. A person suitable for Calc. sulph. has a tendency to be irritable and gloomy, with a jealous nature. Although symptoms are made worse by cold, Calc. sulph. people dislike heat and prefer to feel cool even to the extent of wearing inadequate clothing in winter weather.

Camphora
Camphor; *Laurus camphora*, gum camphor, laurel camphor
This remedy was investigated and proved by Hahnemann who used it to treat a cholera outbreak during the 1830s. The remedy was used again during a further epidemic in 1854 and proved to be highly successful on both occasions. Camphor is obtained from a tree that grows in central China and Japan. Chips of wood are heated with steam, and a liquid is collected from which clear deposits of camphor are precipitated out. Camphor has a characteristic pungent odour and has a range of applications in herbal medicine. In homeopathy, it is used to treat acute conditions and fevers in which there is sweating, a cold clammy pale skin, chills and anxiety. There may be severe symptoms of very low blood pressure, collapse and convulsions. It is sometimes used in circumstances in which other homeopathic remedies have failed to produce an improvement.

Capsicum frutescens
Capsicum; African pepper, red cayenne pepper, chilli pepper, bird pepper
The capsicum plant is a native of South America, West Indies and East Indies, but it is cultivated in many countries throughout the world. Elongated red chilli fruits, which may be used fresh or dried, are much used in Eastern cookery for their fiery properties. They cause sweating and a feeling of heat, dilate blood vessels and promote blood flow. They have been used to treat infectious disorders but are now mainly given for digestive symptoms. Cayenne is one of the most important remedies in herbal practice and is a constituent of many compound medicines. The fruits and seeds are used to prepare the homeopathic remedy, which is used to treat ailments with hot, burning, stinging pains. It is used for indigestion, especially heartburn, piles, or haemorrhoids, diarrhoea, sore throat with painful burning sensation on swallowing, and rheumatic disorders. Symptoms are made worse by cool, draughty conditions and when the person first begins movement. They are made better for warmth and heat, and with sustained exercise and movement. People suitable for this remedy are often fair-haired and blue-eyed and tend to be obese. They are often unfit, disliking physical exercise. Overindulgence in alcohol or rich spicy foods makes them lazy and lethargic, and they tend to have a melancholy disposition. If they go away from home, they soon become depressed and homesick.

Carboneum sulphuratum
Carbon bisulphide
This remedy is used for ailments affecting the nerves, in which there may be weakness, numbness, tremor or paralysis. Also, for some disorders of the eye and vision and for indigestion, abdominal pains, wind, diarrhoea and constipation.

Caulophyllum thalictroides
Caulophyllum; papoose root, squawroot, blueberry root, blue cohosh
This is an attractive perennial plant that is a native species of Canada and North America, growing in moist conditions near creeks or in swamps. It produces greenish-yellow flowers in early summer and, later, large pea-sized seeds that were gathered, roasted and used by the Indian people to make a hot drink. The root of the plant is brown, gnarled and contorted, and this is the part that is used in homeopathy. The preparation made from the root acts as a stimulant on the uterus, and this property was well known to the Indian people, who used the medicine to hasten a slow or painful labour. Caulophyllum was investigated and proved by an American ho-

meopathic doctor, Dr Hale, in the late 1800s, and one of its main uses in homeopathy is to speed up and strengthen weak or painful ineffective contractions of the womb during labour. It is also used to treat absent menstruation and some other conditions of the uterus, such as menstrual and postpartum pain. Caulophyllum is an effective remedy for rheumatic disorders affecting the fingers, hands, wrists, toes, ankles and feet. Typically there are cramp-like stabbing pains that are intermittent in character. Symptoms are worse in women when menstruation is absent or erratic and during pregnancy. All symptoms improve in warm conditions or with the application of heat.

Causticum hahnemanni
Causticum, potassium hydrate

This remedy was prepared, investigated and proved in the early 1800s by Hahnemann, and is used only in homeopathy. It is prepared by a chemical process in which lime that has been newly burnt is combined with potassium bisulphate in water. The mixture is heated and distilled, and the clear liquid distillate is collected and used to prepare the homeopathic remedy. It is used for weakness of nerves and muscles that control the throat and voice box or vocal cords, bladder, eyelids and face on the right side. Typical throat complaints include hoarseness and loss of the voice and there may be a dry, unproductive cough. Bladder complaints include stress incontinence (i.e. a leakage of urine when the person coughs, sneezes, laughs loudly, etc) and wetting the bed, particularly if suffering from a chill. Other symptoms include sore, hot pains as in heartburn and rheumatic complaints. The symptoms are made worse by exposure to cold winds, physical exercise and also during the evening. They improve with warmth and are better for drinking something cold and having a wash. People suitable for Causticum are often thin, pale and with dark eyes and hair. They are able to enter into other people's suffering and feel the effects of grief very profoundly. They tend to feel the cold rather acutely and may be prone to warts on the skin. Causticum people may be rather rigid in their views and tend to have a weak constitution.

Ceanothus americanus
Ceanothus; red root, Jersey tea root, New Jersey tea, wild snowball

This shrub, which grows to a height of about five feet, is a native species of North America and Canada. It produces numerous small white flowers in June and July, and its leaves were used to make tea during the War of Independence when real tea was hard to come by. The plant has thick, reddish-coloured roots that give it one of its common names. The root is used in herbal medicine, but in homeopathy the fresh leaves, gathered when the plant is in flower, are used to prepare the remedy. Ceanothus is given for abdominal pains and enlargement of the spleen and for symptoms on the left side of the abdomen. The pain is of a piercing nature and is made worse by lying on the left side. Exercise and movement exacerbate the symptoms, but they are relieved by rest and lying still. People who benefit from Ceanothus are extremely sensitive to the cold and like to sit as close as possible to a heat source in order to keep warm.

Chelidonium majus
Chelidonium, greater celandine, wartweed, garden celandine

This plant is a native of many countries in Europe and belongs to the same family as the poppy. The plant has a slender branching stem, large leaves that are a yellow-green colour on their upper surface and grey underneath, and yellow flowers. After flowering, long thin pods are produced containing black seeds. The plant produces a yellowish orange poisonous sap that is acrid, caustic and irritant with an unpleasant smell. The fresh flowering plant is used to prepare the homeopathic remedy, which is mainly used to treat liver and gall bladder disorders. The types of disorder treated include gallstones, hepatitis, abdominal pain and indigestion. There may be symptoms of nausea, jaundice, vomiting and digestive upset with an aching pain located under the right shoulder blade. All symptoms are more common on the right side and are made worse by a change in the weather, for heat, in the afternoon around 4 p.m. and in the early morning around 4 a.m. They improve on eating and if firm pressure is applied to the painful area. Also for drinking hot beverages or milk and for passing stools.

People suitable for Chelidonium are often fair-haired and thin with yellowish or sallow skin. They tend to be gloomy and seldom look on the bright side of life and dislike intellectual effort. They are prone to headaches that make them feel heavy and lethargic. Chelidonium types enjoy hot drinks and cheese and may have one hot and one cold foot.

The Chelidonium remedy is also applied externally to remove warts, and this property has given the plant one of its common names, wartweed.

Cicuta virosa
Cicuta; water hemlock

This plant is a native species of Canada, North America, Siberia and some parts of Europe. It has highly poisonous roots that, if eaten, cause convulsions, overproduction of saliva, hyperventilation and profuse perspiration, often with a fatal outcome. The fresh root is used to prepare the homeopathic remedy, which is used as a treatment for injuries and disorders of the central nervous system. Hence it is used to treat spasms, twitchings and muscular jerking, especially when the head and neck are thrown backwards, as may occur in epilepsy, following a head injury, meningitis and eclampsia of pregnancy. The patient may be confused, delirious, agitated and moaning unconsciously. The pupils of the eyes may be dilated. Symptoms are worse for sudden movement, cold and with touch. They improve with warmth and the elimination of abdominal wind. A person who benefits from this remedy may crave unsuitable substances as food.

Cinnamomum
Cinnamon; *Cinnamomum zeylanicum*
There are several varieties of cinnamon but the *Cinnamomum zeylanicum* tree is a native species of Sri Lanka and is also grown in several other eastern countries and the West Indies. The tree grows to about 30 feet in height, producing white flowers and, later, blue-coloured berries. The part used is the bark of the shoots, which is dried and rolled into thin brown quills. There is a characteristic pleasant, aromatic smell, and powdered cinnamon is widely used as a spice in food. In homeopathy, the remedy is used to treat bleeding such as nosebleeds and also vomiting, nausea and diarrhoea. Some of the symptoms may be caused by stress or hysteria.

Clematis erecta
Upright virgin's bower
This poisonous perennial plant is a native of many European countries, growing to about three feet in height and having reddish-green leaves and white flowers. The leaves and flowers are acrid and irritant when crushed, producing inflammation and blistering. In homeopathy, the remedy is used mainly in the treatment of gonorrhoea, including blockage of the urethra and a slow flow of urine because of inflammation or scarring. It may be used to treat other inflammations of the genital and urinary tract, eye disorders and neuralgia.

Cocculus
Indian cockle
This remedy, prepared from the body of the whole animal, is used to treat

symptoms of nausea, sickness, giddiness and vertigo. Often there is accompanying depression, and, in women, symptoms are worse at the time of the period, which tends to be painful and may be early. A person suitable for this remedy is frequently talkative and hates wearing constricting clothing.

Coffea arabica
Coffea; coffee

The coffee tree is a native of Arabia but has been cultivated for many years in other tropical countries. In addition to having been widely used for many centuries as a drink, coffee has been valued medically for its stimulant, analgesic and diuretic properties. The plant has dark green, shiny, evergreen leaves and produces attractive white flowers. Later, berries are formed, which are bright orange-red when ripe, containing the seeds or coffee beans. The beans are roasted for use as a drink, but the unroasted beans are used to prepare the Coffea remedy. Coffea is used to treat insomnia when the brain is over-active and the person cannot relax enough to fall asleep. It is a useful remedy for any form of over-excitability and also severe pain such as toothache and painful labour. The person is very sensitive to noise, touch, disturbance or odours of any kind, and symptoms are made worse by cold winds. They improve with warmth and resting in quiet, calm, peaceful surroundings.

Colchicum autumnale
Colchicum; naked ladies, meadow saffron

This attractive flower grows from a bulbous structure called a corm, which is an underground swollen stem. The pretty light purple flowers appear in September and October (hence 'autumnale') and it grows on limestone soils throughout Europe, parts of Asia, North America and Canada. The plant has been well known since ancient times for its medicinal properties, being especially valued by Greek physicians for the treatment of painful rheumatic and gouty joints. It was known as the 'soul of joints'. It is poisonous, irritant and emetic in larger doses, having an effect on the digestive organs and kidneys. The fresh bulb is used to prepare the homeopathic remedy, which is used to treat severe painful gout, especially of the big toe, and digestive upset including nausea, sickness, diarrhoea and abdominal pains that are relieved if the body is bent forwards. Symptoms are made worse by cold, damp weather, especially in the autumn, and by exercise or being touched. They improve with warmth, and resting in quiet surroundings.

Conium maculatum

Conium maculatum
Conium; hemlock, spotted hemlock, poison hemlock, poison parsley,
  beaver poison, spotted corobane, musquash root

This highly poisonous plant grows widely throughout Europe, parts of
Asia, Canada, the United States of America and South America. It has
been well known and used for centuries and is described in the writings of
the ancient Greeks and Romans, including Pliny and Dioscorides. It was
used as a means of execution of criminals, and Socrates was forced to
drink the fatal poison of hemlock. Roman physicians used hemlock to
treat a number of different disorders, including tumours and swellings of
the joints and skin, cancer of the breast, liver diseases and as a sedative
for spasms and dysfunction of nerves and muscles. Since it induces paralysis, it was used to combat pain and also to control inappropriate sexual
feelings. Hemlock is a tall plant that may reach a height of four feet, producing large, indented green leaves and heads of white flowers. The stalks
are streaked with purply-red, which, one old legend suggests, is a reminder
of the mark on the forehead of Cain, the first murderer. Juice obtained
from the leaves and stems of hemlock is used to prepare the homeopathic
remedy, which is used for enlarged and hardened glands, including the
prostate gland, cancerous tumours and nodules, particularly of the breast,
painful breasts before and during periods or because of pregnancy. The
remedy is also used for nerve and muscle paralysis, especially that which
gradually creeps up the legs and in which there may additionally be a
dislike of strong light. It is used to treat premature ejaculation and dizziness that increases when the person lies down or moves the head. In general, the symptoms are made worse by suppression of sexual needs or an
excess of sexual activity. Watching a moving object and drinking alcohol
also make the symptoms worse. They improve with continued pressure
applied to the painful part, sustained gentle exercise and if there is abdominal flatulence. People who benefit from Conium tend to have rather
fixed and narrow ideas and a lack of interest in the wider world, which
causes depression and a feeling of boredom and apathy. These feelings
may be caused either by an overindulgence in, or too little, sexual activity. Conium people do not cope well if forced to be celibate.

Crocus sativus
Crocus, saffron crocus, saffron

Crocus sativus is a native of the western parts of Asia but has long been
cultivated throughout Europe, especially in Spain. The three long, deep
orange-red stigmas within the crocus flower are the source of saffron,

which has been used medicinally since ancient times. Saffron is mentioned in the Old Testament Song of Solomon (4 :14) and was described by Hippocrates as having aphrodisiac and purgative qualities. It was used to treat uterine bleeding disorders and prolonged and painful childbirth as well as diseases of the liver. Throughout history it has been used to treat a wide variety of physical and mental disorders. In homeopathy the remedy is used to treat disorders of menstruation and nosebleeds and also emotional symptoms of weepiness, depression and mood swings. The symptoms are made worse by warm, stuffy surroundings and listening to music. They improve out in the fresh open air and after eating breakfast.

Crotalus homolus
Crotalus hor.; venom of the rattlesnake

The rattlesnake is familiar to people throughout the world, far beyond its normal habitat in the dry, semi-desert regions of the United States, Canada, Mexico and South America. Its most noteworthy characteristic is the rattling tail, which the snake uses as a warning when it is agitated or about to strike, and the animal has been widely described and depicted in books, films and nature programmes. The snake produces a potent venom that it uses to paralyse its prey, and this was investigated and proved in 1837 by Dr Constantine Hering, an outstanding American homeopathic doctor. In modern homeopathy the remedy is used to treat serious illnesses such as strokes affecting the right side of the body, symptoms of liver failure including jaundice and oedema, cancer and heart disease. The remedy helps to arrest bleeding from a natural orifice of the body and is used to treat septicaemia, shock and collapse. The symptoms are worse for lying on the left side and for wearing constricting, tight clothing. Humid, warm, moist weather aggravates the symptoms but they are better out in the fresh, clean, dry air.

Croton tiglium
Croton oil seeds

This small, shrubby bush is a native species of the coastal regions of India and Asia, and produces fruits that each contain a single seed rich in oil. Croton oil is obtained by compressing the ripe seeds, and in its neat form is highly purgative if taken internally, producing colicky abdominal pains, diarrhoea and vomiting. It may prove fatal if more than one small dose is taken. Applied externally, it produces irritation and blistering of the skin. In herbal medicine it is used to treat severe constipation, often combined with castor oil, and also as a counterirritant in some rheumatic, bronchitic and other disorders. In homeopathy, the remedy is used to treat severe digestive symptoms of colic-type abdominal pains, copious watery diarrhoea and vomiting. Also, it is used for severe skin inflammations in which there is redness, heat and blistering.

Cyclamen europaeum
Cyclamen; sowbread

There are several species of cyclamen, many of which are native to the warmer countries of southern Europe and northern Africa. The plant has a large, swollen, brown root and derives its common name from the fact that these tubers were a source of food for wild pigs. Cyclamen was used by the physicians of ancient Greece and Rome and also Arabia. It was used to treat disorders of the liver and spleen, including jaundice and hepatitis, and to regulate periods in women. The plant produces very pretty pink flowers, each borne on a single firm, fleshy stalk, and varieties of cyclamen are very popular as house plants. The fresh root is extremely acrid and acts as a purgative, and is used for this purpose in herbal medicine. In homeopathy the sap from the fresh root is used to prepare the remedy, which is used for an irregular menstrual cycle in women. It is also helpful in the treatment of searing, hot pains in the muscles or skin and severe migraine-like headaches with disturbance of vision. People who benefit from this remedy may crave bizarre and inappropriate things to eat. They tend to have a melancholy disposition, often feeling sad and depressed or beset by guilt or remorse. Symptoms are made better by exercise and moving around and with crying. They improve in the fresh open air.

Datura stramonium
Stramonium; thorn apple, devil's apple, stinkweed, devil's trumpet, James-town weed, Jimson weed

There are a number of species of *Datura* distributed throughout many countries of the world, and all are poisonous with highly narcotic effects. *Datura stramonium* is found in Europe, North America and Asia, often growing as a weed on waste ground. It is a large, bushy plant, usually about three or four feet in height and producing large white flowers. Later, pebble-sized capsules protected by thorns are produced that open when ripe to reveal black or very dark brown seeds. The flowers have a pleasant scent, but the rest of the plant, especially the leaves, give off an unpleasant, rank smell that is repellent to grazing animals. The plant has been used in herbal medicine for many hundreds of years. Inhalation of the smoke from the burning plant was used as a cure for attacks of asthma, and sometimes a type of cigarette was made from the leaves for this purpose. Preparations of the plant were used externally to relieve painful rheumatism, neuralgic conditions such as sciatica, haemorrhoids, abscesses and boils, and other inflammations. It has also been used for sedation and was eaten by soldiers in medieval Europe before going into battle to calm their fears. Juice extracted from the green parts of the plant before it comes into flower are used to prepare the homeopathic remedy. It is used to treat nervous system disorders and is a useful remedy for children. Symptoms include muscular jerking, spasms and twitches, convulsions because of epilepsy, high fever in children or meningitis and strokes. Also, for physical symptoms suffered by a person who has sustained a severe shock or fright, night terrors in children, states of great anxiety and mental agitation. A child may be terrified of the dark and the imagined creatures of the night. An adult may have a fear of water or is unreasonably afraid that he or she may suffer violence. The person often has a craving for drinks of an acidic nature and has an excessive thirst. Symptoms are worse if the person is left alone and following sleep. Also, when the person tries to swallow liquids or food and if the weather is overcast and cloudy. The symptoms improve if the person has the reassurance and company of other people, particularly if the surroundings are light, airy and warm.

Delphinium staphysagria
Staphysagria; stavesacre, staphisagris, planted larkspur, lousewort
This plant has a long history of medicinal use going back to the civilizations of ancient Greece and Rome, being described by both Dioscorides and Pliny. It was used externally to destroy parasites such as lice and to treat insect bites and stings, and has continued to be employed for this purpose throughout history. It is highly poisonous and even in small doses causes vomiting and diarrhoea, acting as a purgative. Staphysagria is a large, annual plant with hairy stems and leaves, which grows to a height of about four feet and is a native of southern European and Asian countries. It produces spikes of light blue/purple flowers and, later, seed pods containing dark-coloured seeds. The seeds are the part used in both herbal medicine and homeopathy. The homeopathic remedy is used to treat neuralgic pains, toothache, pain from the incision of an operation, pressure headache, inflammation and infection of the eyes or eyelids, such as styes and blepharitis, cystitis and painful sexual intercourse in women. It may also be used for painful teething in young children and for disorders of the prostate gland in men. Usually, the person who benefits has suppressed anger or resentment and is inclined to be irritable. Symptoms are made

worse for suppression of feelings, following a sleep in the afternoon and after eating breakfast. They improve with warmth and by giving voice to the emotions. People suitable for staphysagria appear equable and mild on the outside but internally seethe with suppressed emotions, especially anger. They are inclined to harbour resentment for supposed slights or insults and are somewhat driven, workaholic people. They often have a high libido and suppress their emotions because they are afraid of losing self-control, especially in front of other people. Body secretions may smell unpleasant, and they have a desire for alcoholic drinks and sweetened foods.

Digitalis purpurea
Digitalis; foxglove, fairy thimbles, fairy's gloves, witch's gloves, folk's glove
The striking and attractive foxglove, with its deep pink-purple, long, bell-shaped flowers, is a familiar plant in Britain and other European countries. One of its oldest name, folk's glove, associates it with the 'good folk', or fairies, who were believed to inhabit the woods and groves where the plant commonly grows. The name foxglove is derived from Anglo-Saxon, but the plant was given its Latin adjective of *Digitalis* in the mid-16th century, derived from *digitabulum*, meaning 'thimble'. The plant was used medicinally in ancient times as a cure for wounds and bruising. It was not until 1785, however, that its value in the treatment of dropsy (oedema, or fluid retention, which may accompany heart disease) was discovered by a Dr William Withering. Its main use, both in modern orthodox medicine and homeopathy, is as a major remedy for heart disorders. Liquid extracted from the new fresh green leaves collected in the spring is used to prepare the homeopathic remedy. It is used as a treatment for a slow, faint or irregular heartbeat such as may accompany heart failure and other heart and circulatory disorders. The person often experiences a sinking sensation in the pit of the stomach such as occurs with fear and may feel that the heart is about to cease to beat altogether. There may be additional problems, particularly with the liver or kidneys. The symptoms are made worse by listening to music, eating a meal and sitting in an upright position. They improve out in the fresh open air and by not eating. The person who benefits from this remedy may feel nauseated at the sight of food.

Dioscorea villosa
Dioscorea; wild yam, rheumatism root, colic root, wild yamwurzel
This perennial plant is a native species of Canada and the United States, although there are many other varieties inhabiting most tropical coun-

tries. It has a twining habit with a long, twisted, branched root that is the part used to prepare the homeopathic remedy. Preparations of the root act upon the smooth muscle of the digestive tract, having antispasmodic properties. Hence the remedy is used to treat spasmodic colicky pains, bilious colic, morning sickness during pregnancy, abdominal wind and diarrhoea. Other types of spasmodic pain, such as neuralgia, may benefit from this remedy, and symptoms are relieved by gentle exercise and movement.

Duboisia myoporoides
Duboisia; corkwood elm, corkwood tree

This large shrub or small tree is a native species of Australia, producing large, white flowers and green leaves that are gathered when the plant is flowering to prepare the homeopathic remedy. The preparation made from the leaves acts on the central nervous system, having an hypnotic and sedative effect. Applied to the eye it is a mydriatic, causing dilation of the pupil. In homeopathy, the remedy is used for eye disorders, particularly if there are one or more floating red spots (debris) causing disturbance of vision. Also, for painful, irritated and inflamed eyes such as may be caused by conjunctivitis. It may be used for symptoms of vertigo or where there are symptoms of mental confusion.

Dryopteris filix-mas
Male shield fern

A common type of fern found in the United Kingdom, Europe and many other countries with a temperate climate. The plant has a stocky, short rhizome or underground stem just beneath the surface of the soil, with a tangle of roots protruding from its under surface. This part is collected and dried and used to prepare remedies both in herbal and homeopathic medicine. The root contains a liquid oleoresin and has been known since ancient times for its anthelmintic properties (anti-worm), being particularly useful for the expulsion of a tapeworm. One method, using the root of the fern, is described by Dioscorides, and the remedy continues to be used for this purpose today. If a tapeworm is present there may be little in the way of symptoms but abdominal cramps, slight bleeding and itching. One dose is usually sufficient to expel the parasite, and preparations have also been used in veterinary medicine.

Elaps corallinus
Corallinus; coral snake

The attractive coral snake is a native animal of North and South America, especially Brazil and Canada. The snake has broad red and narrower blue bands of colour down the length of its body that are separated from one another by thin strips of white. The homeopathic remedy is prepared from fresh snake venom and is used as a treatment for troublesome bleeding and strokes. The bleeding disorders that may benefit from Elaps include nosebleeds, heavy menstruation (menorrhagia), piles and strokes affecting the right side of the body. The person may have a feeling of being chilled inside and desire cold drinks. However, cold foods and drinks, humid weather before a thunderstorm and getting too hot in bed make the symptoms worse. Also, they are worse if the person lies on his or her front or walks around. Symptoms are generally better during the night and for staying still. People who benefit from Elaps are usually afraid of snakes and fear being left on their own and do not like the rain. They are frightened of death and the possibility of having a stroke.

Equisetum hiemale, Equisetum arvense
Equisetum; horsetail, scouring rush, pewterwort, bottlebrush, shave-grass, paddock-pipes

The horsetails are a very ancient group of plants descended from species that grew during the Carboniferous geological period. Several species are found in the British Isles. *Equisetum arvense* is the most common of these and is also distributed in many other countries of the world. *Equisetum hiemale* is found in China and other eastern countries. Horsetails produce two kinds of stems, fertile and barren, which are jointed and hollow. There are no leaves but long green spikes at the joints with jagged edges. The fruiting or fertile stem, which is produced early in the season before the barren stems appear, has a cone-like structure at the end containing numerous spores. The stems of horsetails are strengthened with silica, and the plants were formerly used for scouring and cleaning purposes (hence the names pewterwort, scouring brush, bottlebrush, etc). There is a long history of medicinal use going back to ancient times, and the plant is described by Dioscorides as being good for the healing of wounds. While the plant continued to be used for wounds and ulcers, it was also believed to be helpful in the healing of ruptures and for bowel and kidney complaints. In modern herbal medicine, it is used for kidney disorders and fluid retention (oedema) as it has diuretic as well as astringent properties. The fresh parts of the plant are used to prepare the homeopathic remedy, which is used to treat an irritable bladder. The symptoms resemble those of cystitis but without the presence of infection. The bladder feels constantly full with an aching and dragging sensation. There is a continual feeling of the need to pass urine, which is usually released only in small amounts with pain at the end of urination. There may be kidney pain and slight incontinence. Equisetum is a useful remedy for children who wet the bed when suffering from disturbed sleep because of nightmares. The symptoms are worse if pressure is applied to the painful part and with touch, exercise or movement. They improve if the person remains still and lies on the back.

Euonymus atropurpurea
Euonymus; burning bush, wahoo, Indian arrowroot

This shrub is a native species of the United States and grows to a height of about six feet. It produces attractive deep purple flowers and dark green leaves that are edged with a purple tinge. The bark of the roots and stems is used and, in small doses, the preparation has a stimulant effect on the digestive system. However, in large doses it has an irritant and purgative effect. In herbal medicine, it is valued as a liver stimulant promoting the flow of bile juice. The homeopathic remedy is used for digestive complaints with bloatedness and abdominal pain and swelling of the feet and ankles because of retention of fluid (oedema). There may be stomach irritation (gastritis) with diarrhoea or blood in the stools. The remedy is also used for mental symptoms of irritability or confusion.

Euonymus europea
Spindle tree, prickwood, skewerwood, fusanum, fusoria

The spindle tree grows in woods and hedges in the British Isles and other European countries. It produces clusters of white flowers tinged with green in early summer and, later, bright red fruits containing orange seeds. The leaves, fruits and bark are all harmful and are not touched by grazing animals. The fruits cause severe sickness and diarrhoea if eaten, and the seeds are used to prepare the homeopathic remedy. It is used to treat digestive disorders with severe abdominal pains and copious diarrhoea. Also, for symptoms of angina, including constricting chest pains and breathlessness. Symptoms may occur mainly on the left side.

Eupatorium perfoliatum
Eupator; boneset, thoroughwort, agueweed, feverwort

This perennial plant is a native species of North America, being common on damp ground in low-lying situations. It is a very important plant in herbal medicine and has always been valued for its medicinal uses, firstly by the Indian native peoples and later by European and African settlers. It has a thick hairy stem and abundant white flowers throughout the summer months. Preparations made from the plant act as a tonic or stimulant of the digestive system in small doses. However, in large doses it causes sickness and diarrhoea, having a purgative effect. It is also valued for its fever-reducing qualities and, in addition, is diaphoretic, promoting perspiration. The whole green plant and flowers are used to prepare the homeopathic remedy, which is given for feverish conditions such as colds and influenza. Accompanying symptoms include restlessness, severe aches and pains in the bones, hot, dry skin and little perspiration. The person craves ice-cold drinks and foods, such as ice cream, and may have a painful, dry cough. Symptoms are worse for exercise and movement and in the early morning between 7 a.m. and 9 a.m. Also, they are worse outside in fresh clean air. They are better inside and for talking to other people and for vomiting bile.

Ferrum metallicum
Ferrum met.; iron

Iron is a very important mineral in the body, being a part of the haemoglobin molecule. Haemoglobin is the iron-containing pigment in red blood cells that combines with oxygen in the lungs from where it is transported and supplied to all cells and tissues. If there is a deficiency of iron in the blood, which can arise for a number of different reasons, the result is anaemia. The person becomes pale, tired and breathless. especially with any form of exertion, and body systems cannot function properly. Iron is widely used in conventional medicine as well as homeopathy. The source is iron ore, and haematite, a red-coloured bulbous deposit found in association with various rocks, particularly in North America, Canada and Venezuela, is especially rich in this mineral. The homeopathic remedy is used for circulatory disorders and anaemia. The person is frequently tired and listless, looks pale and feels chilled and may have cold hands and feet, but at the same time is often restless. The person soon becomes exhausted and may be breathless with physical exertion. The tiredness may cause irritability, depression and changes of mood. People suitable for Ferrum met. are frequently well built and appear robust but suffer from the symptoms described above. They dislike food rich in fat or cholesterol but enjoy pickled and sour foods. They may be allergic to eggs but like tomatoes.

Fluoricum acidum
Fluor. ac.; hydrofluoric acid

Hydrofluoric acid has several industrial uses, particularly in the manufacture of metals and glassware, being used for cleaning and etching. It is obtained by a distillation process involving sulphuric acid and calcium fluoride with the production of hydrogen fluoride gas. When this gas is passed through water it dissolves to give hydrofluoric acid, which contains fluorine. Fluorine is an important constituent of teeth and bones and is a strengthening substance. The homeopathic remedy is used to treat disorders of connective tissue, bones and teeth. Varicose veins and ulcers, bone pain and tumours and decaying, softened teeth may benefit from Fluor ac. People suitable for this remedy are frequently rather selfish and self-centred and not inclined to commit themselves to others. They are worldly and materialistic and tend to judge success in life in financial terms. Fluor. ac. people lack spiritual and emotional understanding and may have a high sex drive. They manage with little sleep and are very active, seldom feeling cold or tired.

Formica rufa
Red ant

The homeopathic remedy is obtained from the body of the crushed red ant. It is suitable for conditions producing symptoms of hot, burning, stabbing pains such as may affect joints, as in arthritic, rheumatic and gouty disorders. It is also used for severe headaches and numbness affecting the face. There may be an inability to concentrate, vagueness or slight forgetfulness.

Fragaria vesca
Wild strawberry, wood strawberry

This plant is a native species of most European countries, including Britain. It is a low, creeping plant with a tangle of stalks and leaves, and produces white flowers followed by small red berries that are covered with tiny seeds. The flavour of the fruit is delicious and fragrant and has long been valued as food. The fruit, and especially the leaves, have been used for hundreds of years for medicinal purposes, the plant having diuretic, astringent and laxative properties. Preparations made from the plant were used to treat kidney stones and urinary complaints, wounds, gout, tooth decay and diarrhoea. The cut strawberries rubbed on the skin help to relieve sunburn and other skin complaints and remove stains when applied to the teeth. The homeopathic remedy is used to alleviate an allergic reaction to strawberries, especially when this causes a skin rash and itching. It is also used for stones in the kidneys or gall bladder, a build-up of tartar on the teeth and chilblains or sunburn.

Fraxinus americana
American white ash
Ash trees of the genus *Fraxinus* have been used for medicinal purposes in many different countries. Various parts of the plant have been used, especially the bark, leaves, fruit and 'keys'. The bark of the American white ash, which grows in the United States, is used to prepare a homeopathic remedy. It has astringent and tonic properties and is used in homeopathy to treat a prolapsed uterus with dragging lower abdominal pain and also for fibroids.

Gentiana cruciata
Cross-leaved gentian
There are many species of gentian found in most countries throughout the world. In all varieties the plant, and especially the root, is extremely bitter and is used as a tonic medicine. The cross-leaved gentian, with leaves growing in the shape of a cross, has been used in herbal medicine as a treatment for hydrophobia (rabies). In homeopathy, the root is used to prepare the remedy, which is given for a sore throat or hoarseness, gastritis and infections of the stomach, colicky pains, nausea, sickness and diarrhoea and hernia.

Gentiana lutea
Yellow gentian
The yellow gentian is a native species of the mountainous, alpine and sub-alpine pastures of Europe although it does not occur naturally in the British Isles. It has a long root exceeding one foot in length, and the stalk grows to a height of three or four feet. The leaves are a yellow-green colour, and the plant produces attractive, large, deep orange-yellow flowers. The root is collected and dried to make medicinal preparations and has long been valued for its bitter, tonic properties. In homeopathy, it is used as a remedy for digestive problems and gastritis with symptoms of griping abdominal pains, nausea, vomiting and diarrhoea, heartburn and bloatedness.

Glonoinum
Glonoin; nitroglycerine, glyceryl trinitrate
This substance, which occurs as a clear, poisonous, oily liquid, is derived from a chemical process and was discovered in the mid-1800s by an Italian chemist. It is prepared by mixing together certain proportions of sulphuric acid and nitric acid and then adding glycerine. The addition of diatomaceous earth or kiesel-guhr (a natural deposit of sediment com-

posed of the silica skeletons of minute marine creatures called diatoms) to nitroglycerine, produces dynamite. This extremely dangerous explosive was first formulated by the eminent Swedish scientist, Alfred Nobel, in 1867. Nitroglycerine acts very strongly on the heart and blood circulation and is used in conventional medicine as a remedy for the symptoms of angina. In homeopathy the remedy is also used for symptoms affecting the blood circulation and head caused by a sudden, increased rush of blood. Symptoms include a feeling of congestion in the head with a pounding, severe headache, hot flushes and sweats. The person may try to relieve the pain by holding and pressing the head between the hands. Also, it is used in the treatment of heat exhaustion and the early symptoms of heatstroke. The symptoms are made worse by any kind of movement, especially turning the head, and by heat. They are relieved by cold and being out in cool, fresh air.

Helleborus niger
Christmas rose, Christ herb, melampode, black hellebore
The Christmas rose is a highly poisonous plant that is found naturally in the mountainous regions of southern, central and eastern Europe. It is known as a garden plant in the British Isles and derives its name of black hellebore from the colour of the root. It flowers in the depths of winter, from which comes its association with Christmas and Christ. The plant has large, serrated, dark-green leaves and white flowers tinged with pink, but it is the dark-coloured rhizome and root that are used to prepare the herbal and homeopathic remedies. The plant has been known since ancient times and is described in the writings of Pliny. It was used as a cure for various ailments in cattle and other domestic animals, and has strong purgative and narcotic effects. It also has a powerful effect on the kidneys, heart and uterus. In homeopathy, it is used in the treatment of severe headaches with stabbing pain that may be associated with a former head injury. There may be symptoms of mental confusion, mood changes or even convulsions or epilepsy. Slight movements make the symptoms worse, as do cold draughts of air.

Hydrastis canadensis
Hydrastis; golden seal, yellow puccoon, orange root, Indian dye, Indian paint, eye balm, eye root, ground raspberry
This plant is a native species of Canada and the eastern United States, and has a long history of medicinal use, firstly by the Indian peoples, particularly the Cherokees, and later by Europeans. It is a small, perennial plant

growing to a height of about six to twelve inches and producing a greenish white flower and later an inedible fruit resembling a raspberry. There is a knotty, yellow-brown tangled root system from which a dye was extracted and used by the Indians to colour their clothes and skin. The fresh root or rhizome (underground stem) is the part used medicinally. It was used by the Indian peoples to treat digestive disorders, liver complaints, eye irritations, ulcers and cancer, heart conditions and fevers. It has a particular effect on mucous membranes, making it useful in the treatment of catarrh, and has tonic, cleansing and astringent properties. The homeopathic remedy was investigated and proved by the American homeopath Dr Hale in 1875, although the plant had been known in Europe since the mid-18th century. In homeopathy the remedy is used to treat catarrhal complaints such as may occur with infections of the nose and throat and chest. Typically, a thick, yellow catarrh is produced, and there may be a sore throat and other pains. It is also used for digestive disorders in which there may be persistent constipation, nausea and vomiting and loss of appetite and weight. It is particularly useful as a tonic for people who have lost weight because of a long, debilitating illness. The symptoms are worse in the evening and night and out in cold air. They are relieved by rest, quiet and warm surroundings.

Hyoscyamus niger
Hyoscyamus; henbane, henbell, hogbean

Henbane grows widely throughout Europe and western Asia, and has been introduced and become naturalized in North America, Canada and parts of South America, such as Brazil. It is believed that it may have been brought to Britain and other European countries by the Romans, and it is described by both Dioscorides and Pliny. The plant is poisonous, narcotic and sedative, and was used by ancient physicians to induce sleep and relieve pain. Henbane has a varied habit, occurring as both annual and biennial forms. Both are used medicinally, although the biennial form is generally considered to be more useful. The preparations are narcotic, hypnotic and antispasmodic in effect, and are used in conventional medicine to treat spasms of the digestive tract. Juice extracted from the fresh whole flowering plant is used to prepare the homeopathic remedy, which is used for mental and emotional problems.

Symptoms include paranoia and suspicion of others, unreasonable behaviour and jealousy, delusions, aggressive outbursts and the use of foul and sexually suggestive language. Henbane is also used to relieve the physical symptoms of muscular spasms and cramp-like intermittent pains that may accompany epilepsy, disorders of the digestive system and bladder. Symptoms are made worse by lying down and being touched, with being covered up and for any emotional upheaval. They are relieved if the person sits in an upright position.

Iberis amara
Bitter candytuft
This small, flowering annual plant grows throughout Europe and is a familiar garden flower. It grows to a height of about six inches and produces white or pink flowers in the summer months. All parts of the plant are used in herbal medicine, but the seeds alone are gathered and prepared to make a tincture used in homeopathy. The remedy was investigated and proved by the American homeopath Dr Edwin Hale, and it is used to treat heart disorders. It may be given for angina, palpitations, oedema, breathlessness and chest pains. It is also a treatment for bronchitis and asthma and sickness and vertigo.

Iodum
Iodine
Iodine is a nonmetallic element that is an essential substance for the normal functioning of metabolic processes within the body. It is mainly concentrated in the thyroid gland and is a major component of thyroid hormones, which themselves regulate many body processes. A deficiency of iodine causes a gain in weight, swelling of the face and neck, a dry skin and mental apathy. The person feels excessively tired, and the hair starts to fall out. This deficiency is not usually seen in western countries because iodine is added to table salt. Iodine is found naturally in seaweed and deposits of saltpetre (an evaporate mineral found in dry, desert-like conditions, particularly in Chile). Tincture of iodine is used in homeopathy as a remedy for hyperthyroidism (an overactive thyroid gland). The symptoms include weakness and wasting, noticed especially in the limbs, pain and bulging of the eyes, excessive hunger, restlessness, nervousness, sweating, breathlessness, intolerance of heat and rapid heart beat. It is also used for severe, hacking coughs, shortness of breath, laryngitis and throat disorders and pain in the bones. People who benefit from this remedy like to be busy and may be talkative and excitable. However, they may also be forgetful so that their activities may be inefficient and disorganized. Symptoms are made worse by heat in any form and are relieved by cool, fresh air. They also improve for movement and exercise and after meals.

Iris versicolor

Iris versicolor
The blue flag, water flag, poison flag, liver lily, flag lily, snake lily, dagger flower, dragon flower

This attractive but poisonous flowering plant is a native species of North America and Canada, growing in damp, low-lying conditions. It is a popular garden plant in the British Isles, growing to a height of about two or three feet and producing deep blue-purple flowers. Preparations made from the rhizome have a diuretic and stimulant effect and cause sickness and diarrhoea. They are mainly used for liver and digestive complaints. The fresh rhizome or underground stem is used to prepare the homeopathic remedy, which is used for indigestion, vomiting and nausea, diarrhoea, colicky pains and also for migraine where the headache is on the right side.

Kali bromatum
Kali brom.; potassium bromide

This white, crystalline substance, which is obtained from a chemical process, is used in the photographic industry and has also been given as a remedy in conventional medicine. It was given to men to reduce an excessive libido and particularly to male prisoners. It was also given for some other psychiatric disorders and as a treatment for epilepsy. The homeopathic remedy is given as a treatment for severe acne and skin disorders, excessive menstrual bleeding especially during the menopause, impotence, epilepsy, nervous exhaustion and depression. People suitable for Kali brom. tend to be restless and anxious and have a need to be busy. During their teenage years they may require a lot of reassurance and tend to feel guilty about their emerging sexuality. They may have strong religious beliefs and feel that sexual needs are immoral, and this causes mental stress and conflict. They are prone to acne, especially at puberty and during times of hormonal change. In women, symptoms are worse during menstruation. All symptoms improve if the person is fully occupied.

Kali sulphuricum
Potassium sulphate

Potassium sulphate is another of the Schussler tissue salts (*see* Glossary), which is used in homeopathy for catarrhal conditions in which there is a thick white or yellow discharge. This may occur in bronchitis and other infections of the nose and throat. Also, it is used to treat infected skin conditions, such as erysipelas and eczema, in which there is a pus-like discharge. It may be used as a remedy for such infectious illnesses as measles and scarlet fever, which affect the skin, and also for rheumatism. Symptoms are made worse by hot surroundings and heat in any form and are relieved by coldness and fresh air.

Kalium carbonicum
Kali carb; potassium carbonate

Potassium carbonate occurs naturally in all plants, and is obtained from the ash of burnt wood or other vegetation, or by a chemical process. Potassium carbonate was used by the ancient Egyptian civilization in the manufacture of glassware. The remedy is used for complaints affecting the mucous membranes of the upper respiratory system and digestive organs. It is used for coughs and bronchitis with stitch-like pains, menopausal and menstrual problems, pains in the back and head. The person feels cold and fluid is retained (oedema), causing swelling of the face, especially the upper eyelids. The person feels chilled and may be likely to catch colds or influenza. Symptoms are worse for physical exertion, bending the body forwards and for cool conditions. They are worse in the very early morning between 2 and 3 a.m. Symptoms improve in warm, dry conditions and weather. People who are suitable for all the Kalium remedies have a strict sense of duty and firm ideas about right and wrong. They are possessive and may be jealous and difficult to live with. They cope badly with any kind of emotional trauma and may feel as though they have been kicked in the abdomen if they receive upsetting news.

Kalium muriaticum
Kali mur.; potassium chloride

This white or colourless crystalline substance is found naturally as the mineral sylvite, which occurs in beds of evaporite deposits. It is much used as a fertilizer, and in homeopathy is one of the Schussler tissue salts (see Glossary). A deficiency of potassium chloride affects blood-clotting capability. The Kali mur. remedy is used to treat inflammations and infections of the mucous membranes. Typically, there is a thick, mucus discharge, and this may occur with middle ear and throat infections, glue ear in children and tonsillitis. The throat may be very sore and swallowing painful and difficult, and the person may have a fever and swollen glands. Symptoms are worse in cold, damp weather and in cold fresh air. Also, they feel worse for eating fatty foods and, in women, during a period. Symptoms are better for sipping ice-cold drinks and for gently rubbing the painful part.

Kalmia latifolia

Kalmia latifolia
American laurel, broad-leaved laurel, sheep laurel, calico bush, lambkill, kalmia

An attractive but poisonous evergreen shrub that is a native species of some states of the United States of America. It grows to a height of anything up to twenty feet and produces an abundance of pink flowers. The leaves are the part of the plant used medicinally, and they have narcotic and astringent properties and also sedative effects on the heart. The plant was known to the native Indian people and has been used in the treatment of skin diseases, fevers, syphilis, neuralgia, blood disorders, haemorrhages, diarrhoea and dysentery. The homeopathic remedy is made from the fresh leaves of the plant and is used to treat symptoms occurring on the right side of the body, such as facial and other neuralgia, shingles, rheumatic pains, numbness and paralysis, and heart problems such as angina. Symptoms are made worse by cold in any form, touch or pressure, and are relieved by warmth.

Kreosotum
Creosote in spirits

This remedy is used for infected conditions in which there is pus or other discharge that often has an offensive smell. Hence it is used for skin eruptions such as boils, gum disease and tooth decay with bad breath, and infections of the womb, bladder, pelvic organs and prostate gland. The person may suffer from general weakness and debility with nausea, vomiting, diarrhoea and colicky pains. Symptoms may occur mainly on the left side.

Lac caninum
Lac. can.; milk from a female dog, bitch's milk

This is one of the oldest known remedies, being described by a physician of ancient Greece, Sextus, who used it for treating ear infections and sensitivity to light. Pliny referred to its usefulness in treating female reproductive disorders, and this is one of its uses in homeopathy. The homeopathic remedy is used in the treatment of erosion of the cervix, in which cells that line the neck of the womb are worn away. It is also used for sore breasts during breast-feeding or before menstruation. Another major use is in the treatment of severe sore throats, as in tonsillitis, and for diphtheria. The pains or other symptoms often switch from one side of the body to another and may be accompanied by malaise and weakness. The person may feel light-headed, experiencing a floating sensation. People suitable for Lac. can. tend to be highly sensitive, over-imaginative to the point of allowing imagined fears to take over, timid and forgetful. In contrast to this, they are capable on occasion of being unreasonable and aggressive. They have many fears and often experience nightmares, and may have a phobia about snakes. Lac. can. people enjoy spicy salty food and hot drinks. Symptoms are made worse by touch or pressure and improve out in the fresh air.

Lactrodectus mactans
Lactrodectus mac.; female black widow spider

The female black widow is one of the most poisonous of spiders, and its venom can rapidly prove fatal. The venom is injected when the spider bites and produces symptoms of severe, constricting chest pains, sweating, spasm in muscles and blood vessels, fear, collapse and death. The spider is found in a number of countries with a hot climate, particularly in some parts of the United States. The homeopathic remedy is derived from the body of the female spider and is used to treat serious heart complaints including heart attack and angina. It is also used for states of great anxiety and fear with hyperventilation, agitation, breathlessness and collapse. Symptoms are made worse by cold, damp weather and in oppressive conditions before a storm breaks. They are worse at night but improve with reassurance and sitting still and with taking a hot bath.

Lapis albus
Calcium silico-fluoride

This remedy, which is prepared chemically, was investigated and proved by a German homeopathic doctor, Edward von Grauvogl, in the 19th century. It is used to treat hot, stabbing pains in the womb, breasts or stomach and for burning, itchy skin.

Lilium tigrinum
Lilium; tiger lily

This striking flowering plant, which is popular in gardens, is a native species of China and Japan. It produces large, orange flowers that are funnel-shaped with the petals curved back upon themselves. The petals are covered with deep, reddish-coloured spots. The homeopathic remedy, which is made from the whole fresh flowering plant, was investigated and proved in 1869 by the American homeopath Dr Carroll Dunham. It is used for disorders of the female reproductive organs, including a prolapsed uterus with dragging pains, uterine fibroids (benign tumours of the womb) that may affect the bladder, increasing the desire to pass urine, swollen ovaries and ovarian pain, and itching in the genital region. Also, it is given for disorders of the bladder, rectum and veins, and for symptoms of angina. These symptoms include severe constricting chest pain, anxiety and rapid heart beat rate, and a feeling of numbness extending down the right arm. People suitable for this remedy have a very strong sense of right and wrong and set themselves very high standards of behaviour. This may result in conflict between their natural, especially sexual, needs and what they regard as the correct way to behave, leading to feelings of guilt and self-loathing. Their inner turmoil may make them irritable and liable to take offence, especially at remarks that appear to be critical. Lilium people have hot hands and are more comfortable in cool or cold weather. Symptoms are made worse by any form of heat and at night. They improve in cool surroundings and out in the cold fresh air. Symptoms are relieved if the person lies on his or her left side.

Lycopus virginicus
Lycopus; bugleweed, Virginia water, horehound, water bugle, gipsyweed
This attractive plant is a native species of the eastern parts of the United States, growing in damp, low-lying situations in plenty of shade. The plant produces purple-coloured flowers and has smooth, green leaves. It gives off a slightly minty aromatic smell and has astringent, sedative and slightly narcotic properties. It was formerly used to treat bleeding in the lungs, as in tuberculosis, encouraging blood to be coughed up. It has also been used in place of DIGITALIS in the treatment of heart disorders. The whole fresh parts of the plant and flowers are used to prepare the homeopathic remedy, which was first investigated and introduced by the American homeopath, Edwin Moses Hale in the latter part of the 19th century. It is used to treat heart disorders, including abnormalities of the heartbeat and palpitations, aneurysms (balloon-like swellings of artery walls), inflammation of the membranous sac surrounding the heart (pericarditis), raised blood pressure and heart failure. It is also used to treat a disorder of the thyroid gland (goitre) that produces a protrusion of the eyes. Symptoms are made worse by physical activity and exertion, agitation or excitement and heat in any form. The symptoms are usually worse following sleep but are relieved by pressure on the affected part.

Lyssin
Hydrophobinum
This remedy is prepared from the saliva of a dog that has contracted ra-

bies. It is used for serious disorders of the nervous system, especially convulsions that may be related to epilepsy, severe headaches and pre-eclampsia of pregnancy (a condition marked by retention of fluid and swelling of feet and ankles, high blood pressure and the presence of protein in the urine). If not treated, pre-eclampsia may lead to full eclampsia of pregnancy, which is a life-threatening condition marked by convulsions. The fits intensify if the person is in the presence of running water.

Magnesia carbonica
Mag. carb.; magnesium carbonate

Magnesium carbonate, which is a white, powdery substance, has a variety of industrial uses including the manufacture of bricks, cements, paper, paints and materials for insulation. In pharmaceutical manufacture it is used as a bulking material in some types of powder and tablets. The main source is magnesite, which is formed from altered limestones, dolomites or serpentines and is mined in China, the United States and Austria. The homeopathic remedy was investigated and proved by Hahnemann and is used to treat loss of the sense of taste when there is a thick, whitish coating on the tongue, indigestion and heartburn and digestive complaints with diarrhoea or constipation. The person may have a longing for fruity, acidic drinks and an unpleasant taste in the mouth. This is also a remedy for weakness and failure to thrive in babies where there is a lack of muscle tone. Symptoms are made worse by touch, resting, at night and if conditions are windy. They improve for walking about and being out in fresh, clean air. People suitable for Mag. carb. are often dark-haired and pale-skinned and are prone to exhaustion with pains in the legs and feet. They are very sensitive to cold draughts and being touched and may be on edge and irritable. They are prone to having a sour, unpleasant taste in the mouth and are hypersensitive, being apt to feeling ignored and left out by others. They frequently have an intolerance of milk and sweat, etc, smells sour.

Magnesia phosphorica
Mag. phos.; phosphate of magnesia, magnesium phosphate

This white compound is one of the Schussler tissue salts (*see* GLOSSARY) and is prepared chemically from sodium phosphate and magnesium sulphate. Magnesium occurs naturally in the body and is essential for the correct functioning of nerves and muscles. A deficiency can cause cramping pains and spasms and have deleterious effects on the heart and skeletal muscles. The remedy is used to treat neuralgic pains, writer's cramp, spasms and cramps. The pains are shooting and intermittent and may be brought on by a cold draught. Often, they occur mainly on the right side of the body. Colicky pains that are relieved by doubling over or by bending and by heat and firm pressure, benefit from Mag. phos. People who benefit from this remedy are often thin, sensitive and worried and may be academic, workaholic types. Symptoms are worse for cold air, touch, at night and if the person is tired and debilitated. They improve with any form of heat, pressure and warm surroundings.

Manganum aceticum
Acetate of manganese

This remedy was investigated and proved by Hahnemann in the 19th century. It is useful for the treatment of general debility and weakness with loss of appetite and weight, anaemia and, possibly, ulcers of the skin or bed sores. The skin is a bluish colour, and the body is extremely sensitive to touch. The person has great difficulty in eating enough to maintain body weight.

Medorrhinum
A remedy prepared from gonorrhoeal discharge

Gonorrhoea, the sexually transmitted bacterial disease, has plagued humankind since ancient times, and was first given the name of gonorrhoea by Galen, a physician of the Roman civilization. The effects of gonorrhoea can be passed from a mother to her baby during birth. Hahnemann believed that gonorrhoea was responsible for inherited traits or weaknesses in subsequent generations, and he called this a 'miasm', in this case the sycotic miasm (sycosis). Two other miasms were identified, 'psora', connected with the blisters and itching of scabies (*see* PSORINUM), and syphilis (*see* SYPHILINUM). Gonorrhoea has always been a feared and devastating illness and was formerly treated with injections of silver nitrate. In conventional medicine it is treated with modern antibiotics.

The homeopathic remedy is used to treat a variety of physical and mental symptoms. It is used to treat inflammation and infection of pelvic organs, menstrual pain and pain in the ovaries. Some other disorders of the mucous membranes, kidneys, nerves and spine, e.g. neuralgia, may benefit from this remedy. It is especially suitable for people who have a family history of gonorrhoea and some forms of heart disease. Emotional disorders may be treated with Medorrhinum, especially mood swings with the person changing from irritability and extreme impatience to passive withdrawal. In the impatient state the person is always in a hurry and is inclined to be selfish and insensitive. In the withdrawn state the person is dreamy and forgetful and very much in touch with, and moved by, the beauty of nature. In both states, the person tends to be forgetful and may feel neglected, lost or deserted. Symptoms are made worse by damp weather, heat in the early morning between 3 and 4 a.m. and after passing urine. Even slight movements make the symptoms worse, but they improve with lying on the front, in the evening and being beside the sea. Symptoms are also better if the person rests on the hands and knees ('all fours').

Mercurius corrosivus

Merc. cor.; mercuric chloride, mercury chloride $HgCl_2$

Mercuric chloride is a highly poisonous corrosive substance, causing burning and destruction of tissue if swallowed. It has antiseptic properties and is used to treat bulbs and tubers to prevent fungal attack. It is also used industrially in the manufacture of plastics. The homeopathic remedy is used for severe symptoms of ulceration in the digestive and urinary tracts and mouth and throat. It is used for ulcerative colitis with copious diarrhoea containing blood and mucus, and abdominal pains. Also, for severe bladder infections and urethritis with painful and frequent urination, the urine containing blood and mucus. There may be thick discoloured discharges containing pus. Throat and mouth symptoms include ulcerated tonsils covered with a white, pus-containing discharge, facial pain, exhaustion and secretion of excess saliva. Symptoms are worse in the evening and if the person walks about. They are also worse if the person eats fatty meals or acidic foods. Symptoms are better after breakfast and if the person rests.

Mercurius cyanatus

Mercuric cyanide

This homeopathic remedy is used to treat severe symptoms of diphtheria. The throat is extremely sore and the person finds swallowing and speech unbearable, and there is a covering of thick, greyish-white mucus. The person feels cold, and the skin has a blue-coloured tinge because of a lack of oxygen (cyanosis). The person may be on the verge of collapse.

Mercurius dulcis

Merc. dulc.; mercurous chloride, calomel, mercury chloride Hg_2Cl_2

This substance has laxative properties, and calomel was used as a purgative in medieval times. It is now used in the horticultural and agricultural industries as a constituent of certain insecticides and fungicides. Both *Mercurius dulcis* and *Mercurius corrosivus* are found in mineral deposits in the United States of America, Mexico, Germany and parts of central Europe. Merc. dulc. is a useful remedy for children suffering from glue ear and catarrhal problems. The child has swollen glands, and the nasal, ear and throat passages are clogged with discharges of thick, sticky mucus. Breathing may be noisy, and hearing is often affected. Symptoms are worse if the child is engaged in sport or physical exercise and also at night.

Mixed autumn moulds
MAP

This homeopathic remedy is derived from a mixture of three moulds—mucor, aspergillus and penicillum—and it is used to treat symptoms of hay fever that arise in the autumn. These symptoms include a runny nose and catarrh, itchy, red, watery eyes, sneezing and wheezing with a tight feeling in the chest. The usual time for symptoms to appear is in the early months of autumn, especially September.

Moschus moschiferus
Moschus; musk from the musk deer

Musk is a strong-smelling, aromatic secretion produced by the male musk deer in order to attract a female. The secretion has long been used in the production of perfume and has a long-lived effect. Samuel Hahnemann was concerned about the widespread use of musk-based scents, believing that the substance made people more susceptible to disease by weakening their natural immunity. The musk deer is a small deer found in countries of central Asia, inhabiting hilly or mountainous areas. Dried musk is used to prepare the homeopathic remedy, which is mainly given for hysterical, neurotic and emotional symptoms. Physical symptoms include giddiness and fainting, pallor and exhaustion and sweating.

People suitable for this remedy have a tendency towards hypochondria and may feel that everyone is against them. They tend to talk incessantly and have hurried, clumsy movements. They tend to feel chilled, although one half of the body may seem cold and the other hot. Their exhaustion is worse for resting than for moving about, and all symptoms are aggravated by cool, fresh air and emotional upset or excitement. Symptoms improve after burping and for warm surroundings.

Murex
Purple mollusc
This homeopathic remedy is prepared from the body of the shellfish and is useful for menopausal symptoms of irregular bleeding. It is also used to treat emotional and hysterical symptoms and stress. A person suitable for this remedy dislikes being touched and especially having a medical examination.

Mygale lasiodora
Mygale las.; *Mygale avicularia, Aranea avicularia,* Cuban spider
This spider, which is a large variety native to Cuba, has a highly poisonous bite used to immobilize its prey. If a person is bitten, the area becomes inflamed and discoloured, turning purple and green, and the effects spread outwards as the poison drains along the lymph vessels. The person experiences a high fever, tremor, chills, dry skin and mouth, severe anxiety and breathing difficulties and is very thirsty. The person fears that he or she will die. The homeopathic remedy is used to treat involuntary twitching and jerking of the muscles, which may be caused by nerve disorders such as various forms of chorea. The remedy is sometimes used to treat sexually transmitted venereal diseases. Symptoms are worse during the morning but improve when the person is sleeping.

Naja naja
Naja; *Naja tripudians,* venom of the cobra
The cobra, which has the habit of drawing itself erect and extending the skin below its neck to form a hood before it strikes, has long been both revered and feared. The snake is capable of shooting its venom into the eyes of its prey from a distance of six feet away, which causes blindness. The bite of the cobra may prove fatal, affecting the heart and lungs, causing collapse and death. The dried venom, which is bright yellow, is used to prepare the homeopathic remedy. It is used to treat left-sided symptoms, particularly of the heart, but also of the left ovary. Symptoms include crushing, choking pain as in angina, with the pain extending to the left shoulder and down the arm and hand. The pulse may be slow and the person feels breathless and oppressed. Ovarian pain may extend to the upper left-hand side of the body. Asthma that comes on after an attack of hay fever may be treated with Naja. The symptoms are made worse by lying on the left side, by cold draughts and following sleep. They are also aggravated by wearing tight, constricting clothing and drinking alcohol. For women, symptoms are worse following the monthly period.

Natrum carbonicum

Natrum carbonicum
Nat. carb.; sodium carbonate, soda ash
Sodium carbonate was once derived from the ashes of burnt seaweed but is now obtained from a chemical process. It is used industrially in the manufacture of detergents, soaps and glass-making. Sodium carbonate has various uses in conventional medicine, being used in creams and ointments to treat burns, eczema and other skin conditions. Also, it is used in preparations to clear up catarrh and vaginal discharge. The homeopathic remedy was investigated and proved by Hahnemann. It is used to treat a variety of skin disorders such as eczema, chapped, dry, sore skin, cold sores, moles, warts, corns and blisters. Also, for sore throats and catarrh, headache and indigestion. Symptoms are made worse by warm, humid weather, heat in any form, including being out in the hot sun. They are relieved by eating. People suitable for Nat. carb. have a sensitive, kind and intuitive nature, always ready to provide a sympathetic audience to others. They are devoted to their family and friends and give generously of themselves, endeavouring to be cheerful even when feeling unwell or depressed. They tend to be delicate and prone to digestive upsets, especially being intolerant of milk and dairy products. Ankles are another weak point, tending to be easily strained or sprained. Nat. carb. people are highly sensitive to music and are upset by noise and thunderstorms. They are soon exhausted by physical activity.

Natrum phosphoricum
Nat. phos.; sodium phosphate
Sodium phosphate occurs naturally in body cells and is one of the SCHUSSLER TISSUE SALTS (*see* GLOSSARY). It is involved in the regulation of acidity in body tissues and fluids, and in complex metabolic chemical processes utilizing fatty acids. It is derived from a chemical reaction between sodium carbonate and phosphoric acid. It is a useful remedy for symptoms caused by an excess of lactic acid or uric acid. Excess lactic acid may be caused by a diet too rich in milk, dairy products or fatty foods. Also, there may be an excess of gastric or stomach acid, and this may be connected with eating too much sour food. The symptoms are those of acid indigestion with a sour taste in the mouth, wind and abdominal pains. An excess of uric acid is present in people suffering from gout with painful, inflamed stiff joints. Symptoms are made worse by thunderstorms and by eating fatty, sour or sweet foods and with physical exertion. They improve for being out in the fresh, clean air and for cool, airy surroundings. People suitable for this remedy tend to be refined and some-

what timid and prone to blush easily. They are easily exhausted but are inclined to be restless or slightly agitated. They do not accept advice readily and are prone to dissatisfaction and depression.

Natrum sulphuricum
Nat. sulph.; sodium sulphate, Glauber's salt, sal mirabile

Sodium sulphate is a naturally occurring substance within the body and is involved in the regulation of the salt/water balance in tissues and fluids. It is found in natural brines associated with salt lakes or can be manufactured by a chemical process. Sodium sulphate is used in industry in the manufacture of wood pulp and paper, glass, chemicals and detergents. It was investigated and proved by Schussler and is one of the tissue salts (*see* GLOSSARY). It is used in the treatment of liver disorders including jaundice, digestive complaints with indigestion and colicky pains, severe chesty conditions such as bronchitis and asthma, and bladder problems with urinary frequency. It is also used to relieve mental symptoms that arise after a head injury, such as depression or personality changes. Symptoms are made worse by damp, cold weather or surroundings and by lying on the back. The symptoms are worse at night and during the morning. Symptoms are relieved by cool, fresh, dry conditions and being out in the fresh air. Symptoms improve if the person changes position. People suitable for Nat. sulph. may either be very serious, keeping their emotions tightly controlled and putting up a front that may hide severe depression and suicidal thoughts. Or the depression may be more apparent, and they can become emotional on hearing music or contemplating art. These types are less repressed but still tend to suffer from depression. Nat. sulph. people are often somewhat materialistic and are very sensitive to damp weather with a tendency for asthma and chesty complaints with catarrh.

Nicotiana tabacum
Tabacum; tobacco

The tobacco plant derives its Latin name from Jean Nicot, a Portuguese diplomat who was an ambassador for France in South America during the 1500s. He brought tobacco to France in about 1560, but it had long been used by the Indian peoples. The plant has a hairy stem and leaves, giving off a narcotic odour. It contains nicotine, which is a powerful poison causing sickness and nausea, palpitations, sweating, headache and giddiness. It is now well established that smoking tobacco is a major cause of premature death. The homeopathic remedy is prepared from the fresh leaves of the plant and is given as a remedy for nausea and vomiting, such as in travel sickness, vertigo and disorders affecting the organs of balance in the ears. Symptoms are made worse by even slight movements such as turning the head, and for heat and tobacco smoke. They improve in cold surroundings and after vomiting.

Nitric acidum
Nitric ac; nitric acid, aqua fortis

This is a burning, extremely corrosive, clear liquid that gives off choking fumes that cause death by inhalation. Its industrial uses are mainly in the manufacture of agricultural fertilizers and high explosives. It has been used medicinally in extremely dilute form to treat severe infections and fevers, and to dissolve stones in the kidneys or bladder. It has been applied externally to the skin to burn away warts. Nitric acid is derived from a chemical reaction between sulphuric acid and sodium nitrate.

The homeopathic remedy is used to treat sharp, stabbing pains that may be intermittent in nature and are associated with piles, or haemorrhoids, anal fissure, ulcers in the mouth or on the skin, severe sore throat with ulceration, thrush infections and ulcers in the stomach or duodenum. Usually, the affected person suffers from broken, cracked skin with a tendency for ulcers and warts, and usually feels cold. The urine and other bodily secretions have a strong, pungent odour. Symptoms are worse for acidic fruits and drinks, milk, touch or pressure and movement. They are more severe at night and improve with heat and warm, dry surroundings. People suitable for Nitric ac. tend to be selfish, self-centred and apt to hold long grudges against others. They feel that everyone is against them but are themselves apt to fly into a rage and take offence very easily. They like to re-examine events and slights of the past and may be suspicious of other people. When ill, they are very fearful and worry that they may die.

Nux moschata
Nux mosch.; *Myristica fragrans*, nutmeg

The nutmeg tree grows mainly on an Indonesian island called Banda, which is one of the Molucca group, and also in the Far East and India. It was introduced to Constantinople (Istanbul) from India in about 540 AD and soon became widely used both for culinary, cosmetic and medicinal purposes. It was used to treat digestive upsets and headache and rheumatic pain. In herbal medicine, the remedy is given for sharper, clearer eyesight. In large doses, nutmeg produces hallucinogenic symptoms of drowsiness, giddiness and unsteadiness, with unco-ordinated movements and fainting. The homeopathic tincture is made from the inner seeds without their outer tough husks. The remedy is mainly given for mental and emotional disorders and digestive upsets. Symptoms include hysteria, agitation, excitement and exhaustion and drowsiness and confusion that may follow an epileptic attack or stroke. Also, for abdominal pains and indigestion, constipation and inflammation of the gastro-intestinal tract. People who benefit from this remedy have a need for fluids being somewhat dehydrated, but do not feel any great desire to drink. Symptoms are made worse by sudden changes in the weather and damp and cool conditions. They improve for being warm, wearing plenty of clothes and for high humidity.

Ocymum canum
Alfavaca, bush basil
This is a low-growing bushy plant that is a native of India and has a sweet scent. The homeopathic tincture is made from fresh leaves, and it is used as a remedy for renal colic and stones affecting the right kidney. The symptoms are pain and vomiting, a cloudy urine because of a deposit of reddish 'sand', and urinary frequency. There may be infection present and a sharp pain on passing urine, as in cystitis. The urine has a strong, pungent smell.

Oleander
Rose laurel
The fresh leaves are used to make the homeopathic remedy, which was first investigated and proved by Hahnemann. It is given for heart symptoms including palpitations, weakness, great anxiety and fainting. The person may feel giddy or be on the point of collapse. Also, for symptoms of gastroenteritis including diarrhoea, nausea and sickness and abdominal pains. The person often has sore, dry, chapped skin and is liable to suffer from depression, lack of concentration and clumsiness with a tendency for falls and even accidents. Physical symptoms that may benefit from this remedy include vertigo, headache, blurred vision, muscular weakness, and lack of co-ordination.

Oleum petrae
Petroleum
Petroleum, or liquid crude oil, is found trapped in oil-bearing rocks in the earth's crust and is derived from decayed organic material from the Carboniferous geological period. Petroleum is a vital fuel resource upon which people throughout the world are heavily reliant. In conventional medi-

cine, petroleum jelly is used as an external treatment for minor skin abrasions. Purified petroleum is used to prepare the homeopathic remedy, which was first investigated and proved by Hahnemann and which is given for skin complaints. These include dry, cracked, chafed skin, particularly on the fingers, and eczema. These complaints are worse in cold weather, when the skin is subjected to chilling and heating. The remedy is also used for sickness, nausea and vomiting, especially as a result of travel sickness. There is a tendency for headaches to occur, especially in the back of the head. People who benefit from this remedy may be irritable because of having constantly inflamed, itchy, sore skin. They may fly into a rage and tend to have an excitable temperament. They dislike and are upset by fatty foods and their sweat has a strong odour. Symptoms are made worse by cold, windy weather, particularly during the winter months, and by thunderstorms. They improve with warmth and warm, dry weather and following a meal.

Onosmodium
False gromwell
The whole fresh parts of the green plant are needed to make the homeopathic remedy, which is used for mental symptoms including anxiety, tension and irritability. Also, for depression, lack of concentration and clumsiness, with a tendency for accidental and even accidents. Physical symptoms that may benefit from this remedy include vertigo, headache, blurred vision, muscular weakness and lack of co-ordination.

Ornithogalum umbrellatum
Star of Bethlehem
This remedy is used for severe, persistent, digestive upsets and is made from the whole green parts of the plant. There may be burning pains and regurgitation of stomach acid. The abdomen tends to be bloated with air, and there is flatulence. The person may suffer from depression and severe anxiety and is irritable and short-tempered with others. There is a tendency for peptic or duodenal ulcers to occur.

Oxalic acid
Sorrel acid, common wood sorrel, *Oxalis acetosella*
This remedy is derived from the leaves of sorrel, which have long had a culinary use. The leaves have a sour, sharp quality and can be used in place of vinegar. The plant itself is small and delicate and grows in Britain and other European countries. It produces delicate,

white flowers shaped like little bells, which are veined with purple. Preparations made from the plant have cooling and diuretic properties. The homeopathic remedy is used for painful, rheumatic disorders, mainly affecting the left side of the body. The pains are severe and sharp, and the person becomes weak and cold. There is a tendency for small haemorrhages called petechiae to occur, which have the appearance of dark red spots beneath the skin. The person may have a tendency to bleed easily and to vomit blood.

Paeonia officinalis
Peony
This plant is well known in the British Isles as a pretty, deep pink garden flower, but it has been used medicinally since ancient times. It is believed to derive its name from a Greek physician called Paos, who, according to mythology, used it to cure the gods, including Pluto, of wounds sustained during the Trojan War. Many ancient superstitions and charms were connected with the plant, which was believed to have come from the moon and to have divine origins. The root of the peony has been used to prevent nightmare and epilepsy, as a cure for madness and to combat infection after childbirth. The fresh root, which is used to prepare both the herbal and homeopathic remedies, has antispasmodic, sedative and antiseptic qualities. In homeopathy, it is used as a remedy for itchy piles, or haemorrhoids, with discomfort and swelling. Also, it is used for sleep disturbance because of nightmares and indigestion and the need to sleep during the afternoons.

Pareira brava
Ice vine, velvet leaf
This climbing vine is a native species of Peru, Brazil and the West Indies and has very large leaves and flowers. It has a twisted, knotty root, and it is this part that is used to prepare the homeopathic remedy. Preparations made from the root have a stimulant effect on the kidneys and bowels and have diuretic and tonic properties. The homeopathic remedy is used for the treatment of urinary tract infections and disorders including cystitis, urethritis, urine retention and urinary frequency. There may be hot, burning pains on passing urine with abdominal pain or discomfort.

Paris quadrifolia
One berry, true love, herba Paris
This herbaceous, perennial plant flourishes in moist, shady conditions in

woodlands throughout Europe and in Russia. A single stem is produced, which grows to a height of about ten inches or one foot, near the top of which are four pointed leaves. A single flower is produced in early summer, which is a whitish-green in colour and has an unpleasant rank smell. Later, a purple-black fruit is produced, which splits to release its seeds when ripe. The whole plant is used to prepare the homeopathic remedy, and it was first investigated and proved by Hahnemann. The plant is poisonous and has narcotic properties. If eaten in large quantities, it produces vomiting and diarrhoea, giddiness, dry throat, sweating and possibly convulsions and death. In homeopathy, it is used as an eye remedy for conjunctivitis and inflamed, irritated, itchy, watery eyes. Symptoms are mainly on the left side and the person is often excitable and talkative.

Papaver somniferum
Opium poppy, mawseed

The opium poppy is a native of Asia but is widely cultivated in other countries. In the wild, the poppy flowers are a pale mauve colour with a deeper purple spot at the base of the petals. Cultivated flowers have a variety of colours, from white to red/purple. The unripened green seed capsules that develop at the base of the flowers are the part used in herbal medicine and homeopathy. An incision is made into the capsule, and a milky white juice is exuded that darkens as it dries. This is collected by scraping the capsules. The principal constituents of the opium juice are the alkaloids morphine and codeine, which are widely used in conventional medicine for their potent analgesic properties. Opium was used by the physicians of ancient Greece and Rome as a painkiller. It was probably introduced into India and hence to Europe by Arabian physicians. Dark grey poppy seeds, from the red/purple coloured flowers (called mawseed) are used in cooking and do not contain opium or morphine. They are also a constituent of bird seed. Opium has narcotic, sedative, hypnotic and antispasmodic properties. In homeopathy the remedy is used to treat symptoms of mental shock following a severe emotional shock or frightening experience. The symptoms may either be those of withdrawal and apathy, or of great agitation, excitement and sleeplessness with a greatly enhanced acute sense of hearing. It is also given for respiratory and breathing problems, constipation, alcohol withdrawal symptoms (delirium tremens) and following a stroke. Symptoms are worse for sleep and heat and improve with movement and exercise and in cool surroundings.

Parotidinum
The mumps nosode
This homeopathic remedy is derived from mumps-infected parotid salivary gland secretion. It is usually given as a preventative medicine to adults at risk of contracting mumps.

Passiflora incarnata
Passionflower, maypops
There are a number of species of passionflower, which gain their name from the resemblance of the blooms to the crown of thorns worn by Jesus. The plant produces large, sweet-scented flowers that are white or whitish-peach coloured with tinges of purple. Later, large berries with many seeds are produced, which are edible. The green parts of the plant are used to prepare herbal and homeopathic remedies. Preparations derived from the passionflower have sedative, narcotic and antispasmodic properties. In homeopathy, the remedy is used for convulsions, as in epilepsy, and also for illnesses in which there are severe spasms, such as whooping cough, asthmatic attacks and tetanus. Also, for serious mental disturbance, including delirium tremens resulting from alcoholism, and excited manic states.

Pertussin
Coqueluchin
This remedy is a nosode of whooping cough and is derived from material contaminated with the virus. It is given to treat the symptoms of whooping cough but also as a preventative measure for those at risk of contracting the disease.

Phellandrium aquaticum
Water fennel, fine-leaved water dropwort
This plant grows in ditches or on the banks of rivers near to the water; the lower parts may be submerged. The plant produces fruits that yield a yellow liquid from which the herbal and homeopathic remedies are derived. The preparations have expectorant and diuretic properties and are useful for treating chesty, bronchitic complaints. In homeopathy, the remedy is used for chest and respiratory disorders, with symptoms mainly on the right side. Conditions treated include bronchitis and emphysema with breathlessness, a severe cough and the production of thick mucus. Headache is another common symptom.

Phleum pratense

Timothy grass

This is a remedy for hay fever that is triggered by exposure to the pollen of flowering grasses. The person has the typical symptoms of watering, itchy eyes and running nose and sneezing. Breathlessness and asthma may also occur. The remedy is sometimes given to prevent the occurrence of an attack of hay fever.

Phosphoricum acidum

Phos. ac.; phosphoric acid

Phosphoric acid is a clear, crystalline substance that is obtained by a chemical process from a naturally occurring mineral, apatite. Apatite is rich in phosphate and occurs in various igneous (volcanic) and metamorphic rocks (ones altered by high temperatures and pressures) and mineral veins. Phosphoric acid has various industrial uses in the manufacture of fertilizers and detergents. It is used in the food industry as a flavouring for soft drinks and in the refining of white sugar. Also, it is used in the production of various pharmaceutical drugs. In conventional medicine it is used in the treatment of parathyroid gland tumours, acting to reduce blood calcium levels.

The homeopathic remedy was first investigated and proved by Hahnemann and is used to treat emotional and physical symptoms of apathy, exhaustion, listlessness and depression. These symptoms may arise from overwork or study or follow on after a debilitating illness that has caused dehydration. Other symptoms are a loss of appetite, feeling continually cold and shivery, dizziness, especially in the evening, and a feeling of pressure pushing downwards on the head. Phos. ac. is also given for growing pains in children or who suffer from sleep disturbance because of an awareness of sexual feelings. Symptoms are worse for cold, damp, draughty conditions and for loud noises. They improve following restful sleep and with warm surroundings.

Physostigma veneriosum

Calabar bean, chop nut, ordeal bean

This perennial climbing plant grows to a height of about 50 feet and is a native species of West Africa. It was introduced into Britain (and grown in the Botanical Gardens in Edinburgh) in 1846. It produces purple-coloured elongated flowers and later, dark brown seeds in pods about 6 inches in length. The seeds are extremely poisonous and were given as a test for witchcraft by West African peoples. If the accused person vomited after being forced to swallow the seeds, he or she was deemed innocent, but if death was the outcome then the accusation of being a witch was upheld. The poison causes depression of the central nervous system, slowing of the pulse and a rise in blood pressure, and death may follow because of respiratory collapse. Preparations made from the seeds are also miotic, causing a rapid contraction of the pupil of the eye, and its main use in herbal medicine is in the treatment of eye diseases. The ripe beans or seeds are used to prepare the homeopathic remedy, which is given for serious disorders in which there are muscular spasms. These include tetanus, meningitis and poliomyelitis. Also, for other disorders characterized by muscular and nervous degeneration or paralysis including Friedrich's ataxia, motor neurone disease and multiple sclerosis. The remedy may also be given for diarrhoea, vomiting, fever, sweating, prostration, and palpitations in which the pupils of the eye are very much contracted.

Phytolacca deccandra
Phytolacca; Virginian poke root, garget, reading plant, pocon, branching grape, pigeon berry

This plant is a native species of the United States and Canada, but is also found in Mediterranean countries, China and North Africa. It has a striking appearance and produces white flowers followed by clusters of shiny black berries. The orange-coloured fleshy root is the part used to prepare the homeopathic remedy, but both the root and berries are used in herbal medicine. Preparations derived from the plant have purgative, emetic and restorative properties. Native American Indians used poke root to cause vomiting and to encourage movement of the bowels and as a heart stimulant. It was also used as a remedy for skin disorders. Europeans used the plant to treat breast lumps and tumours and for mastitis (inflammation). In herbal medicine it is used to treat skin disorders, ringworm and scabies, chronic rheumatism, granular conjunctivitis (eye inflammation), ulcers and severe menstrual pain.

In homeopathy the remedy is given for small hard lumps or tumours in the breasts, which may be either benign or cancerous, and for mastitis. The breasts may be hot, swollen and painful to touch with stabbing pains. Also, it is used to treat severe sore throats and swallowing difficulty in which there is great pain, redness and inflammation. These symptoms may occur with tonsillitis, pharyngitis and diphtheria. The symptoms are made worse by swallowing, movement, hot drinks and in cold, damp draughty conditions. They improve with warmth and sunny, dry weather, cold drinks and having plenty of rest.

Picricum acidum
Picric acid

This poisonous substance is obtained by chemical reactions between nitric, sulphuric and carbolic acids. Since it was first investigated and proved for homeopathic use in 1868, it has been used to treat extreme exhaustion with mental and intellectual indifference and apathy. It usually occurs after an extended period of intense intellectual activity such as may occur among students cramming for exams. The person feels generally heavy and lethargic and is too tired to engage in conversation or to think clearly. Often, a numbing headache and aching eyes occur, or there may be a boil in the outer part of the ear. These symptoms may also arise as a result of grief. Symptoms are made worse with any physical or intellectual activity and in hot surroundings. They improve with rest and in cool conditions and if the weather is sunny but not hot.

Pilocarpus jaborandi, Pilocarpus microphyllus
Jaborandi

The drug known as Jaborandi is extracted from the leaves of *Pilocarpus*, which are shrubs native to Brazil. The leaves contain a volatile oil, and the most important active constituent of this is an alkaloid substance called pilocarpine. Preparations made from the leaves have diaphoretic properties, causing sweating, and are also stimulant and expectorant. Pilocarpine is mydriatic, causing contraction of the pupil of the eye. In herbal medicine, Jaborandi is used to treat diabetes, asthma, skin disorders such as psoriasis, catarrh and oedema (fluid retention). Also it is used as a tonic in preparations to stimulate new hair growth in the treatment of baldness. The homeopathic remedy is given for various eye and vision disorders, sweating because of the menopause or in hyperthyroidism (an overactive thyroid gland) and mumps.

Plantago major
Common plantain, broad-leaved plantain, waybread, ripple grass

This is a very familiar weed that grows throughout Britain and Europe and was introduced by colonists into the New World continents. The use of plantain in medicine goes back to ancient times, and it is described by Erasmus and Pliny. In Britain, plantain was an ingredient of many old remedies. It has been used in the past to treat wounds and external bleeding, for venomous bites and for disorders of the bowels and kidneys. It was used as a remedy for piles, or haemorrhoids, and to treat diarrhoea. Plantain is still used to treat these ailments in modern herbal medicine and homeopathy. The whole fresh plant is used to prepare the homeopathic remedy, which is sometimes used as the mother tincture. It is given for piles, toothache and tooth abscess and facial neuralgia. It is also used in the treatment of conditions such as diabetes, characterized by large quantities of urine being passed. Most symptoms occur on the left side and are worse for movement, cold and heat and draughts.

Platinum metallicum
Platinum

Platinum was discovered in South America during the 1700s. It is regarded as a very precious metal and is used to make jewellery. It is used in the electrical industry, in dentistry for fillings, and to make surgical pins to repair fractured bones. The homeopathic remedy is used almost entirely for female reproductive disorders that may have associated emotional problems. These include pain in the ovaries, spasm in vaginal muscles, making it difficult for the woman to have sexual intercourse (vaginisimus), heavy menstrual bleeding, absence of periods and genital itching. The woman may experience feelings of numbness, chilling and constriction of muscles and has a great fear of gynaecological examinations and procedures. Symptoms are made worse by touch and physical contact and by tiredness. They are worse in the evening but are relieved by being out in fresh clean air.

Women suitable for platinum set themselves and others extremely high standards of achievement that are not possible to attain. Hence they feel let down by apparent failures and tend to become depressed and irritable, feeling that the past was better than the present. They may become cynical and contemptuous of the efforts of others.

Plumbum metallicum
Plumbum met.; lead

Lead has been useful to humana for centuries and was used extensively by the Romans, especially to make pipes for plumbing systems. Lead continued to be mined and used throughout the ages, and has had many uses, e.g. in roofing, to make weights and lead shot, pencils, pottery glazes, paint and as an additive in fuel for vehicle engines. It has been known for some time, however, that lead is an insidious poison if present above a certain level in the human body. Early symptoms of poisoning are constipation that persists, weakness of muscles, pale skin and a blue line (because of lead sulphide) along the margin of gums and teeth. There is intellectual dullness and impairment and behavioural changes, and these are especially noticeable in children. Later, there are severe abdominal pains of a colicky nature, drooping wrists and feet, tremors, increasing muscular weakness and paralysis. Convulsions and lead encephalopathy affecting the brain may occur, leading to death if not diagnosed and treated.

The homeopathic remedy is used to treat long-term diseases of a sclerotic nature, i.e. leading to hardening of the affected tissues. These conditions include arteriosclerosis and atherosclerosis, Parkinson's disease and multiple sclerosis. Also for colic, constipation, muscular weakness and tremor and retention of urine. Symptoms are made worse by movement and are more severe at night. They improve with warmth and firm pressure or massage on the affected area. People suitable for Plumbum met. may have poor concentration and intellectual capabilities dulled by illness. They may have a poor memory and find it difficult to express themselves clearly. This intellectual impairment may make the person lethargic or short-tempered with others.

Podophyllum peltatum
Podophyllum; May apple, hog apple, American mandrake, duck's foot, wild lemon, racoonberry.

This herbaceous perennial plant is a native of the United States and Canada. The stalks grow to a height of about one or two feet and produce large, divided leaves and white flowers that have an unpleasant scent. Later, yellow fruits are produced that are edible although the leaves and roots are poisonous. The plant has a yellowish-brown rhizome and roots, and these are the parts used both in herbal medicine and homeopathy. Preparations made from the plant have purgative and emetic properties and act strongly on the liver and digestive organs. The plant was used by the native American peoples to eliminate parasitic worms and as a cure for deafness. The homeopathic remedy is given for digestive disorders such as vomiting and diarrhoea in gastroenteritis, gallstones, colicky pain and flatulence. There may be alternate bouts of diarrhoea and constipation. Symptoms are worse first thing in the morning and during hot weather. They are better for massaging the abdomen and for lying on the front.

Primula veris
Cowslip, herb Peter, key flower, mayflower, key of heaven, pargle, peggle

This familiar and pretty wild flower is common in shady woodlands in Europe and Great Britain. It produces delicate yellow flowers, and it is these that are used to prepare the herbal and homeopathic remedies. Preparations made from the plant have a sedative and antispasmodic effect.

The flowers have been used to make cowslip wine, and the leaves were once valued as a salad vegetable. The homeopathic remedy is used for serious symptoms of high blood pressure and threatened stroke. These include confusion and giddiness, headache and a feeling of throbbing heat.

Prunus laurocerasus
Cherry laurel, cherry bay, common laurel

This fairly small evergreen shrub is a native species of Russia but also grows in Europe and some parts of Asia. It produces dark green shiny leaves and white flowers followed by clusters of black, cherry-like fruits. The fresh leaves are used to prepare the herbal and homeopathic remedies and give off a characteristic bitter almonds smell because of the presence of prussic acid. The shrubs are popular in gardens in Europe, having been first introduced in the late 16th century. The leaves are mainly used to produce cherry laurel water in herbal medicine, and preparations have a sedative effect. They are used for coughs and spasms, particularly whooping cough and asthma. The homeopathic remedy is used to treat severe symptoms of breathlessness and cyanosis (a blue tinge to the skin because of lack of oxygen in the blood) with a spasmodic cough. The symptoms are caused by serious disorders of the heart or lungs.

Psorinum

This remedy is derived from the fluid of scabies blisters and was first investigated and proved by Hahnemann. Hahnemann wrote extensively about the development of chronic diseases. He believed that in certain people the blisters produced in scabies were a manifestation of a deeper disorder. While the scabies blisters themselves might heal and disappear, this suppressed disease, or MIASM, still continued to cause disruption within the body and might even be passed on to subsequent generations. The symptoms or disorder associated with the scabies miasm are called psora and mainly affect the skin. The skin is dry, cracked and sore and there may be infections with pus-filled blisters. Also, digestive upsets, particularly diarrhoea and indigestion, exhaustion, depression and a pessimistic outlook on life are believed to be common manifestations of psora. The psorinum remedy is given to treat the symptoms described above and also for some respiratory ailments, especially hay fever, and general debility. Digestive ailments treated include irritable bowel syndrome and diverticulitis. Skin conditions such as eczema, acne, dermatitis, boils and ulceration may all respond to psorinum.

People suitable for this remedy are generally worried, pessimistic and gloomy, with a fear of all that may go wrong in life. They are very sensitive to cold and often feel chilled, even during the height of summer. They often experience a gnawing hunger and have a headache that is relieved by eating. They may feel that friends and family have deserted them. Symptoms are worse for cold winter weather and also for becoming too hot, either in bed or through physical exercise or wearing too many clothes. They improve in summer, with resting with the limbs spread out and with warm surroundings.

Ptelea trifoliata
Wafer ash, swamp dogwood, hop tree, wingseed, shrubby trefoil, ptelea
This small, shrubby tree, which grows to a height of six to eight feet, is a native species of the United States and Canada. The bark of the root is the part used to prepare remedies used in herbal medicine and homeopathy. The bark has a fairly pungent smell and a bitter taste and has a tonic effect, acting mainly on the liver and digestive organs. The homeopathic remedy is used mainly for liver disorders such as hepatitis and enlargement and tenderness. There is discomfort and heaviness in the region of the liver. Also, for digestive disorders, particularly indigestion, and rheumatism. All symptoms are mainly on the right side of the body and are made worse if the person lies on his or her right side.

Pyrogenium
Pyrogenium is a remedy introduced to homeopathy by Dr John Drysdale in 1880. It was a mixture of raw beef and water left to stand for three weeks. After straining, a straw-coloured liquid, called sepsin, was left, which, when mixed with glycerine, was called pyrogen. Dr Drysdale believed that pyrogen had profound effects upon the blood if taken in large amounts, causing septicaemia or blood poisoning. In modern homeopathy, the pyrogenium remedy is given for blood poisoning and septic conditions in which the healing process is rather slow. Characteristically, the person is feverish and has aching bones, a rapid pulse with feelings of heat and burning. The person is uncomfortable and restless and may have considerable pain if suffering from a septic condition such as an abscess. Symptoms are made worse by cold and draughts but improve with moving about.

Radium bromatum
Radium brom.; radium bromide
Radium bromide is derived from radium, which was discovered by Pierre and Marie Curie at the end of the 19th century. Radium is used in conven-

tional medicine in radiotherapy for the treatment of cancer. It is obtained from the radioactive mineral uranite, which is also the main ore of uranium. Radium bromide is obtained by a chemical process from radium, and the homeopathic remedy is used to treat skin complaints in which there is itching and burning. Ailments include eczema, moles, skin ulcers, acne, skin cancer, rosacea (a red, flushed face and enlargement of the skin's sebaceous glands) and dry, chafed, sore skin. Also, for aching painful bones as in lumbago, rheumatic and arthritic disorders and bone cancer. Pains may move from one side of the body to the other, and symptoms are worse at night and on first moving after resting. They improve if the person lies down or moves about for a prolonged period. They are also better for lying down and for having a hot bath.

Rananculus bulbosus
Buttercup, bulbous buttercup, crowfoot, St Anthony's turnip, gold cup, frogsfoot

The familiar bright yellow buttercup is a familiar summer flower in Great Britain and other European countries. Small, bulbous swellings that resemble little turnips occur at the base of the stems. The plant can cause blistering and inflammation of the skin and has been used in a similar way to Cantharis (Spanish fly). The homeopathic remedy is used for skin irritation and blistering, as in shingles and eczema, and for rheumatism with hot, tearing pains. Also, for pleurisy with severe pains during breathing. All symptoms are made worse by cold and damp and if the person feels afraid. The person tends to be generally rundown and unwell.

Raphanus sativus
Black radish, black Spanish radish

There are many varieties of radish that are cultivated as salad vegetables. In herbal medicine, the juice obtained from the radish is used as a cure for gallstones and other stones or gravel. In homeopathy the remedy is used for abdominal flatulence and may be given post-operatively if there is sluggishness or some degree of paralysis of the digestive tract.

Rhatanhy
Krameria triandra, krameria root, Peruvian rhatany, rhantania

This low-growing shrub, which produces attractive large, red flowers, is a native species of Peru, growing in dry sandy soils in mountainous regions up to about 8,000 feet. The plant has strong roots, and it is these that are used to prepare the herbal and homeopathic remedies. Preparations made from the plant have astringent and tonic properties and have been used to treat anal fissure and haemorrhage, diarrhoea, urinary incontinence, and excessive menstrual bleeding. The homeopathic remedy is used to treat constipation with the development of painful haemorrhoids, or piles. The pains feel like glass splinters in the rectum and are very sharp. The person may have an odd sensation as though cold water is flowing over the molar teeth.

Rhododendron chrysanthemum
Rhododendron; yellow rhododendron, snow rose, rosebay

This low shrub or bush has a highly branched, reddish stem and grows to a height of about eighteen inches or two feet. The leaves are oval and resemble those of laurel. Large, attractive, golden yellow flowers are produced, and the plant is a native of the mountainous regions of Siberia, Asia and Europe. In herbal medicine the plant has long been used to treat rheumatic disorders and gout. The fresh leaves are used to prepare the herbal and homeopathic remedies. In homeopathy, the remedy is also used to treat gout, rheumatism and arthritis. Main symptoms are hot, painful swollen joints with severe pains. The remedy is additionally used for stabbing neuralgic pains around the eyes and in the face, pain in the testicles, high fever with confusion and delirium, and severe headaches. People who benefit from this remedy tend to have an anxious temperament. Symptoms are worse during the approach of a thunderstorm and at night. They are also made worse by standing still for a long period of time, by resting and at the start of movement. They improve with warmth and following a meal.

Rosa canina
The familiar dog-rose is an attractive bush producing pretty, delicately perfumed white or pink flowers in summer. Later, scarlet-coloured hips are produced containing the seeds that are used to make rose hip syrup. The hips have astringent and cooling properties and are a good source of vitamin C. They have been used in herbal medicine to treat diarrhoea, coughs and the coughing up of blood, as in consumption (tuberculosis), colic and kidney stones. In homeopathy, the remedy made from the ripe hips is used to treat disorders of the bladder and prostate gland, characterized by difficult and slow release of urine.

Rosmarinus officinalis
Rosemary, compass weed, polar plant, compass plant

This small, evergreen herb is a native of the arid, rocky hills along the

Mediterranean coast but may also grow inland. It has been grown in Britain for centuries and has been important for both culinary and medicinal purposes. It was believed to affect the brain, strengthening the memory, and became associated with the virtues of remembrance, fidelity and friendship. It was included in bridal and funeral wreaths and flowers, burned as incense in religious festivals and believed to have magical properties. It was burnt or hung up as an antiseptic in sick rooms and hospitals, and strewn among clothes and linen to prevent attack by moths. Oil of rosemary was used externally to treat baldness, dandruff and gout in the hands and feet, and in wine for headaches, palpitations and dropsy (fluid retention or oedema). Oil of rosemary is obtained from the flowering sprigs or tops of the plant. The homeopathic remedy is used for memory loss and lack of concentration and for baldness.

Rumex crispus
Yellow dock, curled dock

This dock is commonly found on wasteland and along roadsides in the British Isles and has leaves that are curled and crisp at the edges. It grows to a height of about three feet and has large green leaves. The root is used in herbal medicine and has laxative and tonic properties. The homeopathic remedy is prepared from the whole flowering plant. It is used to treat itching skin conditions, nasal congestion with an abundance of thick, sticky catarrh, and diarrhoea and digestive disorders. Symptoms are made worse by cold and draughts and are better for warmth and heat.

Sabadilla officinarum
Sabadilla; *Asagraea officinalis*, cevadilla, cebadilla, *Veratum sabadilla*

These rushlike plants grow in the southern states of the United States, Mexico and Central America (Venezuela and Guatemala). The seeds are used to prepare herbal and homeopathic remedies, and these have been known in Europe since the 16th century. The preparations can be poisonous if taken internally, causing severe vomiting and diarrhoea. They were formerly used in Europe to kill intestinal parasitic worms and to eliminate lice. They were also used to treat rheumatism, gout and neuralgia. Sabadilla produces respiratory symptoms, resembling those of a cold, i.e. sneezing, running nose, watering, itchy eyes, coughing, headache and a painful sore throat. The homeopathic remedy is used to treat these symptoms and also to eliminate an infestation of threadworms. The symptoms are worse for cold and draughts and better for warmth and wearing warm clothes.

Sabal semilata
Sabal; the sabal palm, saw palmetto, palmetto scrub

This palm-like tree grows to a height of six to ten feet and has a crown of large, serrated leaves. It grows in the coastal regions of South Carolina and Florida and in southern California. Irregularly shaped, oval, dark brown berries are produced containing seeds, and these are a source of fatty oil. They are a valuable food source for wild animals, promoting weight gain. The fresh berries and seeds are used to prepare the remedies used in herbal medicine and homeopathy, and they have sedative, tonic and diuretic properties. The homeopathic remedy is mainly used to treat enlargement of the prostate gland, causing difficult, slow urination with sharp pains. Sexual intercourse may be painful, and there is general tiredness and loss of libido. Also, for inflammation of the testicles and breasts (mastitis) with heat, swelling and tenderness.

 People who are suitable for sabal are afraid of going to sleep, and their symptoms are made worse by cold, damp conditions and the sympathy of others. Symptoms improve with warm, dry weather and surroundings.

Sabina cacumina
Savine; savine tops

The shrub or small evergreen tree *Juniperus sabina* is a native species of the northern states of North America and some European countries. This plant is grown in gardens in Britain, and the fresh spring growth is used to prepare herbal and homeopathic remedies. Preparations derived from the plant are irritant and poisonous in large doses and have powerful effects upon the uterus, causing bleeding. In herbal medicine the remedy is used externally for skin conditions, especially to encourage the drawing out of infection. In homeopathy the remedy is given for rectal and uterine bleeding with pains that may be stabbing or burning. Also, for cystitis, heavy menstrual periods and varicose veins.

Salvia officinalis
Sage, garden sage

Sage is a familiar garden herb that has been cultivated in Europe for many centuries. There are several varieties, but the wild form of sage is found in the warmer parts of Europe and along the Mediterranean coast. Sage has long been valued as a herb for flavouring food and to make a form of 'tea'. It has been used medicinally since ancient times and was used to treat liver diseases, wounds, ulcers and bleeding, especially the coughing up of blood, headache and rheumatic pains, throat infections, as a remedy for snake bites and to strengthen the brain and memory. The homeopathic remedy is made from the fresh leaves and flowers, and preparations derived from sage have astringent and tonic properties and calming effects on the digestive organs. The remedy is used to treat hoarseness and sore throats, mouth ulcers or ulcerated throat and bleeding or infected gums.

Sanguinaria canadensis
Sanguinaria; red puccoon, blood root, coon root, sweet slumber, snake-bite, Indian paint

This attractive, perennial plant is a native species of North America and Canada, growing in rich soils in woodlands. It produces beautiful, white flowers and has thick, bulbous fleshy roots containing orange-red sap. This juice was used by the native Indian peoples as dye for clothes and body paint. The root, green parts of the plant, fruit and seeds are used to prepare herbal and homeopathic remedies. The plant contains a potent alkaloid substance called sanguinarine, which forms colourless crystals. This is toxic in large doses, causing burning in the stomach with vomiting, thirst, giddiness, disturbed vision and possible collapse and death. In smaller doses the preparations have emetic and expectorant properties and also act on the uterus, promoting menstruation. In both herbal and homeopathy, the remedies are used for chest and respiratory ailments, including bronchitis, pharyngitis (inflammation of the pharynx), asthma and polyps (small, fleshy projections) in the nose or throat. Symptoms include dryness and soreness, thirst, chest pain that may extend to the right shoulder, and croup-like cough. Also, for whooping cough, colds and influenza, hay fever, severe migraine-like headaches with visual disturbance and rheumatic pains in the right shoulder. Symptoms often occur mainly on the right side and are worse if the person lies on that side of the body. They are made worse by cold, damp weather, touch and movement and by eating sweet foods. Symptoms improve in the evening and following sleep and if the person lies on the left side.

Sanicula aqua
Sanicula

Sanicula is a spring of water in Ottawa in Canada and Illinois in the United States of America. The water contains various salts and minerals that are themselves used to make homeopathic remedies. The sanicula remedy is mainly given to children with delicate stomachs and a tendency to suffer from constipation or diarrhoea after eating, vomiting and sickness, travel sickness and wetting the bed. Children who need this remedy are usually thin in spite of eating heartily and may have rapidly changing moods. Often there is a tendency for the head and feet to be hot and sweaty. Symptoms are made worse by downward, falling movements but improve if the child rests with little clothing or covering.

Secale comutum
Secale; ergot, spurred rye
The condition known as ergot is a form of fungus that grows on rye, wheat and various other grasslike cereals. The spores of the fungus germinate and grow on the stigmas and ovaries of the head of the grass. They form small, curved, black seed-like bodies (sclerotia, singular sclerotium) that eventually fall off when the ears of the cereal crop are ripe. The sclerotia are collected when immature before the grain is ripe to prepare the homeopathic remedy. Ergot has been known as a poison for many centuries. Cases of poisoning occurred because of eating foods made from contaminated cereals. Ergot contains several potent alkaloid substances, and symptoms of poisoning include burning pains, a crawling feeling on the skin, delirium, convulsions, gangrene, collapse and death. The substances have a powerful effect on the uterus and other smooth muscle, causing it to contract, and also on the central nervous system.

  In modern homeopathy the remedy is used to treat spasms in the arteries, as in Raynaud's phenomena (numbness and blanching, redness and burning in fingers and toes), cramp-like pain in leg muscles, uterine pains and contractions leading to bleeding irregularities, and ineffective contractions during labour. The person has cold, numb skin but feels hot and burning inside. (In orthodox medicine, ergot is used to control postpartum haemorrhage following childbirth or abortion). Symptoms are worse for any form of heat or covering and better in cool, fresh air and surroundings.

Senecio aureus
Golden groundsel, life root, golden senecio, squaw weed
This perennial plant, which grows to a height of one or two feet, is a native of North America and Canada and also grows in Europe. It produces golden yellow flowers, and the whole plant is used to prepare the remedies used in herbal medicine and homeopathy. Preparations made from the plant have astringent and diuretic properties and also act on the uterus, chest and lungs. The homeopathic remedy is used for absent or

suppressed periods that may be accompanied by pain, chesty catarrhal complaints, urinary problems such as kidney stones and cystitis, and bleeding problems, e.g. nosebleeds.

Smilax officinalis, Smilax medica
Sarsaparilla; red-bearded sarsaparilla, Jamaica sarsaparilla

The unusual name of this plant was derived from two Spanish words, *sarza* for 'bramble' and *parilla* for 'vine'. The plant has prickly, thorny stems and is a native of Central and South America. It is thought to have been exported via Jamaica to Europe, but it does not grow in the West Indies. It was once used as a treatment for syphilis, and smoke from the burning plant was considered beneficial in the treatment of asthma. Preparations made from the plant have diuretic and tonic properties and promote perspiration. The fresh root is used to prepare the herbal and homeopathic remedies. In homeopathy sarsaparilla is used to treat bladder, kidney and urinary disorders, especially kidney stones causing renal colic and cystitis. There is a frequent need to urinate, although only small amounts may be passed, and sharp burning pains. The urine frequently appears cloudy, containing small deposits or stones. There may be a slight degree of incontinence of urine, especially if sitting down. The remedy is also used for rheumatism with pains that are worse at night and in cold, damp, draughty conditions. Also, for eczema and dry skin with painful deep cracks and fissures. People who benefit from this remedy feel cold and have a tendency to have dry scaly skin and spots. Skin conditions are worse in the months of spring. Symptoms are worse at night and in cold, damp, draughty conditions. They improve if the person is standing and uncovers the chest and neck.

Solanum dulcamara
Dulcamara; woody nightshade, scarlet berry, bittersweet, felonwort, felonberry, violet bloom

This rambling, trailing plant grows over bushes and hedges, extending for a considerable distance and supported by other plants. It is a native species of many European countries, including Britain. The young stems of the plant are green and furry, but they become more woody and smooth with age. The plant produces purple-blue flowers and, later, berries that are bright red when ripe. The stems taste bitter at first if chewed and then sweet (hence, bittersweet). Felon is an old name for a whitlow (an abscess on a finger or toe) and the name felonwort refers to the fact that the plant was used to cure these. Woody nightshade has a long history of medicinal use going back to ancient times. It has been used to treat a wide variety of disorders, especially skin complaints, asthma and chesty, catarrhal conditions, rheumatism and absent menstruation. The young shoots and twigs, leaves and flowers are used to prepare the homeopathic remedy. This is given for ailments that are made worse, or are brought on, by exposure to cold and damp or sudden cooling, including colds and coughs, catarrhal complaints and conjunctivitis. Also, for skin conditions such as eczema, itchy rashes, ringworm, nettle rash (urticaria) and warts. Symptoms are worse for cold, damp weather and changes of temperature. They improve with exercise, movement, warmth and heat.

Solidago virgaurea
Golden rod, woundwort, Aaron's rod, solidago
This familiar garden plant grows in Europe, Asia and North America. It produces green leaves and golden yellow flowers and has long been valued as a remedy for kidney and urinary disorders, especially kidney stones. The green parts are used to prepare the homeopathic remedy, which is used to treat problems of urine retention and lack of urination and renal colic.

Spigelia anthelmia
Spigelia; pink root, annual worm grass
This perennial plant is a native of the northern countries of South America and the West Indies, and a related type, *Spigelia marylandica*, grows in some states of North America. It was used by the native Indian peoples to expel intestinal parasitic worms, and is narcotic and a potent poison if taken in large amounts. The fresh plant has an unpleasant smell and is gathered and dried to prepare the homeopathic remedy, which is given especially for left-sided symptoms and particularly heart disorders. These include angina and coronary artery disease with severe pain. Also given for neuralgia, left-sided headache and migraine, iritis (inflammation of the iris of the eye), all of which are accompanied by sharp pains. People who benefit from this remedy have a phobia about long, pointed, sharp objects, e.g. needles. Symptoms are worse for lying on the left side, cold air, touch and movement, and during the approach of a thunderstorm. They improve with warm, dry conditions, lying on the right side, in the evening and for having the head raised when resting.

Spongia tosta
Spongia; natural sponge
Natural sponge has been used since the early Middle Ages to treat the

enlargement of the thyroid gland, known as goitre, that results from a deficiency in iodine. The condition may result from a dietary lack of iodine or by some disorder of metabolism or of the thyroid gland itself. In more recent times, scientists discovered that sponges are naturally rich in iodine. Roasted sponge is used to prepare the homeopathic remedy, which is used to treat thyroid gland disorders and goitre. There may be symptoms of palpitations, flushing, sweating, breathlessness, heat intolerance, anxiety and nervousness. Also, for heart disorders, including an enlarged heart or disease of the valves. Symptoms include palpitations, pain, breathlessness, exhaustion and a feeling of being crushed by a heavy weight. The person may be flushed and anxious with a fear of death. The Spongia remedy is useful in the treatment of a hoarse, dry sore throat, as in laryngitis, and particularly where respiratory illnesses such as tuberculosis are associated with the family. Symptoms are worse for movement, touch, trying to talk and for cold drinks and cold surroundings. They improve with warmth and warm meals and drinks, and for sitting propped up. People suitable for Spongia are often thin with a fair complexion and light-coloured hair.

Stannum metallicum
Stannum met.; tin

Tin is obtained from the mineral cassiterite, which occurs as dark-coloured crystals in such rocks as pegmatites and granites and in the alluvial deposits of streams and rivers. Tin is a soft, silver-coloured metal that has long been useful to humankind and has had many industrial uses. Medicinally, it was once given to expel intestinal tapeworms. In modern homeopathy, the remedy is used for severe catarrhal chest complaints, including bronchitis, laryngitis, asthma and inflammation of the windpipe (tracheitis). There is a thick, yellowish catarrh and a hoarse, dry cough. The person is sometimes weak and debilitated, suffering from loss of weight and exhaustion with associated depression and weepiness. The remedy is also given for neuralgic pain and headache, particularly on the left side. The pains may have a gradual onset and also be slow to disappear. Symptoms are made worse if the person lies on his or her right side and drinks warm fluids. They improve for coughing up catarrh and for firm pressure on the painful part.

Sticta pulmonaria
Sticta; lungwort, oak lungs, lung moss, Jerusalem cowslip

This plant, which is familiar in gardens in Great Britain and other European countries, has rough, oval green leaves speckled with white, reminiscent of lungs. The stalks grow to a height of about one foot, and the flowers are a pinky-red at first but purply-blue when fully open. Preparations of the plant have astringent properties and act on the mucous membranes of the respiratory tract. The homeopathic remedy is prepared from the whole fresh plant and is used to treat colds, asthma, lung inflammation and rheumatic disorders. The catarrh is difficult to cough up and persistent. Symptoms are worse at night and for cold, damp conditions. They are worse for lying down and better for warmth.

Strophanthus kombe, Strophanthus hispidus
Kombé seeds

These climbing plants are native to tropical parts of East Africa. The name is derived from two Greek words, *strophos*, 'rope' or 'twisted cord', and *anthos*, 'flower'. They produce seeds that are extremely poisonous, and the poison was used on arrows for hunting by African tribal peoples. The most active constituents are a glucoside substance called strophanthin and an alkaloid, inoeine. Preparations made from the seeds have a similar effect to digitalis, and are used to treat heart and circulatory disorders. The homeopathic remedy is used to treat palpitations, irregular heartbeat and breathlessness. It is a useful remedy for those whose health has been compromised by smoking or drinking alcohol.

Sulphuric acid
This remedy is used for mental exhaustion and depression, the person being restless and agitated. There is a tendency for skin problems to occur, including ulcers and boils. Other symptoms include mouth ulcers, bleeding gums and depression.

Symphoricarpus racemosa
Snowberry, wolf berry, coal berry, wax berry

Preparations made from this North American plant have emetic and purgative properties. The homeopathic remedy is used for cases of severe vomiting and nausea, including morning sickness in pregnancy. There is a loss of appetite and there may also be a loss of weight.

Syphilinum
This remedy is derived from material obtained from a syphilitic lesion. Syphilis is a serious sexually transmitted bacterial disease that has plagued humankind for centuries. Hahnemann believed that syphilis was one of

three main MIASMS, having an inherited element from earlier generations affected with the illness. The homeopathic remedy is used to treat chronic ulcers and abscesses, especially in the genital area. Also for menstrual pains, neuralgia, varicose ulcers, constipation and inflammation of the iris of the eyes (iritis). The person may experience pain in the long bones and have weak teeth. Symptoms are worse for great heat or cold, at night, near the sea and during a thunderstorm. They improve with gentle walking and through the day and for being in a mountainous region.

People suitable for this remedy tend to be anxious and on edge, with nervous mannerisms such as exaggerated blinking or a muscular twitch or tic. They may show obsessive behaviour, such as a need to recheck constantly on something or to keep on washing their hands. They may find it difficult to concentrate and have a poor memory. They may have a problem with alcohol, drugs or smoking.

Tammus communis
Black bryony, blackeye root

This poisonous climbing plant is common in hedges, copses and open woodlands in the British Isles. It has heart-shaped leaves and white flowers, with bright red berries produced in the autumn. The plant has a dark-coloured root that is the part most often used in herbal medicine and homeopathy. Preparations made from the plant have diuretic and blistering properties and are helpful for clearing the discoloration of a bruise (hence blackeye root). The homeopathic remedy is used to treat chilblains with soreness, redness, inflammation and itching.

Terebinthinae oleum
Terebinth; turpentine

Turpentine is obtained from pine and other coniferous trees in the form of an oily, aromatic resin. It has many industrial uses, especially as a cleaning agent, in paint strippers and thinners and in products containing pine oil. It causes burning if swallowed and produces vomiting and diarrhoea. It also causes external burning and blistering if applied to the skin, and choking, sneezing and coughing if the fumes are inhaled. It was once used in the treatment of genital infections, including gonorrhoea. The homeopathic remedy is used to treat similar types of infection involving inflammation and infection of the bladder and kidneys. These include cystitis with frequent urination, blood in the urine and burning pains, and kidney inflammation with stabbing back pains. The urine is usually cloudy or contains blood and may have a strong smell. Also, for other forms of kidney disease with symptoms of puffiness because of retention of fluid (oedema). Symptoms are worse at night and in cold, damp, draughty conditions. They are better for walking about in fresh clean air and for warmth.

Teucrium marum venum
Teucrium mar. ver.; cat thyme, marum

This strongly aromatic plant is a native of Spain but grows in many countries throughout the world. It has branching stalks and forms a bush or shrub about two to four feet in height. The small, oval leaves are sage green in colour and slightly furred, and the flowers are an attractive deep pink. Both flowers and leaves have a pungent aromatic smell, especially when rubbed. The plant has stimulant and astringent properties and has long been used in herbal medicine for a variety of disorders. All the fresh parts of the plant are used to prepare the homeopathic remedy, which is used to treat polyps, which are small growths or tumours on mucous membranes. These may occur in the rectum, bladder or nasal passages. Also, the remedy is used for conditions producing thick catarrh that is persistent and difficult to eliminate. The remedy may be given to treat threadworm infestation in children. Symptoms are worse for cold, damp conditions and sudden weather changes. Also, if the person becomes hot and sweaty in bed. Symptoms improve for being out in the cool, fresh clean air.

Theridion curassavicum
Orange spider of Curaçao and other parts of the West Indies

This is a small spider about the size of a pea that has a body covered with orange spots. There is a larger yellow spot on its under surface, and it is particularly found in Curaçao. It has a poisonous bite and causes unpleasant symptoms of tremor, chilling, sweating, fainting and great anxiety. The whole spider is used to prepare the homeopathic remedy, which was first investigated and proved in the early 1830s by Dr Constantine Hering. The remedy is used to treat ailments of the spine and nerves and bone disorders. All these ailments are very sensitive to movement, vibration and noise, which set off sensations of great pain. Disorders treated include Ménière's disease, a disease of the inner ear with deafness and tinnitus (ringing in the ear) with symptoms of vertigo, nausea and vomiting. Also, toothache, degeneration of bones and spine with inflammation and pain, morning sickness, travel sickness, vertigo, severe headache, chills and fainting. Symptoms are made worse by closing the eyes, by any kind of movement or vibration, bending, touch and during the night. They improve for rest with the eyes open and with warmth and quiet surroundings.

Trillium erectum, Trillium pendulum
Bethroot, Indian balm, birthroot, Indian shamrock, lamb's quarters, wake-robin
Plants belonging to this group are all native species of North America. *Trillium erectum*, which flourishes in rich, moist soils in woodlands and grows to a height of between one foot and sixteen inches, produces white flowers. Preparations made from the plant have astringent, antiseptic and tonic properties and were used by the native Indian peoples for childbirth and haemorrhage, especially from the womb. The homeopathic remedy is used to treat heavy bleeding from the womb, which may be associated with fibroids or the menopause. It may be given to prevent an early threatened miscarriage.

Tuberculinum koch, Tuberculinum bovum
Dead, sterile tuberculous tissue derived from cattle or human beings
This remedy was extensively investigated and researched by Dr Compton Burnett in the late 1800s, following an earlier discovery by Dr Robert Koch, that dead tuberculous material was effective in the prevention and treatment of tuberculosis. The homeopathic remedy is given for chronic conditions characterized by wasting, pallor, a persistent racking cough, drenching sweats at night and pains in the left lung. The glands in the neck are enlarged, and the whites of the eyes (sclera) may appear slightly blue. Symptoms are erratic and may move about. Often there is a family history of tuberculosis or other severe respiratory disorder such as asthma. People who benefit from this remedy are usually thin, fair-haired and blue-eyed, prone to colds and chest ailments and lacking physical strength and stamina. They tend to be restless, seeking constant change in their personal life and surroundings, yearning for excitement, travel and new romantic attachments. They may be afraid of dogs or cats and enjoy milk and the taste of smoked foods.

Valerian officinalis
Great wild valerian; all-heal, setwall, capon's tail
Valerian species grow throughout Europe and northern Asia, and *Valerian officinalis* flourishes in marshy, wet ground in ditches and near rivers and streams. The stems reach a height of three to four feet, producing dark

green leaves and light pink flowers. The rhizome or root is the part used in herbal medicine and homeopathy, and the plant has a long history of medicinal use. It was valued so highly in the Middle Ages as to be given the name all-heal, while its Latin name may be derived from *valere*, meaning 'to be in health'. Preparations made from the plant have powerful effects on the central nervous system, acting as sedatives and antispasmodics. The homeopathic remedy is given for excitable, mental symptoms including agitation and restlessness. Also, for muscular spasms, hysteria, headache and pains that may move from one part to another. The person may suffer from sleeplessness, headaches, diarrhoea and restlessness with gnawing hunger and nausea.

Veratum album
Verat. alb.; white hellebore

This plant grows throughout Europe, although not in the British Isles, and produces a creamy-white flower. The rhizome or root is the part used in herbal medicine and homeopathy, and it is extremely poisonous. If swallowed it causes diarrhoea and vomiting and may result in collapse, convulsions and death. Preparations made from the plant have irritant and cardiac depressant properties. There is a long history of medicinal use going back to the time of Hippocrates, and the remedy was investigated and proved for homeopathy by Hahnemann during the late 1820s.

The homeopathic remedy is used for severe conditions of collapse and shock in which there is pallor, dehydration, chilling and possibly cyanosis (a blue tinge to the skin because of a lack of oxygen in the blood and tissues). The person may be cold with clammy skin because of sweating. Also, for diarrhoea, severe throbbing headache and mental symptoms of extreme agitation or severe depression, suicidal feelings, mania and aggression. It may be given for severe cramping menstrual pain or cramp during pregnancy leading to fainting, and collapse because of mental shock or trauma. Symptoms are made worse by movements and cold drinks, and also during the night. They improve with warmth, heat and hot meals and drinks. They are also better for rest and lying down.

Viburnum opulus
Guelder rose, high cranberry, dog rowan tree, cramp bark, snowball tree, rose elder

The guelder rose is a bush or small tree found in copses and hedges in

England, Europe and North America. It produces abundant heads of white flowers and, later, bright red berries that have a bitter taste. The bark, which contains a bitter glucoside substance called viburnine, is used to prepare remedies in herbal medicine and homeopathy. Preparations of the bark are very effective in the relief of cramp-like pains and spasms. The homeopathic remedy is used to treat menstrual cramps, pain in the ovaries at ovulation and prevention of early threatened miscarriage.

Vinca minor
Lesser periwinkle

This trailing plant grows in Great Britain and other European countries, producing dark-green leaves and purply-blue flowers. Periwinkles have a long history of use in herbal medicine and were used to treat bleeding, cramps, piles and skin inflammations. There are also many ancient superstitions attached to the plant, and it was believed to ward off evil spirits. Preparations made from the plant have astringent and tonic properties. In homeopathy it is used for heavy menstrual bleeding and haemorrhage and for inflammations of the scalp.

Viola tricolor
Wild pansy, love-lies-bleeding, love-in-idleness, heartsease, and many other country names

This pretty flower is abundant throughout the British Isles, with rounded green leaves and purple, yellow and white flowers. The whole plant is used to prepare herbal and homeopathic remedies that have a long history of medicinal use. The plant has been used to treat a wide variety of ailments, including asthma, epilepsy, skin disorders, convulsions, heart and blood disorders. Preparations made from the plant have diuretic properties. In homeopathy, the remedy is used for skin conditions such as infected eczema or impetigo. There is a thick pus-containing discharge and crusts and scabs on the skin. Also, the remedy is used to treat bed-wetting and urinary incontinence.

Vipera communis
Venom of the adder or viper

This attractively patterned snake is a greyish colour with a dark zig-zag pattern down the length of its back. Its bite is painful but rarely serious, causing swelling, inflammation and bleeding in the veins, which then become enlarged. The homeopathic remedy made from the venom of the snake, is used to treat phlebitis and varicose veins and ulcers with swelling, inflammation and pain. The leg feels heavy, as though it might burst. Symptoms are worse for touch, pressure or tight clothing and are relieved by raising the affected part.

Viscum album
Mistletoe

This parasitic plant grows in the British Isles and throughout Europe, trailing over fruit and other trees. It produces white berries that ripen in December, but the leaves and twigs are used to prepare the remedies for herbal medicine and homeopathy. Preparations derived from the plant act on the central nervous system and have tonic, antispasmodic and narcotic properties. It has been used to treat epilepsy, spasms and haemorrhage. Many ancient superstitions are attached to mistletoe, which was a sacred plant for the Druids. In homeopathy, the remedy is used as a last resort to treat extreme conditions of collapse, weak pulse and respiration and low blood pressure.

Vitex agnus castus
Agnus castus; chaste tree; monk's pepper, wild lavender

This aromatic shrub is a native plant of the shores of the Mediterranean and also grows in other part of Europe and North America. It has flexible fine twigs that are used to weave baskets, dark green leaves and fragrant flowers. Dark, purply-red berries are produced containing seeds, and these are used to prepare herbal and homeopathic remedies. The plant was associated with chastity by the ancient Greeks. The plant was used to treat muscular weakness and paralysis and is used in herbal medicine to stimulate hormone production during the menopause. The homeopathic remedy is given for menopausal symptoms and for physical disorders arising from alcohol or drug abuse or sexual excess. Symptoms may include fatigue, depression, loss of sexual desire, apathy and inability to concentrate. Also for postnatal depression with loss of libido and drying up of the breast milk. Symptoms are worse in the morning and for exercise and movement and are relieved by firm pressure on an affected part.

Zincum metallicum
Zinc. met.

Zinc is an essential trace element in the human body, being a constituent of digestive enzymes and essential for normal growth. Zinc is used in conventional medicine as a constituent of creams and ointments for a variety of skin complaints. It is also taken internally for some nervous complaints, spasms and neuralgia. The homeopathic Zinc. met. remedy is prepared from zinc sulphide and is used for conditions of restlessness, agitation and nervous twitching. The person is usually suffering from great mental and physical exhaustion and is irritable and highly sensitive to the least noise, interruption or touch. Symptoms are worse for suppression of natural discharges (e.g. by using a suppressant remedy in the case of a cold). Also, they are made worse by noise, touch, vibration and alcoholic drinks, particularly wine. Symptoms improve when natural body functions take place and are not suppressed.

Appendix:
Herb Action

alterative a term given to a substance that speeds up the renewal of the tissues so that they can carry out their functions more effectively.

anodyne a drug that eases and soothes pain.

anthelmintic a substance that causes the death or expulsion of parasitic worms.

antiperiodic a drug that prevents the return of recurring diseases, e.g. malaria.

antiscorbutic a substance that prevents scurvy and contains necessary vitamins, e.g. vitamin C.

antiseptic a substance that prevents the growth of disease-causing micro-organisms, e.g. bacteria, without causing damage to living tissue. It is applied to wounds to cleanse them and prevent infection.

antispasmodic a drug that diminishes muscle spasms.

aperient a medicine that produces a natural movement of the bowel.

aphrodisiac a compound that excites the sexual organs.

aromatic a substance that has an aroma.

astringent a substance that causes cells to contract by losing proteins from their surface. This causes localized contraction of blood vessels and tissues.

balsamic a substance that contains resins and benzoic acid and is used to alleviate colds and abrasions.

bitter a drug that is bitter-tasting and is used to stimulate the appetite.

cardiac compounds that have some effect on the heart.

carminative a preparation to relieve flatulence and any resultant griping.

cathartic a compound that produces an evacuation of the bowels.

cholagogue the name given to a substance that produces a flow of bile from the gall bladder.

cooling a substance that reduces the temperature and cools the skin.

demulcent a substance that soothes and protects the alimentary canal.

deobstruent a compound that is said to clear obstructions and open the natural passages of the body.

detergent a substance that has a cleansing action, either internally or on the skin.

diaphoretic a term given to drugs that promote perspiration.

diuretics a substance that stimulates the kidneys and increases urine and solute production.

emetic a drug that induces vomiting.

emmenagogue a compound that is able to excite the menstrual discharge.

emollient a substance that softens or soothes the skin.

expectorant a group of drugs that are taken to help in the removal of secretions from the lungs, bronchi and trachea.

febrifuge a substance that reduces fever.

galactogogue an agent that stimulates the production of breast milk or increases milk flow.

haemostatic a drug used to control bleeding.

hepatic a substance that acts upon the liver.

hydrogogue a substance that has the property of removing accumulations of water or serum.

hypnotic a drug or substance that induces sleep.

insecticide a substance that kills insects.

irritant a general term encompassing any agent that causes irritation of a tissue.

laxative a substance that is taken to evacuate the bowel or soften stools.

mydriatic a compound that causes dilation of the pupil.

nervine a name given to drugs that are used to restore the nerves to their natural state.

narcotic a drug that leads to stupor and complete loss of awareness.

nephritic a drug that has an action on the kidneys.

nutritive a compound that is nourishing to the body.

parasiticide a substance that destroys parasites internally and externally.

pectoral a term applied to drugs that are remedies in treating chest and lung complaints.

purgative the name given to drugs or other measures that produce evacuation of the bowels. They normally have a more severe effect than aperients or laxatives.

refrigerant a substance that relieves thirst and produces a feeling of coolness.

resolvent a substance that is applied to swellings to reduce them in size.

rubefacient a compound that causes the skin to redden and peel off. It causes blisters and inflammation.

sedative a drug that lessens tension, anxiety and soothes over-excitement of the nervous system.

sternutatory the name given to a substance that irritates the mucous membrane and produces sneezing.

stimulant a drug or other agent that increases the activity of an organ or system within the body.

stomachic name given to drugs that treat stomach disorders.

styptic applications that check bleeding by blood vessel contraction or by causing rapid blood clotting.

sudorific a drug or agent that produces copious perspiration.

taeniacide drugs that are used to expel tapeworms from the body.

tonic substances that are traditionally thought to give strength and vigour to the body and that are said to produce a feeling of wellbeing.

vermifuge a substance that kills, or expels, worms from the intestines.

vesicant similar to a rubefacient, agent that causes blistering when applied to the skin.

vulnerary a drug that is said to be good at healing wounds.

Classification of Herbs by Action

alterative anemone pulsatilla, bethroot, betony (wood), bitter root, bittersweet, blue flag, brooklime, burdock, burr marigold, caroba, celandine, clivers, clover (red), cohosh (black), dock (yellow), dropwort (water), echinacea, elder, fireweed, fringe tree, frostwort, golden seal, Jacob's ladder, meadowsweet, mezeron, pipsissewa, plantain (common), poke root, polypody root, rosinweed, sarsaparilla (Jamaica), sassafras, soap tree, soapwort, speedwell, spindle tree, tag alder, walnut.

anodyne aconite, camphor, chamomile, coca, figwort, gladwyn, henbane, hemlock, hops, hound's tongue, lettuce (wild), mandrake, poppy (red), poppy (white), sassy bark, stramonium, valerian.

anthelmintic aloes, balmony, camphor, cedar (yellow), cohosh (blue), gentian (yellow), groundsel, hellebore (black), knotgrass, lupin (white), male fern, savine, tansy, walnut, wormseed (American), wormwood.

antiperiodic lilac, willow (white).

antiscorbutic groundsel, lemon, lime fruit, radish, rowan tree, scurvy grass, shepherd's purse, sorrel, spinach, watercress.

antiseptic avens, barberry, beech, bergamot,

bethroot, black root, camphor, cinnamon, costmary, echinacea, elecampane, eucalyptus, garlic, gentian (yellow), horseradish, myrrh, oak, olive, sandalwood, stockholm tar, thyme, violet, woundwort.

antispasmodic anemone pulsatilla, arrach, baneberry, belladonna, bergamot, camphor, chamomile, clover (red), cohosh (blue), cowslip, cramp bark, cumin, daisy (ox-eye), ephedra, eucalyptus, gelsemium, gladwyn, hemlock, henbane, masterwort, mayweed, mistletoe, motherwort, musk seed, oats, passionflower, peony, peppermint, pleurisy root, poppy (white), primrose, red root, rosinweed, rue, scullcap (Virginian), skunkcabbage, spearmint, stramonium, sumbul, thyme, tree of heaven, valerian, vervain, woundwort, yam (wild).

aperient butcher's broom, clivers, club moss costmary, couchgrass, dandelion, elder, feverfew, fringe tree, fumitory, germander (wall), horseradish, jewelweed, olive, parsley, rhubarb, rose (pale), scurvy grass.

aphrodisiac celery, coca, damiana, guarana, musk seed.

aromatic allspice, angelica, angostura, asarabacca, avens, basil, bergamot, betony (wood), birthwort, bugle, calamint, calamus, camphor, caraway, cardamom, cedar (yellow), cicely (sweet), cinnamon, cloves, coriander, dill, eryngo, eucalyptus, fennel, gale (sweet), golden rod, hops, lavender, lovage, magnolia, meadowsweet, melilot, musk seed, orange (bitter), orange (sweet), pepper, pine oils, sage (common), St. John's wort, sandalwood, sassafras, savory (summer), saxifrage (burnet), spearmint, wintergreen, yerba santa.

astringent agrimony, alder, apple, avens, bayberry, bearberry, bethroot, betony (wood), birch, bistort, blackberry, bugle, burnet (greater), cassia, cedar (yellow), chestnut (horse), chestnut (sweet), cinnamon, cohosh (black), columbine, comfrey, costmary, cudweed, dog-rose, elder, elecampane, elm, evening primrose, eyebright, fireweed, frostwort, gale

(sweet), golden rod, hawthorn, horsetail, hound's tongue, houseleek, ivy (ground), Jacob's ladder, knotgrass, lady's mantle, larch, lily (Madonna), loosestrife, lungwort, maple (red), matico, meadowsweet, mullein, myrrh, nettle, oak, olive, pipsissewa, plantain (common), poppy (white), primrose, quince, ragwort, raspberry, red root, rhubarb, rose (pale), rose (red), rosemary, rowan tree, rupturewort, sage (common), sassy bark, scullcap (Virginian), self-heal, St. John's wort, silverweed, solomon's seal, speedwell (common), strawberry, tag alder, tea, thistle (scotch), tree of heaven, vervain, vine, walnut, willow (white), wintergreen, witch hazel.

balsamic larch.

bitter angostura, bugle, birch, calumba, feverfew, gentian (yellow), nux vomica, simaruba, snapdragon, wormwood, yerba santa.

cardiac asparagus, bitter root, butterbur, foxglove, hawthorn, kola nuts, lily of the valley, mescal buttons, strophanthus, tree of heaven.

carminative allspice, angelica, anise, balm, basil, bergamot, calamus, caraway, cardamom, cassia, catmint, cayenne, celery, cicely (sweet), cinnamon, cloves, coriander, cumin, dill, fennel, feverfew, ginger, golden rod, horsemint (American), juniper, lavender, lovage, mace, marjoram, masterwort, melilot, nutmeg, orange (bitter), orange (sweet), parsley, pennyroyal, pepper, peppermint, pleurisy root, saffron, sage (common), savory (summer), saxifrage (burnet), spearmint, thyme, valerian.

cathartic black root, bloodroot, blue flag, bogbean, broom, bryony (white), castor oil plant, croton, fireweed, gladwyn, hedge-hyssop, hydrangea, ivy, jewelweed, mountain flax, pleurisy root, poke root, sabadilla, saffron (meadow), senna, stavesacre.

cholagogue spindle tree.

cooling basil, cucumber, lemon, mandrake, plantain (common), ragwort, sorrel, witch hazel.

demulcent almonds, barley, borage, chick-weed, coltsfoot, comfrey, couchgrass, elm, fig, flax, hound's tongue, Iceland moss, Irish moss, lily (Madonna), liquorice, marshmallow, mullein, olive, parsley piert, peach, pellitory-of-the-wall, pine (white), pumpkin, quince, rice, salep, slippery elm, Solomon's seal, sundew.

deobstruent agrimony, bladderwrack, bogbean, butcher's broom, carrot, liverwort (English), plantain (common), water dock.

depurative figwort.

detergent balmony, blackcurrant, golden seal, ragwort, soap tree, soapwort, walnut, water betony, water dock.

diaphoretic aconite, anemone pulsatilla, angelica, balm, blackcurrant, black root, boneset, box, buchu, burdock, burr marigold, butcher's broom, camphor, caroba, carrot, catmint, chicory, clematis, clivers, cohosh (blue), cuckoopint, dwarf elder, elder, elecampane, eryngo, fumitory, garlic, gelsemium, germander (wall), groundsel, heartease, hedge-hyssop, horehound, horsemint (American), horseradish, ipecacuanha, ivy, jaborandi, Jacob's ladder, knapweed (greater), laurel, lettuce (wild), lily of the valley, lobelia, lovage, marigold, marjoram, motherwort, mugwort, pennyroyal, pimpernel (scarlet), pine (white), pleurisy root, poppy (white), ragwort, rosemary, rosinweed, saffron, samphire, sarsaparilla (Jamaica), sassafras, saxifrage (burnet), senega, sheep's sorrel, skunk-cabbage, slippery elm, smartweed, speedwell (common), stockholm tar, thistle (holy), turpentine, vervain, woodruff.

diuretic apple, arnica, asparagus, bella-donna, bittersweet, blackcurrant, blue flag, bluebell, broom, buchu, burdock, burr marigold, butterbur, cacao, caroba, cedar (yellow), celandine, celery, clematis, club moss, coffee, cohosh (black), cohosh (blue), coolwort, couchgrass, cucumber, daisy (ox-eye), damiana, dandelion, dropwort (water), dwarf elder, elder, elm,

eryngo, figwort, foxglove, fringe tree, fumitory, garlic, germander (wall), golden rod, groundsel, goutwort, hair cup moss, hawthorn, heartease, henbane, hops, horsemint (American), horseradish, horsetail, houseleek, hydrangea, ivy (ground), jewelweed, juniper, kava-kava, knotgrass, kola nuts, larch, lettuce (wild), lupin (white), mastic, matico, meadow-sweet, mezeron, mugwort, mustard (black), nettle, parsley, parsley piert, peach, pellitory-of-the-wall, pimpernel (scarlet), pipsissewa, plantain (common), poplar, pumpkin, radish, rest-harrow, rosinweed, rupturewort, sandalwood, sarsaparilla (jamaica), sassafras, savine, saw palmetto, saxifrage (burnet), scurvy grass, senega, sheep's sorrel, shepherd's purse, smartweed, soap tree, sorrel, St. John's wort, stockholm tar, strawberry, sunflower, tobacco, vine, watercress, wintergreen, yam (wild).

emetic asarabacca, black root, bloodroot, daffodil, elder, fireweed, groundsel, hedge-hyssop, ipecacuanha, jewelweed, laurel, lobelia, mandrake, mayweed, mescal buttons, mustard (black), poke root, primrose, rosinweed, sabadilla, saffron (meadow), spearwort (lesser), stavesacre, tag alder, thistle (holy), tobacco, vervain.

emmenagogue aloes, arrach, bloodroot, cassia, catmint, cedar (yellow), cohosh (black), cohosh (blue), cornflower, cotton root, ergot, feverfew, gale (sweet), gentian (yellow), hellebore (black), horsemint (American), lupin (white), marjoram, marjoram (sweet), mayweed, motherwort, mugwort, myrrh, pennyroyal, rue, saffron, savine, senega, smartweed, tansy, thistle (holy), wintergreen.

emollient almonds, borage, cacao, cucumber, fenugreek, fig, flax, Irish moss, liquorice, marshmallow, melilot, mullein, olive, ragwort, slippery elm.

expectorant balsam of Peru, beech, bethroot, bloodroot, boneset, calamint, cedar (yellow), cicely (sweet), cohosh

Classification of Herbs by Action

(black), coltsfoot, comfrey, cuckoopint, cup moss, dropwort (water), dwarf elder, elder, elecampane, eryngo, garlic, ginger, honeysuckle, horehound, ipecacuanha, jaborandi, Jacob's ladder, larch, lobelia, loosestrife, maidenhair, myrrh, peach, pimpernel (scarlet), pine (white), pleurisy root, polypody root, poppy (red), poppy (white), red root, rosinweed, St. John's wort, senega, skunk-cabbage, slippery elm, soap tree, speedwell (common), stockholm tar, sundew, sunflower, tobacco, violet, watercress, yerba santa.

febrifuge aconite, avens, balm, blackcurrant, bogbean, boneset, calumba, chestnut (horse), gelsemium, gentian (yellow), guarana, holly, lilac, pepper, poplar, verbena (lemon), wormwood.

galactogogue castor oil plant, vervain, wintergreen.

haemostatic puffballa, shepherd's purse.

hepatic dodder, spindle tree.

hydragogue bitter root, bryony (white).

hypnotic corkwood tree, henbane, mandrake, poppy (white).

insecticide laburnum, larkspur, musk weed, pyrethrum (dalmatian).

irritant bryony (white), cedar (yellow), croton, ivy (poison), mustard (black), pellitory, rue, turpentine.

laxative almonds, asparagus, boneset, castor oil plant, chicory, dock (yellow), dodder, elder, fig, golden seal, honeysuckle, mountain flax, mulberry, olive, pellitory-of-the-wall, rose (pale), sassy bark, senna, spinidle tree, strawberry, violet, walnut.

mydriatic belladonna, corkwood tree, henbane.

narcotic belladonna, bittersweet, box, cherry laurel, chestnut (horse), guarana, hellebore (black), henbane, ivy (poison), laurel, lettuce (wild), mescal buttons, mistletoe, mullein, nightshade (black), paris (herb), passionflower, poke root, poppy (red), sassy bark, skunk-cabbage, stramonium, tobacco.

nephritic hydrangea.

nervine anemone pulsatilla, arrach, celery, club moss, cramp bark, guarana, kola nuts,

hops, lavender, lime tree, mistletoe, motherwort, mugwort, musk seed, oats, scullcap (Virginian), St. John's wort, sumbul, valerian, vervain.

nutritive almonds, barley, cacao, fig, Iceland moss, Irish moss, mulberry, oats, parsnip, rice, salep, saw palmetto, slippery elm, spinach, watercress.

parasiticide balsam of Peru, larkspur.

pectoral anise, bethroot, dog-rose, euphorbia, flax, horehound, Irish moss, liquorice, lungwort, maidenhair, polypody root, slippery elm, sundew.

purgative aloes, angostura, asarabacca, barberry, bindweed (greater), castor oil plant, celandine, croton, cucumber, damiana, dodder, dwarf elder, elder, groundsel, hellebore (black), kamala, liverwort (English), mandrake, mercury (dog's), mountain flax, rhubarb, senna.

refrigerant blackcurrant, borage, catmint, chickweed, dog-rose, houseleek, lemon, lime fruit, mulberry, parsley piert, pellitory-of-the-wall, plantain (common), rice, sheep's sorrel, sorrel.

resolvent bittersweet, saxifrage (burnet), St. John's wort.

rubefacient bryony (black), buttercup (bulbous), cayenne, croton, horsemint (American), horseradish, ivy (poison), pellitory, pine oils, rue, spearwort (lesser), turpentine.

sedative aconite, asparagus, belladonna, box, camphor, cherry laurel, clover (red), corkwood tree, cowslip, cramp bark, ergot, evening primrose, foxglove, gelsemium, goutwort, hemlock, lettuce (wild), motherwort, mullein, passionflower, peach, poppy (white), red root, saw palmetto, skunk-cabbage, tobacco, verbena (lemon), witch hazel.

sternulatory asarabacca, soap tree, soapwort.

stimulant allspice, angelica, angostura, arnica, asarabacca, balsam of Peru, bayberry, beech, birthwort, blue flag, boneset, buchu, butterbur, cacao, calamus, caraway, cardamom, carrot, catmint, cayenne, celery, chives, cinnamon, cloves, coca, coffee, coriander, cornflower, cuckoopint, cumin, damiana, dill, elder, elecampane, ephedra, ergot, eryngo, eucalyptus, fennel, feverfew, garlic, germander (wall), ginger, ginseng, golden rod, guarana, horsemint (American), horseradish, ipecacuanha, ivy, ivy (ground), ivy (poison), jabarandi, kava-kava, kola nuts, larch, lavender, lime tree, lobelia, lovage, mace, magnolia, marigold, marjoram, marjoram (sweet), masterwort, mastic, matico, mezeron, mugwort, mustard (black), myrrh, nettle, nutmeg, nux vomica, oats, pennyroyal, pepper, peppermint, poplar, raspberry, rosemary, rue, sage (common), sassafras, scurvy grass, senega, shepherd's purse, smartweed, snapdragon, soap tree, spearmint, spindle tree, stockholm tar, sumbul, tansy, tea, thistle (holy), valerian, watercress, wintergreen, yerba santa.

stomachic angelica, avens, cassia, chamomile, cicely (sweet), dill, fennel, gentian (yellow), ginseng, golden seal, juniper, laurel, musk seed, nutmeg, orange (bitter), orange (sweet), peppermint, rhubarb, saxifrage (burnet), wormwood.

styptic avens, bluebell, knotgrass, lady's mantle, matico, self-heal.

sudorific avens, nightshade (black), vervain.

taeniacide cucumber, kamala, male fern, pumpkin.

tonic agrimony, alder, angelica, angostura, asarabacca, avens, balmony, barberry, bayberry, bergamot, bethroot, bitter root,

black root, blackberry, bogbean, boneset, burnet (greater), butterbur, calamus, calumba, cassia, catmint, cayenne, celery, chamomile, chestnut (horse), chestnut (sweet), chicory, clivers, coca, coltsfoot, coolwort, cornflower, daisy (ox-eye), damiana, dandelion, dock (yellow), elecampane, elm, eyebright, fireweed, foxglove, fringe tree, frostwort, fumitory, gentian (yellow), germander (wall), ginseng, golden seal, guarana, hawthorn, holly, hops, horehound, hydrangea, Iceland moss, ivy (ground), kava-kava, knapweed (greater), kola nuts, lemon, lilac, lily of the valley, lime tree, mace, magnolia, marjoram, marjoram (sweet), mayweed, mescal buttons, mistletoe, motherwort, mugwort, myrrh, nettle, nux vomica, oak, orange (bitter), orange (sweet), parsley, peony, pipsissewa, pleurisy root, polypody root, poplar, rose (red), rosemary, rosinweed, sage (common), sarsaparilla (Jamaica), saw palmetto, scullcap (Virginian), self-heal, silverweed, simaruba, soapwort, solomon's seal, speedwell (common), spindle tree, strophanthus, sumbul, tag alder, tansy, thistle (holy), thyme, vervain, willow (white), wintergreen, witch hazel, wormwood, woodruff, yerba santa.

vermifuge aloes, castor oil plant, cohosh (blue), lilac, male fern, pink root, primrose, sabadilla, stavesacre, walnut, wormseed (American).

vesicant mezereon.

vulnerary arnica, comfrey, knotgrass, mare's tail, water betony.

Chemical Glossary

acid a substance that can form hydrogen ions when dissolved in water. Aqueous solutions of acids typically have a sharp taste and turn litmus paper red. Most organic acids have the C(O)OH grouping but they may have other acid groups, e.g. the sul-

phonic group—$S(O_2)OH$. Acids can vary in strength according to the degree of ionization in solution.

alcohol an organic compound with one or more hydroxyl (-OH) groups attached directly to a carbon atom. This is a large as-

Chemical Glossary

semblage of compounds that form part of waxes, esters, aldehydes, ketones and volatile oils. Alcohols may be in the solid or liquid form depending on the size of the carbon chain.

aldehydes organic compounds with a carbonyl group joined directly to another carbon atom. Aldehydes may be either solids or colourless liquids.

alkali the name given to a substance that gives a solution in water with a pH of greater than seven. They may also be called a base.

alkaloid probably the most important chemicals found in plants, as they usually have a medical action. They are organic substances, found in association with organic acids in most plant groups, particularly the flowering plants. Alkaloids are alkaline and combine with acids to form crystalline salts which are water-soluble in most cases. The alkaloids themselves are generally insoluble in water but dissolve well in alcohol or ether. Alkaloids include a number of important drugs, e.g. morphine, caffeine, atropine, quinine and nicotine and many of these chemicals are very poisonous with characteristic physiological effects.

anthraquinones glycoside compounds present in some plants and that are used to prepare dyes and purgative drugs.

bitters the name given to herbs that have a bitter taste. It may be due to a combination of chemicals within the plant. The herbs include angostura, yellow gentian, nux vomica and wormwood and they can be used as appetite stimulants, relaxant drugs and for their anti-inflammatory action.

carbohydrates these compounds are formed in plants as a result of photosynthesis. They include sugars, starches and cellulose which all have an important nutritional value. A polysaccharide is made up of hundreds of sugar molecules linked together, and they form part of compounds such as mucilage or pectin which help protect the alimentary canal. Carbohydrates are one of the main classes of naturally-derived organic compounds.

coumarins glycoside compounds widely distributed in plants. They provide the distinctive smell of many grass species.

ester organic compounds produced when an acid and an alcohol react. They often have distinctive fruity odours and are found naturally in fruits. An ester is generally a volatile liquid but may exist in a solid form.

fatty acids an organic compound made up of a hydrocarbon chain and a terminal carboxyl group (-COOH). The chain can range in length from one to thirty carbon atoms and branches can occur in the compound. Fatty acids are classified as saturated or unsaturated depending on the presence of a double bond in the chain structure. In nature, fatty acids form part of glycerides, that make up part of many important tissues and are important in many energy-releasing processes in the body.

flavonoid glycosides compounds made up of glycoside sugars and a flavone compound. The flavones are a group of chemicals, that give a yellow pigmentation to plants. This group of compounds is widely distributed through the plant kingdom, and they can have diuretic antispasmodic or stimulating effects on the body.

glucoside a term given to glycoside chemicals that contain glucose as the sugar.

glycoside molecules made up of two sections, a sugar and another chemical group. This name is given to all compounds independent of the sugar within them. As a class, glycosides are colourless, crystalline and bitter and are very common in plants. There are various classes of glycosides including cardiac glycosides, e.g. foxglove/digitalis and purgative glycosides, e.g. the anthraquinone chemicals in senna and rhubarb.

gum complex polysaccharides, that contain several different sugar and acid groups. They are generally soluble in water and produce viscous solutions, that are sometimes called mucilages. They are normally insoluble in organic solvents and are found in variable quantities in plant tissues.

hydrocarbons compounds made up of carbon and hydrogen alone. There are various categories of compounds, depending upon the arrangement of carbon atoms in the molecule and the number of double bonds in the molecule.

isomer compounds can have the same chemical composition and molecular weight but differ in their physical structure and hence are termed isomers. These isomers can have different physical and physiological qualities. Isomers can differ in the order in which the atoms are joined together (structural isomers) or they differ in the spatial orientation of atoms in the molecule (stereo-isomerism). In plants, two isomeric forms of an active chemical may exist with one form having beneficial medical effects, and the other having no impact or a deleterious impact on the body. Care must be taken where several isomers of a chemical exist to utilize the correct form.

mucilage a gum-like substance found in the cell walls or seed coats of plants. They are polysaccharides that have a soothing effect on inflamed tissues, and they are used as an ingredient in some cosmetic preparations.

phenols slightly acidic compounds with at least one hydroxyl (-OH) group bonded to a carbon atom in an aromatic ring. They are widely found in natural plant constituents, e.g. tannins, anthocyanine glucoside pigments and salicylic acid. Salicylic acid frequently combines with a sugar to form a glycoside that has antiseptic properties, e.g. in crampbark, meadowsweet and white willow.

resin a naturally-produced acidic polymer obtained from trees. It is thought to help protect the tree from physical or mechanical damage, and attack by fungi and insects, in a similar way to how gums or mucilage protect green plants. It is a high molecular weight class of compounds usually produced by coniferous trees.

saponins glycosides that form a lather when shaken with water. They are found in two groups; the steroidal saponins that mimic the precursors of female sex hormones and the tri-terpenoid saponins that mimic the adrenocorticotropic hormone ACTH. They occur in a wide variety of plant groups and also act as a poison affecting fish.

starch a complex polysaccharide carbohydrate made by green plants during photosynthesis and which forms one of the plants' main energy stores. It is composed of water-soluble amylose and amylopectin, which forms a mucilaginous paste in water. Starch grains formed in the plant vary in size and shape according to the plant that produced them. Starch is used in industry as a food thickener, an adhesive and for sizing paper and cloth.

sugars a group of water-soluble carbohydrates with a sweet taste. They can contain six or twelve carbon units in each molecule and the simple sugar units or monosaccharides can combine to form more complex sugar groups. It is a crystalline substance, found in many forms in plants.

tannins a group of complex organic chemicals found in the leaves, unripe fruits and bark of trees. They generally taste astringent and may be a protective mechanism against the grazing of some animals. They have commercial uses in treating cattle hides to produce leather, in producing ink and as mordants in the textile industry.

terpenes a group of unsaturated hydrocarbons, made up of multiples of isoprene units. The group includes vitamins A, E and K, carotene and other carotenoid pigments and squalene, the precursor to cholesterol. The terpenes are of great scientific and industrial importance. They are very reactive chemicals, with characteristic and pleasant odours that are used in perfumery.

volatile oil these compounds are formed from an alcohol and a hydrocarbon. They are found in many plants and can give a plant a characteristic taste and flavour. Many volatile oils have medicinal properties and are used as antifungal, antiseptic or aromatic oils taken internally or externally. They are very important oils in herbal medicine.

waxes fatty acid esters of alcohols with a high molecular weight. They are normally solid and have water-repellent properties. Waxes form a protective coating on animal skin, fur or feathers and also reduce water loss in leaves and fruits. The waxes are used for various commercial uses including polishes, textiles and pharmaceuticals.

Medical Glossary

amenorrhoea an absence of menstruation which is normal before puberty, during pregnancy and while breast-feeding is being carried out and following the menopause. Primary amenorrhoea describes the situation where the menstrual periods do not begin at puberty. This occurs if there is a chromosome abnormality (such as Turner's syndrome) or if some reproductive organs are absent. It can also occur where there is a failure or imbalance in the secretion of hormones. In secondary amenorrhoea, the menstrual periods stop when they would normally be expected to be present. There are a variety of causes including hormone deficiency, disorders of the hypothalamus, psychological and environmental stresses, during starvation, anorexia nervosa or depression.

arthritis inflammation of the joints or spine, the symptoms of which are pain and swelling, restriction of movement, redness and warmth of the skin. There are many different causes of arthritis including osteoarthritis, rheumatoid arthritis, tuberculosis and rheumatic fever.

asthma a condition characterized by breathing difficulties caused by narrowing of the airways (bronchi) of the lung. It is a distressing condition with breathlessness and a paroxysmal wheezing cough and the extent to which the bronchi narrow varies considerably. Asthma may occur at any age but usually begins in early childhood, and is a hypersensitive response that can be brought on by exposure to a variety of allergens, exercise, stress or infections. An asthma sufferer may have other hypersensitive conditions such as eczema and hay fever, and it may be prevalent within a family. It may or may not be possible for a person to avoid the allergen(s) responsible for an asthma attack. Treatment involves the use of drugs to dilate the airways (bronchodilators) and also inhaled corticosteroids.

atheroma a degenerative condition of the arteries. The inner and middle coats of the arterial walls become scarred and fatty deposits (cholesterol) are built up at these sites. The blood circulation is impaired and it may lead to such problems as angina pectoris, stroke and heart attack. The condition is associated with the western lifestyle. i.e. lack of exercise, smoking, obesity and too high an intake of animal fats.

atrophy wasting of a body part due to lack of use, malnutrition or as a result of ageing. The ovaries of women atrophy after the menopause and muscular atrophy accompanies certain diseases.

boil (or furuncle) a skin infection in a hair follicle or gland that produces inflammation and pus. The infection is often due to the bacterium *Staphylococcus*, but healing is generally quick upon release of the pus or administration of antibiotics. Frequent occurrence of boils is usually investigated to ensure the patient is not suffering from diabetes mellitus.

bronchitis occurring in two forms, acute and chronic, bronchitis is the inflammation of the bronchi. Bacteria or viruses cause the acute form that is typified by the symptoms of the common cold initially, but develops with painful coughing, wheezing, throat and chest pains and the production of purulent (pus-containing) mucus. If the infection spreads to the bronchioles (bronchiolitis) the consequences are even more serious as the body is deprived of oxygen. Antibiotics and expectorants can relieve the symptoms.

Chronic bronchitis is identified by an excessive production of mucus and may be due to recurrence of the acute form. It is a common cause of death among the elderly and there are several parameters of direct consequence to its cause: excessive smoking of cigarettes; cold, damp climate; obesity; respiratory infections. Damage to the bronchi and other complications may occur giving rise to constant breathlessness. Bronchodilator drugs are ineffective in treatment of the chronic form.

bruises injuries of, and leakage of blood into, the subcutaneous tissues, but without an open wound. In the simplest case minute vessels rupture and blood occupies the skin in the immediate area. A larger injury may be accompanied by swelling. A bruise begins as blue/black in colour, followed by brown and yellow as the blood pigment is reabsorbed.

burns burns and scalds show similar symptoms and require similar treatment, the former being caused by dry heat, the latter moist heat. Burns may also be due to electric currents and chemicals. Formerly burns were categorized by degrees (a system developed by Dupuytres, a French surgeon) but are now either superficial, where sufficient tissue remains to ensure skin regrows,

or deep where grafting will be necessary.

Severe injuries can prove dangerous because of shock due to fluid loss at the burn. For minor burns and scalds, treatment involves holding the affected area under cold water. In more severe cases antiseptic dressings are normally applied and in very severe cases hospitalization is required. Morphine is usually administered to combat the pain. If the burns exceed nine per cent then a transfusion is required.

calculus stones formed within the body, particularly in the urinary tract (gravel) or gall bladder (see gallstones). They are formed from mineral salts, e.g. calcium oxalate and they generally cause pain as they may block the ureter or bile ducts. Treatment is by removing or crushing the stone surgically, by drugs and diet (in gallstones a low fat diet eases pain and prevents formation of more stones) and also by the use of herbal remedies.

cancer a widely-used term describing any form of malignant tumour. Characteristically, there is an uncontrolled and abnormal growth of cancer cells that invade surrounding tissues and destroy them. Cancer cells may spread throughout the body via the blood stream or lymphatic system, a process known as metastasis, and set up secondary growths elsewhere. There are known to be a number of different causes of cancer including cigarette smoking, radiation, ultraviolet light, some viruses and possibly the presence of cancer genes (oncogenes). Treatment depends upon the site of the cancer but involves radiotherapy, chemotherapy and surgery, and survival rates in affected people are showing encouraging improvements.

chilblain a round, itchy inflammation of the skin that usually occurs on the toes or fingers during cold weather, and is caused by a localized deficiency in the circulation. Chilblains may sometimes be an indication of poor health or inadequate clothing and nutrition. Keeping the feet and hands warm, paying attention to the diet and exercise to improve the circulation help to prevent chilblains.

cholera an infection of the small intestine caused by the bacterium *Vibrio cholerae*. It varies in degree from very mild cases to extremely severe illness and death. The disease originated in Asia but spread widely last century when there were great cholera epidemics in Britain and elsewhere. During epidemics of cholera, the death rate is over fifty per cent and these occur in conditions of poor sanitation and overcrowding. The disease is spread through contamination of drinking water by faeces of those affected by the disease, and also by flies landing on infected material and then crawling on food.

Epidemics are rare in conditions of good sanitation but when cholera is detected, extreme attention has to be paid to hygiene including treatment and scrupulous disposal of the body waste of the infected person. The incubation period for cholera is one to five days and then a person suffers from severe vomiting and diarrhoea (known as 'cholera diarrhoea' or 'rice water stools'). This results in severe dehydration and death may follow within twenty four hours. Treatment involves bed rest and the taking by mouth of salt solutions, or these may need to be given intravenously. Tetracycline or other sulphonamide drugs are given to kill the bacteria. The death rate is low (five per cent) in those given proper and prompt treatment but the risk is greater in children and the elderly. Vaccination against cholera can be given but it is only effective for about six months.

chorea a disorder of the nervous system characterized by the involuntary, jerky movements of the muscles mainly of the face, shoulders and hips. *Sydenham's chorea* or *St. Vitus' dance* is a disease that mainly affects children and is associated with acute rheumatism. About one third of affected children develop rheumatism elsewhere in the body, often involving the heart, and the disease is more common in girls than in boys. If the heart is affected there may be problems in later life but treatment consists of rest and the giving of mild sedatives. The condition usually recovers over a period of a few months. *Huntington's chorea* is an inherited condition that does not appear until after the age of forty and is accompanied by dementia. *Senile chorea* afflicts some elderly people but there is no dementia.

cirrhosis a disease of the liver in which fibrous tissue resembling scar tissue is produced as a result of damage and death to the cells. The liver becomes yellow-coloured and nodular in appearance, and there are various types of the disease including alcoholic cirrhosis and postnecrotic cirrhosis caused by viral hepatitis. The cause of the cirrhosis is not always found (cryptogenic cirrhosis) but the progress of the condition can be halted if this can be identified and removed. This particularly is applicable in alcoholic cirrhosis where the consumption of alcohol has to cease.

cold (common cold) widespread and mild infection of the upper respiratory tract caused by a virus. There is inflammation of the mucous membranes and symptoms include feverishness, coughing, sneezing, runny nose, sore throat, headache and sometimes face ache due to catarrh in the sinuses. The disease is spread by coughing and sneezing and treatment is by means of bed rest and the taking of mild analgesics.

conjunctivitis inflammation of the mucous membrane (conjunctiva) that lines the inside of the eyelid and covers the front of the eye. The eyes become pink and watery and the condition is usually caused by an infection that may be bacterial, viral or the microorganism *Chlamydia* may be responsible. Treatment depends upon cause but a number of drugs are used often in the form of eyedrops.

constipation the condition in which the bowels are opened too infrequently and the faeces become dry, hard and difficult and painful to pass. The frequency of normal bowel opening varies between people but when constipation becomes a problem, it is usually a result of inattention to this habit or to the diet. To correct the condition a change of lifestyle may be needed including taking more exercise, fluid and roughage in the diet. Laxatives and enemas are also used to alleviate the condition. Constipation is also a symptom of the more serious condition of blockage of the bowel (by a tumour), but this is less common.

convulsions also known as fits, these are involuntary, alternate, rapid, muscular contractions and relaxations throwing the body and limbs into contortions. They are caused by a disturbance of brain function and in adults usually result from epilepsy. In babies and young children they occur quite commonly but, although alarming, are generally not serious. Causes include a high fever due to infection, brain diseases such as meningitis and breath-holding, that is quite common in infants and very young children. Convulsions are thought to be more common in the very young because the nervous system is immature. Unless they are caused by the presence of disease or infection that requires to be treated, they are rarely life-threatening.

cramp prolonged and painful spasmodic muscular contraction that often occurs in the limbs but can affect certain internal organs. Cramp may result from a salt imbalance as in heat cramp. Working in high temperatures causes excessive sweating and consequent loss of salt. It can be corrected and prevented by an increase of the salt intake. Occupational cramp results from continual repetitive use of particular muscles, e.g. writer's cramp. Night cramp occurs during sleep and is especially common among elderly people, diabetics and pregnant women. The cause is not known.

croup a group of diseases characterized by a swelling, partial obstruction and inflammation of the entrance to the larynx, occurring in young children. The breathing is harsh and strained producing a typical crowing sound, accompanied by coughing and feverishness. Diphtheria used to be the most common cause of croup but it now usually results from a viral infection of the respiratory tract (laryngotracheo bronchitis). The condition is relieved by inhaling steam and also by mild sedatives and/or pain killers. Rarely, the obstruction becomes dangerous and completely blocks the larynx in which case emergency tracheostomy or nasotracheal intubation may be required. Usually, the symptoms of croup subside and the child recovers, but then he or she may have a tendency towards attacks on future occasions.

delirium a mental disorder typified by confusion, agitation, fear, anxiety, illusions and sometimes hallucinations. The causal cerebral disfunction may be due to deficient nutrition, stress, toxic poisoning or mental shock.

depression a mental state of extreme sadness dominated by pessimism and in which normal behaviour patterns (sleep, appetite, etc.) are disturbed. Causes are varied upsetting events, loss, etc. and treatment involves the use of therapy and drugs.

diarrhoea increased frequency and looseness of bowel movement, involving the passage of unusually soft faeces. Diarrhoea can be caused by food poisoning, colitis, irritable bowel syndrome, dysentery, etc. A severe case will result in the loss of water and salts that must be replaced and anti-diarrhoeal drugs are used in certain circumstances.

diphtheria a serious, infectious disease caused by the bacterium *Corynebacterium diphtheriae,* and commonest in children. The infection causes a membranous lining on the throat that can interfere with breathing and eating. The toxin produced by the

279

bacterium damages heart tissue and the central nervous system and it can be fatal if not treated. The infection is countered by injection of the antitoxin with penicillin or erythromycin taken to kill the bacterium. Diphtheria can be immunized against.

dropsy old-fashioned name for oedema.

dysentery an infection and ulceration of the lower part of the bowels that causes severe diarrhoea with the passage of mucus and blood. There are two forms of dysentery caused by different organisms. Amoebic dysentery is due to *Entamoeba histolytica* that is spread via infected food or water and occurs mainly in the tropics and subtropics. The appearance of symptoms may be delayed but in addition to diarrhoea there is indigestion, anaemia and weight loss. Drugs are used in treatment.

Bacillary dysentery is caused by the bacterium *Shigella* and spreads by contact with a carrier or contaminated food. Symptoms appear from one to six days after infection and include diarrhoea, cramp, nausea, fever and the severity of the attack varies. Antibiotics may be given to kill the bacteria but recovery usually occurs within one to two weeks.

dysmenorrhoea painful menstruation. There are two main types, primary and secondary. Primary or spasmodic dysmenorrhoea is extremely common, but is normally mild and short-lived in duration. In a small proportion of women, the pain is severe enough to cause partial or total debility. The pain generally occurs in the lower abdomen or back and is cramping, often coming in waves that is due to uterine contractions. It is associated with dizziness, nausea, vomiting, headache, fainting and pale complexion with obvious distress. Secondary or congestive dysmenorrhoea is pain with a congested ache and cramps in the lower abdomen. It is generally due to specific pelvic conditions, e.g. chronic pelvic infection, endometriosis, fibroid tumours and the presence of an interuterine contraceptive device (IUCD).

eczema an inflammation of the skin that causes itching, a red rash and often small blisters that weep and become encrusted. This may be followed by the skin thickening and then peeling off in scales. There are several types of eczema, *atopic* being one of the most common. (Atopic is the hereditary tendency to form allergic reactions due to an antibody in the skin). A form of atopic eczema is infantile eczema that starts at three or four months and it is often the case that eczema, hay fever and asthma is found in the family history. However, many children improve markedly as they approach the age of ten or eleven. The treatment for such conditions usually involves the use of hydrocortisone and other steroid creams and ointments.

epilepsy a neurological disorder involving convulsions, seizures and loss of consciousness. There are many possible causes or associations of epilepsy, including cerebral trauma, brain tumour, cerebral haemorrhage and metabolic imbalances as in hypoglycaemia. Usually an epileptic attack occurs without warning, with complete unconsciousness and some muscle contraction and spasms. Some drugs are used in treatment although little can be done during the fit itself.

erysipelas an infectious disease, caused by *Streptococcus pyogenes*. It produces an inflammation of the skin with associated redness. Large areas of the body may be affected and other symptoms may include vesicles, fever and pain with a feeling of heat and a tingling sensation. In addition to being isolated, patients are given penicillin.

fistula an abnormal opening between two hollow organs or between such an organ or gland and the exterior. These may arise during development so that a baby may be born with a fistula. Alternatively, they can be produced by injury, infection or as a complication following surgery. A common example is an anal fistula, that may develop if an abscess present in the rectum bursts and produces a communication through the surface of the skin. An operation is normally required to correct a fistula, but healing is further complicated in the case of an anal fistula because of the passage of waste material through the bowels.

gallstones stones of varying composition, that form in the gall bladder. Their formation seems to be due to a change in bile composition rendering cholesterol less soluble. Stones may also form around a foreign body. There are three types of stone cholesterol, pigment and mixed, the latter being the most common. Calcium salts are usually found in varying proportions. Although gallstones may be present for years without symptoms, they can cause severe pain and may pass into the common bile duct to cause, by the resulting obstruction, jaundice.

gleet discharge due to chronic gonorrhoea.

gonorrhoea the most common venereal disease that is spread primarily by sexual intercourse but may be contracted through contact with infected discharge on clothing, towels, etc. The causative agent is the bacterium *Neisseria gonorrhoeae* and it affects the mucous membrane of the vagina, or in the male, the urethra. Symptoms develop approximately one week after infection and include pain on urinating with a discharge of pus. Inflammation of nearby organs may occur (testicle, prostate in men; uterus, Fallopian tubes and ovaries in women) and prolonged inflammation of the urethra may lead to formation of fibrous tissue causing stricture. Joints may also be affected and later complications include endocarditis, arthritis and conjunctivitis.

If a baby is born to a woman with the disease, the baby's eyes may become infected, until recently a major cause of blindness (called *Ophthalmia neonatorum*). Treatment is usually very effective through the administration of penicillin, sulphonamides or tetracycline.

gout a disorder caused by an imbalance of uric acid in the body. Uric acid is normally excreted by the kidneys but sufferers of gout have an excess in their bloodstream that is deposited in joints as salts (urates) of the acid. This causes inflammation of the affected joints and painful gouty arthritis with destruction of the joints. The kidneys may also be damaged, with formation of stones. Deposits of the salts (called *tophi*) may reach the stage where they prohibit further use of the joints, causing hands and feet to be set in a particular position. Treatment of gout is through drugs that increase the excretion of the urate salts or slow their formation.

gravel this name refers to small stones formed in the urinary tract. They normally are made up of calcareous material and crystalline matter and passage of stones from the kidneys is normally linked to severe pain and, possibly, the presence of blood in the urine.

haemorrhoids (piles) varicose and inflamed veins around the lower end of the bowel situated in the wall of the anus. They are classified as internal, external and mixed depending upon whether they appear beyond the anus. They are commonly caused by constipation or diarrhoea, especially in middle and older age, and may be exacerbated by a sedentary life style. They may also occur as a result of childbearing. Symptoms of haemorrhoids are bleeding and pain, and treatment is by means of creams, injections and suppositories. Attention to diet (to treat constipation) and regular exercise are important, but in severe cases, surgery to remove the haemorrhoids may be necessary.

hysteria a type of neurosis that is difficult to define and in which a range of symptoms may occur. These include paralysis, seizures and spasms of limbs, swelling of joints, mental disorders and amnesia. The person is vulnerable to suggestion. Two types are recognized, *conversion hysteria* that is characterized by physical symptoms and *dissociative hysteria* in which marked mental changes occur. *Mass hysteria* affects a group, especially those gathered together under conditions of emotional excitement. A number of people may suffer from giddiness, vomiting and fainting that runs through the whole crowd. Recovery occurs when those affected are separated from the others under calmer conditions. Treatment for hysteria is by means of psychotherapy, involving suggestion.

influenza a highly infectious disease caused by a virus that affects the respiratory tract. Symptoms include headache, weakness and fever, appetite loss and general aches and pains. Sometimes there is the complication of a lung infection that requires immediate treatment. There are three main strains of influenza virus, designated A, B and C. The viruses quickly produce new strains which is why an attack of one is unlikely to provide protection against a later bout of the disease. Epidemics occur periodically and in Britain virus A is responsible for the majority of outbreaks.

jaundice a condition characterized by the unusual presence of bile pigment (bilirubin) in the blood. The bile produced in the liver passes into the blood instead of the intestines and because of this there is a yellowing of the skin and the whites of the eyes.

There are several types of jaundice: *obstructive* due to bile not reaching the intestine due to an obstruction e.g. a gallstone; *haemolytic* where red blood cells are destroyed by haemolysis; *hepatocellular* due to a liver disease such as hepatitis which results in the liver being unable to use the bilirubin. *Neonatal jaundice* is quite common in newborn infants when the liver is physiologically immature but it usually lasts only a few days. The infant can be exposed to blue light that converts bilirubin to biliverdin, another (harmless) bile pigment.

laryngitis inflammation of the mucous membrane that lines the larynx and vocal cords. It is due to viral infection in the main, but also bacteria, chemical irritants, heavy smoking or excessive use of the voice. *Acute* laryngitis accompanies infections of the upper respiratory tract and the symptoms include pain, a cough, difficulty in swallowing. *Chronic* laryngitis may be due to recurrence of the acute form, but is often attributable to excessive smoking worsened by alcohol. Changes occurring in the vocal cords are more permanent and the symptoms are as for the acute form, but longer lasting.

leucorrhea a discharge of white or yellow-coloured mucus from the vagina. It may be a normal condition, increasing before and after menstruation but a large discharge probably indicates an infection somewhere in the genital tract. A common cause is the infection called thrush but it may also be due to gonorrhoea in which case the treatment will differ.

malaria an infectious disease caused by the presence of minute parasitic organisms of the genus *Plasmodium* in the blood. The disease is characterized by recurrent bouts of fever and anaemia, the interval between the attacks depending upon the species. The parasite is transmitted to man by the *Anopheles* mosquito, (common in subtropical and tropical regions) being present in the salivary glands and passed into the bloodstream of a person when the insect bites. Similarly, the parasite is ingested by the mosquito when it takes a blood meal from an infected person. Efforts to control malaria have centred on destruction of the mosquito and its breeding sites. Once injected into the blood, the organisms concentrate in the liver where they multiply and then re-enter the bloodstream destroying red blood cells. This releases the parasites causing shivering, fever, sweating and anaemia. The process is then repeated, with hours or days between attacks. Drugs are used both to prevent infection, although these may not be totally effective, and to cure the disease once present.

nephritis inflammation of the kidney, that may be due to one of several causes. Types of nephritis include glomerulonephritis (when the glomerulus is affected), acute nephritis, hereditary nephritis, etc.

neuralgia strictly, pain in some part or the whole of a nerve (without any physical change in the nerve) but used more widely to encompass pain following the course of a nerve or its branches, whatever the cause. Neuralgia often occurs at the same time each day and is frequently an agonizing pain. It occurs in several forms and is named accordingly, e.g. sciatica, trigeminal neuralgia (affecting the face) and intercostal neuralgia (affecting the ribs). Treatment often involves the application of ointments, and the taking of pain-killing drugs. If such treatments do not bring relief, it is possible to freeze the nerve or destroy part of it by surgery.

oedema an accumulation of fluid in the body, possibly beneath the skin or in cavities or organs. With an injury the swelling may be localized or more general as in cases of kidney or heart failure. Fluid can collect in the chest cavity, abdomen or lung (pulmonary oedema). The causes are numerous, e.g. cirrhosis of the liver, heart or kidney failure, starvation, acute nephritis, allergies or drugs. To alleviate the symptom, the root cause has to be removed. Subcutaneous oedema commonly occurs in women before menstruation, as swollen legs or ankles, but does subside if the legs are rested in a raised position.

palsy the term used formerly for paralysis and retained for the names of some conditions.

pleurisy (*or* **pleuritis**) inflammation of the pleura resulting in pain from deep breathing, and resulting shortness of breath. There is a typical frictional rub heard through a stethoscope. Pleurisy is often due to pneumonia in the adjacent lung and is always associated with disease in the lung, diaphragm, chest wall or abdomen e.g. tuberculosis, abscesses, bronchial carcinoma, etc.

pneumonia a bacterial infection of the lungs resulting in inflammation and filling of the alveoli with pus and fluid. As a result the lung becomes solid and air cannot enter. The symptoms vary depending upon how much of the lung is unavailable for respiration, but commonly there will be chest pain, coughing, breathlessness, fever and possibly cyanosis. Pneumonia may be caused by several bacteria, viruses or fungi, but bacterial infection is commonest. Bronchopneumonia affects the bronchi and bronchioles; lobar pneumonia the whole lobes of the lung(s). Antibiotic treatment is usually effective although it helps to know which is the infecting organism, to provide the most specific treatment.

prolapse a moving down of an organ or tissue from its normal position due to the supporting tissues weakening. This may happen to the lower end of the bowel (in children) or the uterus and vagina in women who have sustained some sort of injury during childbirth. In the latter case prolapse may result in the uterus itself showing on the outside. Surgery can shorten the supporting ligaments and narrow the vaginal opening.

psoriasis a chronic skin disease for which the cause is unknown and the treatment is palliative. The affected skin appears as itchy, scaly red areas, starting usually around the elbows and knees. It often runs in families and may be associated with anxiety, commencing usually in childhood or adolescence. Treatment involves the use of ointments and creams.

rheumatism a general term used to describe aches and pains in joints and muscles.

rickets a disease affecting children that involves a deficiency of vitamin D. Vitamin D can be manufactured in the skin in the presence of sunlight but dietary sources are important especially where sunlight is lacking. The disease is characterized by soft bones that bend out of shape and cause deformities.

Bones are hardened by the deposition of calcium salts and this cannot happen in the absence of vitamin D. Treatment consists of giving vitamin D, usually in the form of calciferol, and ensuring that there is an adequate amount in the child's future diet. Vitamin D deficiency in adults causes the condition called osteomalacia.

scarlet fever an infectious disease, mainly of childhood, caused by the bacterium *Streptococcus*. Symptoms show after a few days and include sickness, sore throat, fever and a scarlet rash that may be widespread. Antibiotics are effective and also prevent any complications e.g. inflammation of the kidneys.

sciatica pain in the sciatic nerve, and therefore felt in the back of the thigh, leg and foot. The commonest cause is a prolapsed intervertebral disc pressing on a nerve root, but it may also be due to ankylosing spondylitis and other conditions.

scurvy a deficiency disease caused by a lack of vitamin C (ascorbic acid) due to a dietary lack of fruit and vegetables. Symptoms begin with swollen, bleeding gums and then subcutaneous bleeding, bleeding into joints, ulcers, anaemia and then fainting, diarrhoea and trouble with major organs. Untreated, it is fatal, but nowadays it is easily prevented, or cured should it arise, through correct diet or administration of the vitamin.

smallpox a highly infectious viral disease that has nonetheless been eradicated. Infection results, after about two weeks, in a high fever, head and body aches and vomiting. Eventually red spots appear that change to water and then pus-filled vesicles that on drying out leave scars. The person stays infectious until all scabs are shed. Fever often returns, with delirium. Recovery is usual, but complications often ensue, e.g. pneumonia. The last naturally-occurring case was in 1977.

stone another name for calculus.

strangury the desire to pass water, that can only be done in a few drops and with accompanying pain. It is symptomatic of an irritation of the base of the bladder by a stone, cancer at this site, or cystitis or prostatitis.

syphilis an infectious, sexually-transmitted disease, caused by the bacterium *Treponema pallidum* that shows symptoms in three stages. Bacteria enter the body through mucous membranes during sexual intercourse and an ulcer appears in the first instance. Within a short time the lymph nodes locally and then all over the body enlarge and harden and this lasts several weeks.

Secondary symptoms appear about two months after infection and include fever, pains, enlarged lymph nodes and a faint rash that is usually noticed on the chest. The bacterium is found in enormous numbers in the primary sores and any skin lesions of the secondary stage. The final stage may not appear until many months or years after infection and comprises the formation of numerous tumour-like masses throughout the body (in skin, muscle, bone, brain, spinal cord and other organs such as the liver, stomach, etc.). This stage can cause serious damage to the heart, brain or spinal cod resulting in blindness, tabes dorsalis, and mental disability.

Congenital syphilis is much rarer than the former, *acquired*, type. It is contracted by a developing foetus from the mother, across the placenta and symptoms show a few weeks after birth. Treatment of syphilis is with penicillin, but it should be administered early in the development of the disease.

torpor a state of physical and mental sluggishness that accompanies various mental disorders, some kinds of poisoning and may be present in elderly people with arterial disease.

tuberculosis a group of infections caused by the bacillus (bacterium) *Mycobacterium tuberculosis* of which pulmonary tuberculosis of the lungs (consumption or phthisis) is the best known form. The pulmonary disease is acquired through inhalation of air containing the organism from an infected person, or dust laden with bacteria. People infected in this way can show no symptoms but still be carriers. In the lungs, the infection causes formation of a *primary tubercle* that spreads to lymph nodes to form the *primary complex.*

The disease may wax and wane for years as the body's natural immune system acts against the infection. If the infection is severe, symptoms include fever, wasting, night sweats and the coughing up of blood. The bacteria may enter the blood stream and spread throughout the body setting up numerous tubercles in other tissues (*Miliary tuberculosis*). The organism may also be acquired by eating contaminated food, especially milk, in which case the production of a primary complex in abdominal lymph nodes can lead to peritonitis. Rarely, the infection is acquired via a cut from contact with an infected person or animal. Tuberculosis affects people throughout the world (about six thousand new cases each year in England and Wales). Many people acquire the infection and recover without suspecting its presence and the disease is curable with antibiotics, e.g. streptomycin. In addition, BCG vaccina-

tion as a preventive measure is given to children in the U.K., in addition to X-ray screening to detect carriers.

ulcer a break on the skin surface or on the mucous membrane lining within the body cavities that may be inflamed and fails to heal. Ulcers of the skin include bedsores and varicose ulcers (that are caused by defective circulation). Ulcers of the alimentary tract include duodenal ulcers, gastric ulcers and peptic ulcers.

varicose veins that have become stretched, distended and twisted. The superficial veins in the legs are often affected although it may occur elsewhere. Causes include congenitally defective valves, obesity, pregnancy and also thrombophlebitis (inflammation of the wall of a vein with secondary thrombosis in the affected part of the vein). Elastic support is a common treatment although alternatives are sclerotherapy and phlebectomy.

whooping cough (*pertussis*) an infectious disease caused by the bacterium *Bordetella pertussis.* The mucous membranes lining the air passages are affected and after a one to two week incubation period, fever, catarrh and a cough develop. The cough then becomes paroxysmal with a number of short coughs punctuated with the 'whooping' drawing in of breath. Nosebleeds and vomiting may follow a paroxysm. After about two weeks the symptoms abate but a cough may continue for some weeks. Whooping cough is not usually serious and immunization reduces the severity of an attack. However, a child may be susceptible to pneumonia and tuberculosis during the disease.

Terms Used in Homeopathy

aggravations a term first used by Dr Samuel Hahnemann to describe an initial worsening of symptoms experienced by some pa-

tients, on first taking a homeopathic remedy, before the condition improved. In modern homeopathy this is known as a *healing crisis.* To prevent the occurrence of aggravations, Hahnemann experimented with further dilutions of remedies and, in particular, vigorous shaking (SUCCUSSING) of preparations at each stage of the process.

allopathy a term first used by Dr Samuel Hahnemann meaning 'against disease'. It describes the approach of conventional medicine, which is to treat symptoms with a substance or drug with an opposite effect in order to suppress or eliminate them. This is called the 'law of contraries' and is in direct contrast to the 'like can cure like', the 'law of similars' or *similia similibus curentur* principle, which is central to the practice of homeopathy.

centesimal scale of dilution the scale of dilution used in homeopathy based on one part (or drop) of the remedy in 99 parts of the diluent liquid (a mixture of alcohol and water).

classical the practice of homeopathy based on the work of Dr Samuel Hahnemann and further developed and expanded by other practitioners, particularly Dr Constantine Hering and Dr James Tyler Kent.

constitutional prescribing and constitutional types the homeopathic concept, based on the work of Dr James Tyler Kent, that prescribing should be based on the complete make-up of a person, including physical and emotional characteristics, as well as on the symptoms of a disorder.

decimal scale of dilution the scale of dilution used in homeopathy based on one part (or drop) of the remedy in nine parts of the diluent liquid (a mixture of alcohol and water).

healing crisis the situation in which a group of symptoms first become worse after a person has taken a homeopathic remedy, before they improve and disappear. The healing crisis is taken to indicate a change and that improvement is likely to follow. It is usually short-lived (*see also* AGGRAVATIONS).

homeopathy the system of healing based on the principle of 'like can cure like' and given its name by Samuel Hahnemann. The word is derived from the Greek *homeo* for 'similar' and *pathos* for 'suffering' or 'like disease'.

laws of cure, law of direction of cure three concepts or 'laws' formulated by Dr Constantine Hering to explain the means by which symptoms of disease are eliminated from the body.

(1) Symptoms move in a downwards direction.

(2) Symptoms move from the inside of the body outwards.

(3) Symptoms move from more important vital organs and tissues to those of less importance.

Hering was also responsible for the view in homeopathy that more recent symptoms disappear first before ones that have been present for a longer time. Hence symptoms are eliminated in the reverse order of their appearance.

materia medica detailed information about homeopathic remedies, listed alphabetically. The information includes details of the symptoms that may respond to each remedy, based on previous research and experience. Details about the source of each remedy are also included. This information is used by a homeopathic doctor when deciding upon the best remedy for each particular patient and group of symptoms.

miasm a chronic constitutional weakness that is the aftereffect of an underlying suppressed disease that has been present in a previous generation or earlier in the life of an individual. The concept of miasm was formulated by Samuel Hahnemann who noted that some people were never truly healthy but always acquired new symptoms of illness. He believed that this was because of a constitutional weakness that he called a miasm, which may have been inherited and was caused by an illness in a previous generation. These theories were put forward in his research writings entitled *Chronic Diseases*. Three main miasms were identified, PSORA, SYCOSIS and SYPHILIS.

modalities a term applied to the responses of the patient, when he or she feels better or worse, depending upon factors in the internal and external environment. These are unique from one person to another, depending upon the individual characteristics that apply at the time, although there are common features within each constitutional type. Modalities include responses, fears and preferences to temperature, weather, foods, emotional responses and relationships, etc, which all contribute to a person's total sense of wellbeing. Modalities are particularly important when a person has symptoms of an illness in prescribing the most beneficial remedy.

mother tincture (symbol O) the first solution obtained from dissolving a substance in a mixture of alcohol and water (usually in the ratio of 9/10 pure alcohol to 1/10 distilled water). It is subjected to further dilutions and SUCCUSSIONS (shakings) to produce the homeopathic remedies.

nosode a term used to describe a remedy prepared from samples of infected diseased tissue, often to treat or prevent a particular illness. They were first investigated by Wilhelm Lux, not without considerable controversy. Examples are *Medorrhinum* and *Tuberculinum*.

organon *The Organon of Rationale Medicine*. is one of the most important works of Samuel Hahnemann, published in Leipzig in 1810, in which he set out the principles and philosophy of modern homeopathy. The *Organon* is considered to be a classic work and basic to the study of homeopathy.

polycrest a remedy suitable for a number of illnesses, disorders or symptoms.

potency the dilution or strength of a homeopathic remedy. Dr Samuel Hahnemann discovered that by further diluting and SUCCUSSING (shaking) a remedy, it became more effective or potent in bringing about a cure. It is held that the process of diluting and shaking a remedy releases its innate energy or dynamism, even though none of the original molecules of the substance may remain. Hence the greater the dilution of a remedy, the stronger or more potent it becomes. Hahnemann called his new dilute solutions 'potentizations'.

potentiate the release or transfer of energy into a homeopathic solution by succussing or vigorous shaking of the mixture.

principle of vital force 'vital force' was the term given by Samuel Hahnemann to the inbuilt power or ability of the human body to maintain health and fitness and fight off illness. Illness is believed to be the result of stresses, causing an imbalance in the vital force, which assail all people throughout life and include inherited, environmental and emotional factors. The symptoms of this 'disorder' are illness and are held to be the physical indications of the struggle of the body's vital force to regain its balance. A person with a strong vital force will tend to remain in good health and fight off illness. A person with a weak vital force is more likely to suffer from long-term, recurrent symptoms and illnesses. Homeopathic remedies are believed to act upon the vital force, stimulating it to heal the body and restore the natural balance.

provings the term given by Samuel Hahnemann to experimental trials he carried out to test the reactions of healthy people to homeopathic substances. These trials were carried out under strictly controlled conditions (in advance of the modern scientific approach), and the symptoms produced, the results, were meticulously recorded. Quinine was the first substance that Hahnemann investigated in this way, testing it initially on himself and then on close friends and family members. Over the next few years he investigated and proved many other substances, building up a wealth of information on each one about the reactions and symptoms produced. After conducting this research, Hahnemann went on to prescribe carefully the remedies to those who were sick. Provings are still carried out in modern homeopathy to test new substances that may be of value as remedies. Usually, neither the prescribing physician nor those taking the substance—the 'provers'—know the identity of the material or whether they are taking a placebo.

psora one of three MIASMS identified by Samuel Hahnemann, believed to be because of suppression of scabies (an itchy skin infection caused by a minute burrowing mite). Psora was believed to have an inherited element or to be because of suppression of an earlier infection in a particular individual.

Schussler tissue salts Wilhelm Heinrich Schussler was a German homeopathic doctor who introduced the biochemic tissue salt system in the late 1800s. Schussler believed that many symptoms and ailments resulted from the lack of a minute, but essential, quantity of a mineral or tissue salt. He identified twelve such tissue salts that he regarded as essential and believed that a cure could be obtained from replacing the deficient substance. Schussler's work was largely concentrated at the cell and tissue level rather than embracing the holistic view of homeopathy.

similia similibus curentur the founding principle of homeopathy that 'like can cure like' or 'let like be treated by like', which was first put forward by Hippocrates, a physician of ancient Greece. This principle excited the interest of Paracelsus in the Middle Ages, and was later restated and put into practice by Hahnemann with the development of homeopathy.

simillimum a homeopathic remedy that in its natural, raw state is able to produce the same symptoms as those being exhibited by the patient.

succussion vigorous shaking of a homeopathic remedy at each stage of dilution, along with banging the container holding it against a hard surface causing further release of energy.

sycosis one of the three major MIASMS identified by Samuel Hahnemann and believed to result from a suppressed gonorrhoeal infection. Sycosis was believed to have an inherited element or to be because of suppression of an earlier infection in a particular individual.

syphilis the third of the three major MIASMS identified by Samuel Hahnemann believed to result from a suppressed syphilis infection. Syphilis was believed to have an inherited element or to be because of suppression of an earlier infection in a particular individual.

trituration the process, devised by Samuel Hahnemann, of rendering naturally insoluble substances soluble so that they can be made available as homeopathic remedies. The process involves repeated grinding down of the substance with lactose powder until it becomes soluble. The substance usually becomes soluble at the third process of trituration. Each trituration is taken to be the equivalent of one dilution in the centesimal scale. Once the substance has been rendered soluble, dilution can proceed in the normal way.